NCLEX® High-Risk

The Disaster Prevention Manual for Nurses Determined to Pass the RN Licensing Examination

Marian C. Condon, DEd, RN, CNc
Professor
Department of Nursing
York College of Pennsylvania
York, Pennsylvania

Karen S. March, PhD, RN, CCRN, ACNS-BC
Professor
Department of Nursing
York College of Pennsylvania
York, Pennsylvania

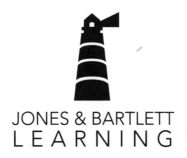

JONES & BARTLETT
LEARNING

World Headquarters

Jones & Bartlett Learning
40 Tall Pine Drive
Sudbury, MA 01776
978-443-5000
info@jblearning.com
www.jblearning.com

Jones & Bartlett Learning Canada
6339 Ormindale Way
Mississauga, Ontario L5V 1J2
Canada

Jones & Bartlett Learning International
Barb House, Barb Mews
London W6 7PA
United Kingdom

Jones & Bartlett Learning books and products are available through most bookstores and online booksellers. To contact Jones & Bartlett Learning directly, call 800-832-0034, fax 978-443-8000, or visit our website, www.jblearning.com.

Substantial discounts on bulk quantities of Jones & Bartlett Learning publications are available to corporations, professional associations, and other qualified organizations. For details and specific discount information, contact the special sales department at Jones & Bartlett Learning via the above contact information or send an email to specialsales@jblearning.com.

The authors, editor, and publisher have made every effort to provide accurate information. However, they are not responsible for errors, omissions, or for any outcomes related to the use of the contents of this book and take no responsibility for the use of the products and procedures described. Treatments and side effects described in this book may not be applicable to all people; likewise, some people may require a dose or experience a side effect that is not described herein. Drugs and medical devices are discussed that may have limited availability controlled by the Food and Drug Administration (FDA) for use only in a research study or clinical trial. Research, clinical practice, and government regulations often change the accepted standard in this field. When consideration is being given to use of any drug in the clinical setting, the health care provider or reader is responsible for determining FDA status of the drug, reading the package insert, and reviewing prescribing information for the most up-to-date recommendations on dose, precautions, and contraindications, and determining the appropriate usage for the product. This is especially important in the case of drugs that are new or seldom used.

Production Credits

Publisher: Kevin Sullivan
Acquisitions Editor: Amy Sibley
Associate Editor: Patricia Donnelly
Editorial Assistant: Rachel Shuster
Associate Production Editor: Lisa Cerrone
Marketing Manager: Rebecca Wasley

V.P., Manufacturing and Inventory Control: Therese Connell
Composition: Paw Print Media
Cover Design: Scott Moden
Cover Image: © Taewoon Lee/ShutterStock, Inc.
Printing and Binding: Courier Stoughton
Cover Printing: Courier Stoughton

Library of Congress Cataloging-in-Publication Data
NCLEX high-risk : the disaster prevention manual for nurses determined to pass the RN licensing examination / Marian C. Condon, Karen S. March.
   p. ; cm.
Includes bibliographical references.
ISBN 978-0-7637-7339-7 (pbk.)
1. Practical nursing—Examinations, questions, etc. 2. Nursing care—Examinations, questions, etc. I. Condon, Marian C. II. March, Karen S.
[DNLM: 1. Nursing—Examination Questions. 2. Nursing—Examination Questions. WY 18.2 N3363 2011]
RT62.N3364 2011
610.73076—dc22
                                                                                    2010008076

6048

Printed in the United States of America
14 13 12 11 10   10 9 8 7 6 5 4 3 2 1

Dedication

This book is dedicated to my beloved sons, Patrick and Adam Hooper: *Labor was worth it, sweethearts—you are the lights of my life.* It is also dedicated to the many graduate nurses I've been privileged to assist in their quest to finally pass the NCLEX. I would like to direct special thanks to Betty DeMeester Webster and Michelle Metz Robinson, who were my very first clients, and to the 25 graduate nurses who allowed me to interview them in 1992 and 1993 as part of my doctoral dissertation research: *You were my first teachers, and it was you who launched me on the journey of understanding that has culminated in the publication of this book. You will always hold a special place in my heart.*

—M.C.C.

I would like to dedicate this book to graduate nurses of the past, present, and future, who inspired my commitment to this project, and to Brad and Zach, who have provided love, encouragement, support, and most of all, patience, throughout the weeks and months of writing. I do what I do because of you.

—K.S.M.

Contents

Letter to Nursing Students

Dear Senior Nursing Student or Graduate Nurse,

Please do not assume that because you've made it through nursing school, you are pretty much guaranteed to pass the NCLEX®. Unfortunately, there is no such guarantee—every year, bright, capable new nurses undergo the humiliating and painful experience of taking the RN licensing examination and not being successful.

From my interactions with the many GNs I've tutored in an effort to help them retake NCLEX successfully, I know that most either put little or no time into preparing for their first attempt, or they wasted their prep time on passive learning strategies that proved ineffective. Also, I know that many were unaware of the risk factors for failure on NCLEX and did not realize they needed to take extra precautions to ensure that they would pass.

This book is written especially for GNs who are at higher than average risk for having to retake the NCLEX. I invite you to take a look at the risk factors listed in *Should You Buy This Book?*, and if one or more apply to you, I urge you to take the process of preparing for NCLEX very, very seriously.

All best wishes for a fulfilling career in nursing,

Marian Condon

Should You Buy This Book?

If any of the risk factors listed below apply to you, the answer is, "Yes!"

- You've had to struggle to keep your GPA up (< 3.4).
- You got one or more Cs in a science course or a nursing course.
- You did better clinically than on classroom tests.
- You consider yourself to be a *hands-on* learner as opposed to a *book* learner.
- You tend to get the gist of things but have trouble with details.
- You did poorly on a predictive exit exam such as Evolve REACH (formerly HESI).
- English is not your native language.
- You've already failed the NCLEX® one or more times.

Foreword

As one of her earliest NCLEX® clients, I was delighted when Dr. Marian Condon invited me to write a foreword to this excellent and much-needed book. Here's my story: I took the NCLEX for the first time in the mid-1980s and did not pass. While the majority of my classmates were rejoicing over having achieved RN status, I was left feeling embarrassed and mad at myself. I was dreading the thought of retaking the boards and felt extremely pressured because I knew that if I failed again, I would lose my graduate nurse (GN) status at the hospital and would have to assume the role of nursing assistant. Thus, I was devastated when the dreaded large envelope again arrived in the mail. I resigned from my job as a GN and wondered about my future.

When Dr. Condon, who had been one of my favorite nursing instructors, learned of my second failure, she called and asked whether I would like her to tutor me, using a new method she was developing to help students perform better on tests. I felt honored, grateful, and even a bit curious. While I do not remember all of the details of our sessions together, I do recall that I quickly learned that the main reason for my failures was not test anxiety, as I'd thought, but the fact that I lacked some essential nursing knowledge. With Dr. Condon's help, I not only passed the boards on my third attempt, but exceeded what was then the passing score by 248 points!

Never let anyone tell you that a history of having failed NCLEX one or more times means you'll never be a successful nurse. Since becoming an RN, I have held staff nurse positions in a variety of hospitals, earned a master's degree in nursing, and worked for 10 years as a clinical nurse specialist in a neonatal intensive care unit. I am currently a nurse coordinator in a nursing program. Ironically, I now find myself sharing with my own nursing students the same study techniques that Dr. Condon taught me over 25 years ago.

Best wishes to all who are reading this!

Betty DeMeester Webster, RNC, MS
Baltimore, Maryland

Acknowledgments

We would like to thank our family members and friends for their patience in allowing us to hole up unmolested on weekends and holidays so we could work on *The Book* and for graciously sharing their households with *The Book* for what must have seemed like an awfully long time.

We would also like to thank our colleagues in the Department of Nursing at York College for putting up with our distraction and seeming inability to talk about anything but *The Book,* and for telling us the truth when we asked for their opinion of a page or a chapter. Special thanks are due to Professors Brigitte Haagen and Janice Ambrose, who lent us their expertise during the practice test development process. We would also like to thank Captain Pamela Gray, USN (Ret.), RN, MSN, FNP, who provided invaluable feedback on the early chapters. And, of course, we absolutely must thank all our helpers at Jones & Bartlett Learning: Amy Sibley, Rachel Shuster, and Lisa Cerrone.

Introduction:
How to Get the Most Out of This Book

Marian C. Condon

WHAT YOU WILL LEARN IN THIS CHAPTER

- Why you should read the chapters in order.
- Why you should bother with Keep Track boxes and Nugget Lists.
- Why you should make preparing for NCLEX® an absolute priority.
- Why you should access a source of additional questions, if necessary.
- How to know whether you need a tutor.

WHY YOU SHOULD READ MOST OF THE CHAPTERS IN ORDER

This book is not merely a source of practice NCLEX questions; it is a blueprint for successful NCLEX preparation, written especially for nurses who are at risk for failure. It is based on a specific methodology that has proven itself consistently, even with nurses who have failed NCLEX several times. Because a good deal of thought has gone into the manner in which this book is organized, you will get more out of it if you read most of the early chapters in order.

Chapter 1, "Are You at Risk for Failing NCLEX?" provides the information you need to evaluate your own degree of risk and aims to boost your motivation to complete the considerable amount of work thorough NCLEX preparation requires. Chapter 2, "Are You Using the Right NCLEX Prep Strategies?," will provide insight into your thinking style and will help you to make a judgment about how well the study habits you have acquired over years of schooling have been serving you.

Chapter 3, "NCLEX-RN®: Purpose, Format, and Scope," is a must-read before you begin tackling the practice questions in this book because it explains their structure and nature. You can save Chapter 4, "CAT-Anatomy: How Computer-Adaptive Testing Works," and Chapter 5, "Registration, Results, and Test-Center Smarts," until the end of your preparation period if you wish, but do not forget to read both before you actually take NCLEX. Chapter 4 will bring you up to speed about the nature of the NCLEX and why it is substantially different from any other test you have taken, and Chapter 5 will tell you how to register to take the NCLEX and avoid last-minute errors that could hurt your performance.

It is essential that you read Chapter 6, "Test Yourself: How Good Are You at Doping Out Test Questions?," to hone your analytical skills and identify deficiencies in your knowledge base before you start using the practice tests in Chapters 7–25. If you start answering practice questions in volume before you have learned to analyze them properly, you will only be reinforcing your current, likely suboptimal approach to reading and analyzing questions. The field of cognitive behavioral psychology is based on the principle that cognitive processes become more habitual and reflexive as they are used over and over again. If you wish to reason out test questions more analytically and effectively, the time to start doing that is as soon as possible.

WHY YOU SHOULD KEEP TRACK OF YOUR PROGRESS

At the end of the practice test in Chapter 9 you will find a box called, "Keep Track."

Keep Track

- Percent correct. (Divide the number of questions you answered correctly by the total number of questions you answered.) _____

- Number of questions you missed due to a reading error: _____

- Number of questions you missed due to errors in analysis: _____

- Number of assessment questions you missed: _____

- Number of lab value questions you missed: _____

- Number of drug/treatment questions you missed: _____

You will use the Keep Track boxes to record various aspects of your performance on the practice tests included in this book, and ultimately to gauge the progress you are making in your preparation for the NCLEX. After you've completed each of the practice tests and examinations provided, you will compute your overall score expressed as a percent. You will also review the questions you answered *incorrectly* and keep track of whether you missed them because you *read* them incorrectly (overlooked an important piece of information in the scenario or failed to understand exactly what was being asked) or because you *analyzed* them incorrectly (failed to consider every answer choice in light of each bit of information provided in the scenario). All of this will be explained thoroughly in Chapter 6. As you complete study session after study session and look back over your Keep Track boxes, you will (if all is going well) see a trend toward missing fewer and fewer questions because of faulty reading and analysis. You will also be using your Keep Track boxes to monitor your progress regarding three categories of nursing knowledge that will be well represented on NCLEX: knowledge related to *assessment*, knowledge related to *lab values*, and knowledge related to *drugs and treatments*. Finally, you will be using the Keep Track boxes to record your scores on topic-specific and comprehensive practice tests. Reviewing your scores on topic-specific practice tests will give you valuable feedback as to whether you need to do more preparation in a given area. Noting trends in your performance on comprehensive practice tests will let you know with considerable certainty whether you are ready to take NCLEX. Taking the time to maintain your performance records is vitally important. When you pass the NCLEX, you will be very glad you did.

WHY YOU SHOULD CREATE AND REVIEW NUGGET LISTS

In Chapter 8, "How to Map Your Progress and Use What You Don't Know to Pass the NCLEX," you will learn how to use practice tests to identify information that was missing from your knowledge base, and you will learn how to master that information quickly and easily. One of the most important tools in your information-acquiring arsenal will be the Nugget List. A nugget is a piece of information you didn't know or a concept you didn't understand. A Nugget List is a two-column list consisting of nuggets expressed as questions in the left-hand column and the corresponding answers in the right-hand column.

Nugget List	
Chapter number _____ Topic _____	

You will prepare a Nugget List for each practice test you complete and study the new material by covering the answer column and attempting to come up with the correct answers to the nugget questions.

As you add more and more nuggets to your knowledge base, you will notice that your scores on the practice tests are improving. That trend, combined with a trend toward missing fewer and fewer questions due to reading and analysis errors, will boost your confidence considerably and provide you with motivation to keep working hard.

WHY YOU SHOULD MAKE PREPARING FOR NCLEX AN ABSOLUTE PRIORITY

This book is a surefire guide to successful preparation for the NCLEX, but merely having purchased it will not guarantee your success. Adequate NCLEX preparation takes effort—often a *lot* of effort—and that is particularly true for graduate nurses who are at some degree of risk for failure. You absolutely must carve out the time you need to prepare adequately from your busy life.

On the whole, my most challenging NCLEX clients have been those who had both jobs and families. This was not because they were any less motivated than other clients, but because it was so difficult to find both time to study and a quiet place in which to study without interruption. Family responsibilities and lack of cooperation from family members can be significant barriers to NCLEX success. Most nurses are female, and women who have spouses, partners, and/or children can sometimes find it difficult to put their own needs before those of family members and be assertive about those needs. If you have a partner and/or children, you may find it necessary to point out to your nearest and dearest that they have a financial stake in your NCLEX success. If you are employed, you may have to decrease your hours or quit work altogether if that is possible for you. Happily, if you work in a hospital or other type of healthcare facility, your employer will likely be willing to cooperate with whatever you need to do in order to achieve RN status.

WHY YOU SHOULD ACCESS A SOURCE OF ADDITIONAL QUESTIONS, IF NECESSARY

As you will find out as you progress to later chapters, the NCLEX prep method upon which this book is based requires you to use NCLEX-type questions both to hone your analytical skills and to identify and plug holes in your knowledge base. It is likely that the questions presented in the latter chapters of this book will be sufficient for your needs, but should you find (as you review your Keep Track logs) that you need more, do not hesitate to access them. Chapter 2 lists a number of companies that market various online NCLEX preparation packages. If you live near your school, you may have free access to questions marketed by a company from which your school has purchased NCLEX prep products. It is essential, however, that whatever your source of questions, you continue to use the methods presented in this book. Continue to keep track of your progress and create and review Nugget Lists (see Chapter 10).

HOW TO KNOW WHETHER YOU NEED A TUTOR

My primary function with my NCLEX clients is to teach them the preparation method presented in this book, which I know will work for them. Many are able to carry on by themselves once they understand the method, and require few or no additional consultations with me. Others, however, aren't particularly good book-learners and find it helpful if I explain various principles of pathophysiology or pharmacology to them. And with quite a few clients, particularly those who've failed NCLEX more than once, I find that it's necessary for me to spend some time pointing out and correcting errors in the reasoning they have brought to bear on practice test questions.

I think it is likely that the majority of nurses who purchase this book will be able to pass the NCLEX without the assistance of a personal tutor, providing they are making good progress in learning to analyze questions and filling the gaps in their knowledge base. If you find, however, that you are not seeing steady progress, or if you just can't understand heart failure or ketoacidosis or some other important concept, you may wish to ask a knowledgeable person for assistance. Likely candidates are nursing program faculty and agency clinical nurse specialists.

Chapter 1

Are You at Risk for Failing NCLEX®?

Marian C. Condon

WHAT YOU WILL LEARN IN THIS CHAPTER

- Why having even a few Cs on your transcript may put you at risk
- Why having done better clinically than in the classroom may put you at risk
- Why being a hands-on learner may put you at risk
- Why getting the gist of things and having trouble with details may put you at risk
- Why having done poorly on a predictive test may put you at risk
- Why having been educated in a country other than the United States puts you at risk
- Why having already failed NCLEX® once puts you at risk for failing again
- What it's like to fail NCLEX and why you don't want to do it
- Why being at risk for failure does *not* mean you won't ever be a good nurse

RISK FACTORS

The information I am about to give you on risk factors for failure on the National Council Licensure Examination for Registered Nurses® (NCLEX-RN) comes from three basic sources: my 1994 doctoral dissertation, *The Meaning of Failure on NCLEX for Graduate Nurses* (Hooper, 1994), the general nursing literature on the NCLEX, and the considerable amount of information I've acquired over my 15 years of tutoring graduate nurses who failed the examination and were desperate to pass on their next try. As I got to know each new group of clients, I inevitably found that they shared a number of characteristics with the other clients that I'd had. Many had some degree of difficulty with one or more of nursing's prerequisite science courses in anatomy and physiology, biology, chemistry and microbiology, or pharmacology and pathophysiology. Most had managed to pass those courses but got a C+ or a lower grade in one or more of them. Quite a few of my clients had also gotten a C+ or lower in one or more nursing courses. Another characteristic that my clients have tended to share is a history of having done better in the clinical component of nursing courses than they did in the classroom component, mostly because of lackluster performance on multiple-choice tests. I believe having difficulty with tests is related to another characteristic that virtually all of my NCLEX clients have reported: being hands-on learners who acquire knowledge

---

®NCLEX and NCLEX-RN are registered trademarks of the National Council of State Boards of Nursing, Inc.

more easily in actual clinical situations than from books, lectures, etc. I've also noticed that individuals who fail NCLEX tend to get the gist (general idea) of things easily but have trouble with details. Here are two other very critical risk factors you need to know about: If you received your basic nursing education in a non-English speaking country and wish to practice in the United States, you are at high risk for failing the NCLEX on your initial attempt and, unfortunately, on subsequent attempts as well. Finally, if you've already failed the NCLEX one or more times, you are at high risk for failing on your next attempt, too.

GPA and Grades in Certain Subjects

You do not have to have a really low GPA to be at risk for failing the NCLEX. Most of my clients have had GPAs in the low- to mid-B range, and nurse researchers have found that to be true also. For example, Griffiths, Papastrat, Czekanski, and Hagen (2004) reported that the GPAs of the unsuccessful NCLEX candidates they studied ranged from 3.0 to 3.4. My observations about my clients' tendencies to have had difficulty in basic science courses, such as pharmacology and pathophysiology, and in one or more nursing courses is also congruent with the findings of many nurse researchers, but I will mention only two here. Vandenhouten (2008) found that graduate nurses who failed the NCLEX had lower grades in pharmacology and certain nursing courses than graduate nurses who passed. Beeson and Kissling (2001) found that earning less than stellar grades in pathophysiology courses and the third-level medical–surgical nursing course was also associated with failure on the NCLEX.

Hands-On Learners

Almost without exception, my clients describe themselves as hands-on learners who learn best by doing. They tell me they find it difficult to fully grasp concepts related to nursing until they have encountered them in real patient care situations in which they are actively involved. As I mentioned previously, my clients also tell me they performed better clinically in nursing courses than on classroom tests. Hearing clients say they found tests challenging but still managed to perform well clinically never surprises me because I learned very early in my tutoring career that failing the NCLEX absolutely does *not* mean that an individual cannot be a good nurse—more about that in the last section of this chapter.

Gist People Versus Detail People

The first question I ask when a new NCLEX client comes into my office is, What do you think stopped you from passing the NCLEX? The answer I hear over and over again is, I don't know. Most clients say they have no idea why they failed, although a few say they suffer from test anxiety. Most, but not all, tell me they thought they had prepared adequately—that they had studied hard for the NCLEX. The next question I ask new clients is, How do you feel about your knowledge base? Only a few clients have told me they thought their nursing knowledge base was weak; most say they feel good about their knowledge and that there must be some other explanation for their failure. I then ask them another question, Do you understand heart failure? Most say yes, and when I ask them to explain it to me, they say something very much like this: heart failure is when the heart muscle gets too weak to pump enough blood to all the organs in the body. That answer captures quite nicely the gist of what heart failure is—so far, so good. But then I probe for more detailed information. I ask, Can you tell me the difference between the signs and symptoms of left- and right-sided heart failure? Many of my clients have not been able to answer that question well, even though they had just told me, with absolute sincerity, that they understood heart failure. Years of tutoring have taught me that most of my clients tend to equate getting the gist of a concept with having an adequate level of mastery of it when, in reality, having adequate mastery requires a grasp of detailed information. I believe that the tendency to mistake getting the gist of something for true mastery is one of the two primary sources of my clients' difficulty not only with NCLEX but with other tests they've had to take in the course of their nursing education.

Global Versus Analytical Cognitive Style

I've long suspected, although I cannot prove, that my clients' cognitive style has a lot to do with their difficulties with NCLEX. The term *cognitive style* refers to the manner in which an individual prefers to process information—his or her typical mode of thinking, remembering, and problem solving. Although a number of different schemas for describing and classifying cognitive style have been developed, the one that addresses the dichotomy that has been termed *analytical* versus *global* is the one that rings most true to me regarding the issue of failure on the NCLEX. The analytical and global styles are conceptualized as polar opposites that lie at either end of a continuum. All of us have a unique style that falls somewhere along that continuum; we might be right in the middle, or we might be a little, or a lot, closer to one end or the other.

A number of characteristics differentiate individuals who have a strongly analytical cognitive style from those who have a strongly global style (Wooldridge & Haimes-Bartolf, 2008). In terms of actual visual perception, analytical individuals are quite good at detecting geometric shapes (where's Waldo?) that are embedded or hidden in a background. Global people, however, do not do nearly as well in perceiving embedded shapes because global individuals become distracted by the background. For global folks, parts tend to be fused with the background and are therefore hard to detect. The difference may become clearer to you if you think of analytical people as tree people and global people as forest people.

Whether our cognitive style is relatively more global or more analytical has a lot to do with how we learn. People with a markedly global style tend to grasp main ideas easily (they get the gist of things) but are less likely to notice details. Consequently,

FIGURE 1-1 Analytical–Global Continuum

Highly Analytical   **Highly Global**

You are....where?

they tend to be less skilled at analytical processes, which involve noticing and thinking separately about the elements (details) that make up larger concepts. Highly analytical people, in contrast, are very oriented to details and to shades of difference among things. An applicable metaphor is that a highly analytical person would easily see and be able to describe the difference among, say, McIntosh, Red Delicious, and Rome apples, and a highly global person would tend to think of them all as simply apples. Because they perceive shades of difference easily and are good analyzers, analytical individuals tend to do better than global individuals on multiple-choice tests (Wooldridge & Haimes-Bartolf, 2008).

Cognitive style is also connected to personality. People who are more global than analytical tend to be highly interpersonal, friendly, and warm. They are people-oriented individuals who are good at reading social cues and are willing to disclose their own feelings to others. People who are highly analytical, on the other hand, tend to be less interpersonally oriented and skilled because they are relatively more oriented to problem solving and intellectual and practical challenges that require these traits.

By now, you no doubt understand why I suspect that most nurses who are at risk for failure on the NCLEX are more global than analytical in terms of their cognitive style. Most of my clients have been friendly, warm gist people with a history of not doing so well on multiple-choice tests. The good news is that anyone can learn to become a more proficient analyzer. The strategies presented in Chapter 6 will help you sharpen your analytical ability.

Documented Learning Disabilities

If you have attention-deficit/hyperactivity disorder or some other disability that compromises your ability to take in, process, retain, and respond to information (McCleary-Jones, 2008), do not despair of passing NCLEX. If you're reading this paragraph, you've completed or nearly completed a nursing program, and if you can do that, you can pass the NCLEX. I have successfully worked with a number of clients who have had diagnosed and undiagnosed (in my opinion) learning disabilities, and all have benefited greatly from using the NCLEX-prep methods that will be presented in later chapters of this book. O'Neil (1991) found that senior nursing students with diagnosed learning disabilities who had been coached in test-taking skills were more likely to pass NCLEX than matched students who had not been coached.

Predictive Tests

A number of standardized exit tests have been developed that are intended to predict whether senior nursing students will be successful on the NCLEX. These tests are typically made available to senior nursing students near the end of their program and include instruments such as Evolve Reach (formerly the HESI Exit Exam) and the ATI RN Comprehensive Predictor. Schools are increasingly using these inventories, particularly Evolve, in an effort to identify senior nursing students at risk for failure in the hope that they will take remedial action to increase their chances of passing the NCLEX. Schools absolutely must ensure that a reasonably high percentage of their graduates pass the NCLEX because if a school's pass rate falls too far below the state average and remains there for several years, the school may eventually lose its accreditation and have to close. Some schools take this threat so seriously that they refuse to allow students who got low scores on the exit test to register to take the NCLEX. Admission to the RN licensing exam is tightly controlled, and only individuals who have been certified by their school as eligible to test are permitted to register for it. Although how well the various exit tests actually predict success or failure on the NCLEX is hotly debated in the nursing literature, I think you would be foolish to pass up an opportunity to get an estimate of your readiness to take the NCLEX. Thus, I have two recommendations for those of you who are about to graduate from nursing school: (1) take a predictive test, and (2) take the results seriously. Among my more recent clients, approximately half have taken an exit test and half have not. Most clients who took an exit test did not do particularly well on it, but unfortunately they did not take that warning seriously. Instead, they rationalized their poor performance, saying the exit test had no actual predictive value because they had not studied for it the way they would study for the actual NCLEX. If you've already taken an exit test and did not achieve a score strongly associated with success on the NCLEX, don't bother retaking the exit test to achieve a better score unless your school requires you to do that. There is evidence in the nursing literature (Spurlock & Hunt, 2008) that it's your initial score that matters and that subsequent scores are not very highly correlated with performance on NCLEX. Instead, use your exit test results, along with the diagnostic sections of this book, to identify the weaknesses in your knowledge base.

Internationally Educated Nurses

If you received your basic nursing education in a country other than the United States, and particularly if English is not your native language, you may be at very high risk for not passing the NCLEX on your first try and at even higher risk for not passing on subsequent tries. Of the internationally educated nurses who took the NCLEX in 2008, fewer than half (45.3%) passed on their first attempt, and among those who failed, only 25% passed on their next attempt. All NCLEX candidates must take the examination in English, and insufficient proficiency in the English language is thought to be one of the principal reasons why English as a second language (ESL) nurses have such difficulty with NCLEX (Cunningham, Stacciarini, & Towle, 2004). There are two levels of language proficiency: proficiency at the basic interpersonal level and proficiency at the cognitive academic level. Individuals whose language ability is at the cognitive academic level of proficiency are much better able to detect subtle differences in meaning among similar words and to understand words and phrases used to convey complex concepts than are individuals proficient only at the basic interpersonal level. Also, candidates who are proficient in interpersonal English but not cognitive academic English may mentally transpose the order in which words occur in English sentences to match the customary order in their native language, and that shift may alter the meaning of the English sentence. Unfortunately, ESL nurses tend to not understand the difference between the two levels of mastery; most who can converse easily in English falsely believe that their language skills are sufficient for the NCLEX when, in reality, they lack the cognitive academic proficiency necessary for success.

Nurses who were born and educated in other cultures may also have a cultural bias that makes answering certain types of NCLEX questions difficult for them. For example, a nurse educated in Japan, where patients are sometimes not told of a serious or terminal diagnosis, might incorrectly answer an NCLEX question based on the

Western presumption that patients are entitled to accurate information about their health status.

Because the NCLEX is a timed test, nurses whose first language is not English may also be handicapped by the time they need to translate English into their native language. When extra time is needed for translation, less time remains for thinking critically about questions.

I strongly recommend that ESL nurses and nurses educated in countries other than the United States go through the CGFNS Certification Program, which is voluntary. The initials CGFNS stand for Commission on Graduates of Foreign Nursing Schools. The commission offers a certification program designed to increase foreign-born nurses' chances of passing the NCLEX. The program includes three components: a credentials review, a one-day test of nursing knowledge that is modeled on NCLEX, and an English language proficiency test. Nurses who go through the certifying process are provided with an estimate of the likelihood that they will pass the NCLEX and recommendations for remediation if they are found to be at high risk for failure. The CGFNS Certification Program has an excellent record of preparing international nurses to take and pass the NCLEX. A study of foreign-born nurses who took NCLEX between April 2006 and March 2007 indicated that 90.8% of CGFNS certificate holders passed, and only 40.7% of noncertificate holders passed (Yocum & Davis, n.d.).

A number of strategies for assisting internationally educated nurses to pass the NCLEX have been suggested, including providing them with specific information about Western healthcare-related values and pointing out potentially confusing words and phrases.

Previous Failure on NCLEX®

Nurses who fail the NCLEX on their first attempt are often horrified to find that they are unsuccessful on their next attempt as well. It is sad but true that on average only about half of the NCLEX repeat test takers in a given year pass; in 2008 the pass rate was 86.7% among first-time test takers who were educated in the United States but only 53.3% among repeat test takers (National Council of State Boards of Nursing, 2009). The situation for nurses educated outside the United States is even worse; only 25% of those who failed on their first attempt pass on their next attempt.

I have tutored many nurses who have failed the NCLEX multiple times, and in the course of interviewing them about their preparation strategies, I've found that although most nurses tried harder and harder to pass after each failure, they also continued to study for the NCLEX in the same way they had before—and got the same results. I will say more in the next chapter about the unsuccessful preparation strategies my clients have typically used, and I'll explain why those strategies don't work.

WHAT IT'S LIKE TO FAIL

The experience of failing the NCLEX is disappointing for just about everyone, but for some it is also embarrassing, humiliating, and financially devastating. How severe the failure experience is for a given nurse depends on his or her circumstances. Some nurses take the NCLEX before they've found a job and some take it afterward. Failing tends to be less severe for the former group than for the latter because if a nurse fails the NCLEX *before* being hired by an agency, the failure is known only to that nurse and others to whom he or she has chosen to reveal it. When nurses take and fail NCLEX *after* they've gained employment, however, the situation is quite different.

In most states, graduate nurses (GNs) who wish to begin practicing before they've passed the NCLEX do so under a temporary practice permit that they obtain from their state board of nursing. After they have been issued a practice permit, they are allowed, in most states, to carry out almost all RN duties under supervision. Although practice permits are generally good for 1 year, agencies usually want their new graduates to take and pass the NCLEX as soon as possible and push them to do so. After a GN has taken and failed the NCLEX, however, the practice permit is revoked, and the GN may no longer practice in the quasi-RN role. Failure under those circumstances is much more public because it is known to the GN's nurse manager and coworkers. GNs who have failed NCLEX once are demoted, often to the role of nursing technician, because they may no longer practice legally in their former role. Such a demotion usually involves a significant cut in pay, which can have serious consequences if the GN is responsible for car payments, rent, etc. Policies regarding GNs who fail multiple times vary from agency to agency. They may be allowed to continue in their tech position, either in the same unit or a different one, or their employment may be terminated.

I have heard graduate nurses describe failing NCLEX as the worst thing that ever happened to them. Many have told me they felt acute embarrassment and shame because they thought they'd disappointed their parents, partners, former nursing instructors, preceptors, and coworkers. Many, particularly those who have failed more than once, come to question their own intelligence and fitness for a career in nursing. GNs are often at a loss as to where to go for help in passing the NCLEX on their next try. Many have told me they felt too humiliated to seek assistance from faculty at their school, and although agency personnel may try to help them, most have no particular ability to do so. GNs who get caught in a spiral of repeated NCLEX failures become increasingly depressed and hopeless, and, sadly, some finally give up on their dream of becoming an RN.

BEING AT RISK FOR FAILING NCLEX® DOES NOT MEAN YOU WILL NEVER BE A GOOD NURSE

Hearing clients say that they found tests challenging but still managed to perform well clinically never surprises me because I learned very early in my tutoring career that failing the NCLEX absolutely does *not* mean that an individual cannot be a good nurse. You see, back in 1994 when I did my doctoral dissertation on nurses who had failed the NCLEX (which was a paper-and-pencil test then), the newly graduated nurses I studied had been working in hospitals for as long as 6 weeks before finding out they had not passed NCLEX. Most were absolutely shocked by the news of their failure because even those working in challenging areas, such as ICUs and emergency departments, had been receiving glowing performance evaluations from their clinical preceptors. You may be surprised to know that the author of a doctoral dissertation (Heupel, 1986) found that there was an inverse relationship between how well the 23 nurses she studied had done on their boards and the performance ratings that were given to them by their supervisors. What that means is that the nurses who had done less well on the

NCLEX received higher ratings from their supervisors than their counterparts who had done better on NCLEX. Now, that research was done during the 1980s on a rather small sample of nurses who had taken a now-outdated version of the NCLEX, so the results must be viewed with caution. Unfortunately, it would be impossible to replicate Heupel's study today with a larger sample because NCLEX is now a pass–fail exam and there would be no scores to compare.

I have long suspected that when novice nurses who are hands-on learners enter the real world of nursing, they easily absorb the knowledge they need to practice well in their chosen area—knowledge they may not have been able to acquire from classroom lectures, reading assignments, and the necessarily limited amount of clinical experience provided by nursing schools.

If nurses who have a hard time passing the NCLEX do tend to have cognitive styles that are relatively more global than analytical, one aspect of their global perspective may help them succeed when they make it into actual nursing practice—their innate orientation to people. Global individuals tend to be warm, caring, and sensitive to the emotional states, needs, and concerns of other people. Such characteristics foster a number of skills that are important in nursing practice: meeting the psychosocial needs of patients and their families, collaborating with other members of the health-care team, and serving in formal and informal leadership positions.

I would not be assisting nurses who failed the NCLEX to become licensed in our profession if I did not know from direct experience that they have the potential to become excellent practitioners. I have had the opportunity to follow the careers of a number of my former clients, and all are practicing with great success in the agencies in which they are employed.

REFERENCES

Beeson, S. A., & Kissling, G. (2001). Predicting success for baccalaureate nurses on the NCLEX-RN. *Journal of Professional Nursing, 17*(3), 121–127.

Cunningham, H., Stacciarini, J. M. R., & Towle, S. (2004). Strategies to promote success on the NCLEX-RN for students with English as a second language. *Nurse Educator, 19*(1), 15–19.

Griffiths, M., Papastrat, K., Czekanski, K., & Hagen, K. (2004). The lived experience of NCLEX failure. *Journal of Nursing Education, 43*(7), 322–325.

Heupel, C. (1986). Selection policy for nursing licensure. *Dissertation Abstracts International, 47*(12). (UMI No. 8706928)

Hooper, M. (1994). *The meaning of failure on NCLEX for graduate nurses.* Unpublished doctoral dissertation, Pennsylvania State University, Harrisburg.

McCleary-Jones, V. (2008). Strategies to facilitate learning among nursing students with learning disabilities. *Nurse Educator, 33*(3), 105–106.

National Council of State Boards of Nursing. (2009). *Number of candidates taking NCLEX-RN examination and percent passing, by type of candidate.* Retrieved March 4, 2009, from https://www.ncsbn.org/Table_of_Pass_Rates_20082.pdf

O'Neil, A. J. (1991). The effectiveness of an intervention to promote successful performance on NCLEX-RN for baccalaureate students at risk for failure. *Journal of Nursing Education, 30*(8), 360–366.

Spurlock, D., & Hunt, L. (2008). A study of the usefulness of the HESI exit exam in predicting NCLEX-RN failure. *Journal of Nursing Education, 47*(4), 157–166.

Vandenhouten, C. L. (2008). *Predictors of success and failure on the NCLEX-RN for baccalaureate graduates.* Unpublished doctoral dissertation, Marquette University. Retrieved June 18, 2009, from http://epublications.marquette.edu/dissertations/AAI3306523

Wooldridge, B., & Haimes-Bartolf, M. (2008). The field dependence/field independence learning styles: Implications for adult student diversity, outcomes assessment and accountability. In P. Blakely & A. T. Tomlin (Eds.), *Adult education: Issues and development* (pp. 231–251). New York: Nova Science.

Yocum, C. J., & Davis, C. R. (n.d.). *Certification program validity study April 2006–March 2007.* Retrieved March 4, 2009, from http://www.cgfns.org/sections/tools/stats/validity.shtml

Chapter 2

Are You Using the Right NCLEX Prep Strategies?

Marian C. Condon

WHAT YOU WILL LEARN IN THIS CHAPTER

- How my clients who failed NCLEX typically studied
- Why their strategies were ineffective
- What two things you absolutely must do if you want to pass NCLEX
- When you should start studying for NCLEX
- The pros and cons of taking a review course
- The truth about test anxiety

INEFFECTIVE PREP STRATEGIES

One of the things I always ask new clients is how they've gone about preparing for NCLEX. Whether they've failed once or multiple times, they almost always tell me they used one or more of the following methods:

- They read and reread content from textbooks, handouts, and course notes.
- They used transparent markers to highlight content.
- They recopied notes they'd already made.
- They made additional notes based on content from NCLEX-prep books or review courses.
- They answered practice questions from NCLEX-prep books and then looked up the answers.

Now you may be thinking that these strategies are the same ones you've been using or will be using. If you've been a strong student and you've done well on one of those tests that predict performance on the NCLEX, those strategies may work for you. But, if you read the list of risk factors for failure on the NCLEX in the last chapter and thought, "Oh, no! That's me!" it is likely that they will not. The problem with the prep strategies my clients used is twofold: (1) they are all relatively passive learning strategies that do not reliably support retention and understanding of material, and (2) they do not involve the high-level cognitive (critical thinking) processes that nurses must practice and master if they want to pass the NCLEX.

Rereading, Highlighting, and Copying Notes

One problem with strategies such as rereading, highlighting, and copying notes is that you will wind up spending quite a bit of your precious study time reviewing material you've already mastered. Nurses who are at risk of failing the NCLEX almost always have significant gaps in their knowledge base, and it is critical that they use their study time to find out what they *don't* know and concentrate specifically on that. Reading review sections is fine, but be sure to review only material you know yourself to be weak on. A second problem with rereading, copying notes, etc. is that those processes do not necessarily lead to memorization of the material. You will find more information on this point later in this chapter and in Chapter 8, How to Use What You *Don't* Know to Pass the NCLEX.

Answering Questions in NCLEX Books

Answering questions in NCLEX-prep books is an excellent strategy, and I highly recommend it. However, merely looking up the answers to questions you answered incorrectly is not going to help you pass the NCLEX. Remember, gist people (the global learners described in Chapter 1) tend to overlook details and to feel that they've mastered a concept or content area when all they really have is the general idea. You need to make sure you've actually mastered the nursing facts, principles, and concepts on which each of the questions you missed was based. By mastered, I mean two things: I mean that you've *committed to memory* any related facts and principles not already lodged solidly in your head, and I mean that you *understand* any related concepts well enough to explain them verbally or in writing. Chapter 8 contains detailed instructions regarding how to proceed when you find you have answered an NCLEX-prep question incorrectly.

Retaining Information

To pass NCLEX, you will have to be able to recall a great deal of information related to nursing practice, analyze it, and then apply it to various test question scenarios. Thus, you must be absolutely certain that you've committed the necessary information to memory. Most of my clients who failed NCLEX had used the passive learning strategies previously described, and most of them also sincerely believed that their knowledge base was adequate, when in reality, it was not. When we read information multiple times, reread it while highlighting, or reread it while copying it into other notes, that information begins to feel increasingly familiar to us, and we may come to believe that we have memorized it sufficiently to be able to recall it, but that is not necessarily the case. Being able to recognize facts or principles as familiar when we see them in print is not the same as being able to recall them from memory in sufficient detail to apply them to an NCLEX question. Storing detailed information in memory to the point where it becomes recallable is a more difficult process cognitively than storing it only to the point where it will seem familiar (Intelegen, 2005). You can easily test this principle for yourself.

> *Exercise*
> Read and reread the following list of 10 objects. Then, cover them and see if you can find them among the larger list of objects on the next page.
>
> Cow   Button   Fan   Tooth   Feather   New   Book   Globe   String   Hood

Without looking at the list of words on the previous page, read the following larger list of words and circle each word that you recognize from the original list. Cover the list when you are finished.

Owl	Hood	Feather	Bush	Stove	Button	Rug	Eye	Chair
Cow	Snow	Fan	Lamp	Frog	New	Tooth	Fresh	Candle
Hard	String	Fern	Newt	Sting	Book	Plane Grass	Globe	Mouth

Now, without looking at either of the previous lists see whether you can recall all 10 words from the original list:

1. _____   6. _____
2. _____   7. _____
3. _____   8. _____
4. _____   9. _____
5. _____   10. _____

Now do you believe that recall is harder than recognition?

TWO THINGS YOU MUST DO IF YOU WANT TO PASS THE NCLEX

If you are determined to pass the NCLEX, you absolutely must do two things: you must determine objectively whether your knowledge base is adequate (if you are a gist person, it probably isn't), and you must find out just how good you are at analyzing test questions and applying your nursing knowledge to them.

One of the first things I do when I work with new clients is estimate the extent of their knowledge base. I ask them to take a comprehensive test from an NCLEX prep book and keep track of how many questions they missed and what domain of nursing (medical–surgical, pediatrics, leadership, etc.) each missed question was in. As I continue to work with clients, I use additional comprehensive tests to gauge their readiness to take the NCLEX again. I also evaluate new clients' test-taking skills. I present them with several fairly complicated NCLEX-type questions and ask them to think out loud as they try to answer them. I find that most do not analyze the scenarios (stems) very well or do a very good job of thinking critically about the four answer choices.

This book provides you with the tools you need to evaluate both your test-taking ability and your knowledge base. In Chapter 3, NCLEX-RN: Purpose, Format, and Scope, you will find out how NCLEX-type questions are structured and about rules the nurse–experts who write NCLEX questions must follow. In Chapter 6, Test Yourself: How Good Are You at Doping Out Test Questions?, you will be given an opportunity to evaluate your own test-taking expertise and take advantage of extensive tutorials designed to hone your test-taking and critical thinking skills. You will use Chapter 7, Test Yourself: How Good Is Your Knowledge Base?, to identify deficiencies in your arsenal of information, and you will use the topic-focused Practice Tests (Chapters 9–23) and Comprehensive Practice Exams (Chapters 24 and 25) to make absolutely sure you know everything you need to know to pass the NCLEX.

WHEN TO START STUDYING FOR NCLEX

Some senior nursing students start preparing for NCLEX during their last semester of school, and others wait until after they have graduated. Students' decisions about when to start studying are often driven by their school's policy regarding NCLEX-prep and readiness materials. Most nursing programs make standardized NCLEX-prep materials available to senior students, and some even mandate that students utilize them. Materials that may be offered to or mandated for students include topic-focused and comprehensive practice tests, topic-focused achievement tests, and comprehensive NCLEX-readiness tests, also known as exit tests. Topic-focused practice tests contain questions organized around specific domains of nursing practice (medical–surgical, psych–mental health, leadership, etc.) or even more narrowly around particular types of patient problems (cardiovascular, renal, endocrine, etc.). Practice tests focused specifically on such areas as pharmacology, medication administration, communication, and leadership are also common. Topic-focused achievement tests are generally organized around clinical domains and are more carefully constructed than practice tests because they are intended to be usable by schools as formal outcome criteria. NCLEX-readiness tests are designed to predict students' likelihood of achieving a passing score on the NCLEX.

Schools vary in the ways in which they use the previously described materials. Some make practice tests, achievement tests, and predictive tests available but optional, and others make achievement tests or readiness tests mandatory. Some schools even use standardized achievement tests as summative outcome criteria in certain courses; if students cannot pass the test, they do not pass the course. As mentioned in Chapter 1, many schools require senior students to take an NCLEX-readiness test early in their last semester and then develop and implement a remedial study plan based on their results, and a few nursing programs even withhold permission to take the NCLEX until the student has retaken the readiness test with a more favorable result.

Although starting to extensively prepare for the NCLEX while still in school is certainly a good idea for many students, doing so may not be feasible for all, particularly those who fit the at-risk-for-failure profile presented in Chapter 1. If you've had to struggle a bit with your nursing courses, it may be necessary for you to apply most or all of your available study time to the courses you need to pass in order to graduate. Indeed, it is documented in the nursing literature that senior nursing students who have experienced some academic difficulty often decline to participate in optional NCLEX-prep activities (Dibartolo & Seldomridge, 2008). I do, however, wish to reiterate what I told you in Chapter 1: I recommend strongly that you take whatever NCLEX readiness test is available at your school. Such tests can provide you with valuable information about the areas of weakness in your knowledge base, and unless your school mandates otherwise, you can always postpone serious remedial work until after you graduate.

If you choose to forgo NCLEX-prep activities during your last semester of school, you will need to give yourself plenty of time to prepare adequately after you graduate. Although you should take the NCLEX relatively soon after graduation so that the information you acquired in school will be fresh in your mind, you do not want to take the exam until you've had time to really prepare and ensure that you are equipped to pass. If you've accepted an offer of employment, you may wish to consider postponing the date on which you begin your new position so you will not have to orient to a new job while still studying for the NCLEX. You will have a lot to learn as a new nurse and may even have to take some certification courses in one or more areas, particularly if you've been hired into a specialty unit. I've had a number of clients who were (1) working full time, (2) studying for Advanced Cardiac Life Support or other such certification, and (3) preparing for the NCLEX all at the same time—a stressful scenario you want to avoid if you possibly can.

REVIEW COURSES

NCLEX-prep packages are marketed to individuals, nursing programs, or both by a number of companies. Most offer an array of package options that vary in terms of cost, whether the content review is available live or online, and the time period for which online materials will be available to purchasers. The types of tests included in such packages usually include content-specific and comprehensive practice tests, content-specific achievement tests, and comprehensive NCLEX-readiness tests.

Companies that market NCLEX-prep courses include, but are not limited to, the following:

- Assessment Technologies Institute (ATI; www.atitesting.com) markets online review courses, practice tests, achievement tests, and readiness tests.
- Evolve Learning System (http://evolve.elsevier.com) markets online review courses, practice tests, achievement tests, and readiness tests to individuals and schools. Evolve Reach testing and remediation tests were formerly marketed under the name HESI (Health Education Systems Inc.).
- Kaplan (www.kaplannursing.com) markets on-site, live classroom, and online review courses, practice tests, achievement tests, and a readiness test.
- National Council of State Boards of Nursing Learning Extension (http://www.learningext.com) markets an online review course that includes practice tests, achievement tests, and a readiness test.
- National League for Nursing (NLN; www.nln.org) markets the Total Assessment Program (TAP) for NCLEX Success to schools of nursing. TAP includes an on-site, live review program, practice tests, achievement tests, and a readiness test. NLN also markets an online review course to individuals (www.rx4nclexsuccess.com) that includes practice tests, achievement tests, and a readiness test.

Some of the clients I have assisted over the years had taken a formal NCLEX-review course and some had not. Although I would never dissuade anyone from taking an on-site or online course, the fact remains that quite a few of my clients took one and failed anyway. There is no guarantee that merely sitting passively in a classroom and listening to several days of content review or participating in an online review will result in sufficient retention of material to provide you with an adequate knowledge base. If you do decide to purchase a review course, I advise you to bring the active learning process outlined in Chapter 8 to bear on the test-prep questions that are made available to you.

TEST ANXIETY

The belief that test anxiety is at the root of some, if not most, instances of failure on NCLEX is very common. Teaching students how to control their test anxiety in relation to NCLEX has been cited in the nursing literature as a useful prep strategy (McDowell, 2008), and when I ask my clients to name the single factor most responsible for their failure on NCLEX, most say it was text anxiety that did them in. Thus, I suspect that you may be wondering whether it would be worthwhile for you to focus on reducing your test anxiety as part of your preparation for NCLEX. My view is that because text anxiety is an unpleasant stressor, controlling it will support your general health and is therefore desirable, but I don't think that minimizing your test anxiety will, in itself, affect your performance on NCLEX. Although I don't doubt for a moment that many of my clients have indeed felt quite anxious while taking NCLEX and other tests, I do *not* agree that their anxiety was the primary or even secondary cause of their failure. My reasons for taking this position are very simple: (1) I've tutored many graduate nurses who failed the NCLEX, and every one of them was a not-so-good test-question analyzer who was also handicapped by knowledge base deficits, and (2) my method has never included strategies specifically aimed at reducing test anxiety. In my view, test anxiety is a result, rather than a cause, of having had difficulty with tests over a significant period of time. The real cause is, of course, a weak knowledge base in combination with underdeveloped analytical skills. When my clients have gotten up to speed in those two areas, they've succeeded in passing the NCLEX whether they were anxious while taking it or not. Having said that, however, I do have a recommendation for those of you who would like to take steps to decrease the anxiety you experience while taking tests of various kinds. There is a self-treatment modality known as Emotional Freedom Techniques (EFT) that I've personally found to be very effective at short-circuiting transitory negative mood states, such as worry and feeling a little bit down. EFT is a treatment modality from the field of energy psychology, which is relatively new and not yet recognized by most mainstream mental health organizations. Although there is controversy about how EFT works, even its most dedicated critics admit that it does work for some people, some of the time. One of my friends, who is a psychotherapist, reports that the technique has been helpful to some of her clients who were open to it. You can learn about EFT at http://www.emofree.com.

REFERENCES

Dibartolo, M., & Seldomridge, L. (2008). A review of intervention studies to promote NCLEX-RN success of baccalaureate students. *Nurse Educator, 5*(33), 78S–83S.

Intelegen. (2005). *Long term memory*. Retrieved May 2, 2009, from http://www.web-us.com/memory/generic_ltm_memory.htm

McDowell, B. (2008). KATTS: A framework for maximizing NCLEX-RN performance. *Journal of Nursing Education, 47*(4), 183–186.

Chapter 3

NCLEX-RN: Purpose, Format, and Scope

Marian C. Condon

WHAT YOU WILL LEARN IN THIS CHAPTER

- What the initials NCLEX stand for
- How the NCLEX is developed and administered
- How the content is decided upon
- Who writes the questions
- How the questions are structured—format and level of complexity
- What you will be expected to know—the test plan

HOW THE EXAM IS DEVELOPED AND ADMINISTERED

The initials NCLEX stand for National Council Licensure Examination. NCLEX-RN, the licensing examination for registered nurses (RNs), is developed by the National Council of State Boards of Nursing (NCSBN). The NCSBN is made up of the nursing boards of all 50 states plus the District of Columbia and the four U.S. territories. The NCLEX-RN Test Plan (discussed later in this chapter) is the official blueprint of the current exam's content and scope and is based on the most recently conducted practice analysis, along with input from a panel of nurse–experts. Practice analyses, which involve surveying thousands of newly licensed RNs to collect data regarding areas of knowledge and skill and how frequently they apply them in practice, are done every 3 years, and the licensing exam is then revised as necessary (NCSBN, 2009). The NCSBN has engaged a company called Pearson VUE to administer the NCLEX at test centers located throughout the United States and its territories.

HOW THE QUESTIONS ARE WRITTEN AND STRUCTURED

All NCLEX questions, known as *items*, are written by experienced RNs who have received instruction in how to write high-quality items for the NCLEX. When completed, items are reviewed extensively by a number of different groups to ensure they are clear, accurate, current, and reflective of entry-level practice expectations. Items are also screened for gender, ethnic, or cultural stereotyping and bias, elitism, and controversial nursing concepts or practices. All items are pretested before they are included in the NCLEX test bank. Pretest items are presented to test takers but are not scored, and only pretested items that meet statistical reliability and validity criteria are eventually admitted to the actual pool of items from which scored NCLEX questions are drawn (NCSBN, 2009).

Format

Most NCLEX questions are written in the multiple-choice format with which you are familiar by virtue of your experience in your nursing program. There is a scenario, called the *stem*, a question based on the scenario, and four answer choices. The correct choice is called the *key*, and the three incorrect choices are called *distracters*. You may also encounter another sort of multiple-choice question, the *multiple-response* question. In multiple-response questions, there may be more than four distracters, and there may be more than one key. When presented with a multiple-response question, you will be instructed to select all keys that apply.

The nurse is preparing a patient for cardiac catheterization. Which of the following teaching points are pertinent for the nurse to include before the procedure? SELECT ALL THAT APPLY.
A. "You will have to lie flat for several hours after the procedure."
B. "You will receive medication to relax you but you will be awake."
C. "You will feel a very cool sensation when the dye is injected."
D. "You will be placed on a hard table that moves during the procedure."

The NCLEX will also contain questions in four additional format types: Hot-Spot, Chart/Exhibit, Drag-and-Drop, and Fill-in-the-Blank.

Hot-Spot questions consist of an illustration on which you will be expected to identify a specific location. The specific location might be something such as the chest-wall area on which you would place your stethoscope to listen to an apical pulse, an appropriate site for an intramuscular injection, a rhythm-strip waveform associated with a specific electrical event in the heart, etc.

The nurse must defibrillate a patient who is in ventricular tachycardia. Place an "X" over areas of the torso to indicate correct paddle placement.

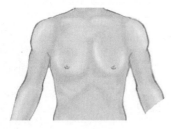

Chart/Exhibit questions are used to test your ability to interpret or utilize information from various forms or data sources used in healthcare agencies. For example, you might be asked to interpret lab results from a simulated lab report or waveforms from a simulated rhythm strip. Other sources of information that might be simulated include flow sheets, prescription forms, medication administration records, order sheets, etc.

The nurse is caring for a patient who was admitted with the following lab work:

Laboratory test	Result
Complete blood count	
Hematocrit (HCT)	42%
Hemoglobin (HGB)	14%
Red blood cells (RBC)	5.0 million/µL
Mean cell volume (MCV)	88 µ/m^3
Mean cell hemoglobin (MCH)	29 pg
Mean cell hemoglobin concentration (MCHC)	36.2%
White blood cells (WBC)	6000/µL
Platelets (Plt)	280,000/µL
Serum electrolytes	
Carbon dioxide	28 mEq/L
Chloride	99 mEq/L
Potassium	2.8 mEq/L
Sodium	138 mEq/L
Serum digoxin	2.5 ng/mL

Upon review, the nurse notes that the patient suffers from which of the following conditions?
A. The patient is neutropenic.
B. The patient is anemic.
C. The patient is hyperkalemic.
D. The patient is digoxin toxic.

   Drag-and-Drop questions, also known as Ordered Response questions, require you to indicate the order in which you would do or attend to something. For example, you might be presented with a nursing procedure and four steps that are a part of it and be asked to indicate the order in which you would carry out the steps. Or you might be presented with descriptions of four patients, each of whom is experiencing a different problem, and be asked to indicate the order in which you would attend to them.

The nurse finds a patient lying flat in bed and struggling to breathe. He is tachypneic and his skin is dusky in color. Place the actions the nurse would carry out in order from first to last:
A. Raise the head of the bed.
B. Call the rapid response team.
C. Start oxygen via nasal cannula at 2 L/min.
D. Take vital signs.

Fill-in-the-Blank questions are just what they sound like. On the NCLEX, questions that require numeric calculation (such as drug dosage questions) are written in this format. You will use the online calculator to arrive at your answer and then type it into the blank answer line. You can access the same NCLEX tutorial that is made available to candidates on test day from the Pearson VUE Web site at http://www.pearsonvue.com/nclex/#tutorial. On the site, you can practice answering questions written in all the alternate formats discussed in this section.

Levels of Complexity

Most NCLEX questions are written at two of the higher levels of cognitive complexity, application and analysis, which are both components of a cognitive skill indispensible to nurses: critical thinking. To say questions are written at the levels of application and analysis means that candidates will have to think at those levels to answer the questions correctly. Here's some background information that will help you better understand cognitive complexity and the reasons NCLEX questions are written at the higher levels.

Knowing, understanding, applying, and analyzing represent increasingly complex cognitive processes. Knowing is considered to be the least complex process because to say that you know something, such as a fact or principle, means only that you can recognize or recall it. To say accurately that you know something, you do not necessarily have to understand it. For example, it is possible to know that Lasix is classified as a loop diuretic without having any understanding of what a loop diuretic does or how it works. A test question concerning Lasix that is written at the level of knowledge might look like this:

The drug Lasix (furosemide) is classified as a _____ drug.
A. psychotropic
B. cardiotonic
C. potassium-sparing diuretic
D. loop diuretic

A candidate who had merely memorized the fact that Lasix is classified as a loop diuretic would have answered that question correctly.

A question regarding Lasix and other loop diuretics written at the level of comprehension will require you to demonstrate a level of thought beyond knowledge; it will require you to understand the nature of loop diuretics—what they do and how they do it, as illustrated in the following question:

The drug Lasix (furosemide) affects which of the following?
A. serotonin and dopamine levels in the brain
B. ion exchange in the myocardium
C. ion exchange in the renal tubule
D. epinephrine levels in the bronchioles

Questions written at the level of application require even more complex thought; they require candidates to use their knowledge and understanding of facts, rules, and principles in making decisions or solving problems related to patient care, as illustrated in the following example:

The nurse is caring for a patient with a diagnosis of heart failure. The nurse properly withholds a scheduled dose of Lasix (furosemide) based on which of the following findings?
A. a decreased level of consciousness
B. elevated blood pressure
C. a hematocrit of 22.4
D. a serum potassium level of 2.8

To answer that question correctly, you must apply your knowledge that the normal range for serum potassium is 3.5–4.5 and your understanding of what loop diuretics do (cause potassium to be excreted from the body) to the question to arrive at the conclusion that Lasix should be held because it is causing hypokalemia.

Analysis is the highest cognitive level at which NCLEX questions are written. The process of analysis involves considering multiple variables and their relationship to and interactions with one another. Questions written at the level of analysis may require you to prioritize, determine causes and effects, perceive recurring themes, etc. The following question is written at the level of analysis:

The nurse is talking with a 17-year-old client who has been admitted to an inpatient psychiatric facility with a diagnosis of depression. The client tells the nurse that she has been thinking a lot about death lately because her father was killed in an accident 2 weeks ago. Which of the following actions should the nurse take?
A. Ask the client to describe her relationship with her father.
B. Assure the client that she will recover from her grief.
C. Ask the client to tell the nurse more about her thoughts about death.
D. Convey to the client condolences regarding the death of her father.

To choose the correct answer, C, you must consider and apply your knowledge and understanding of the implications of multiple variables—the client's age, her diagnosis, the fact that her father died recently, and her statement that she had been "thinking a lot about death lately." You would recall that adolescents sometimes attempt or commit suicide for reasons that do not seem logical to an adult and that depressed people may be at risk for developing suicidal thoughts, and you would know it is quite reasonable and common for a person who has just experienced the death of a close relative to be thinking about death. And, of course, you would know and understand that nurses must always prioritize patient safety. As you consider each factor in light of the others (analysis), you conclude that the correct course of action is to explore the patient's thoughts about death to determine whether she is experiencing suicidal ideation.

To practice entry-level nursing safely and effectively, and to pass the NCLEX, you must know and understand certain facts and principles related to nursing and the physical and social sciences upon which nursing is based, and you must be able to apply them while carrying out the various steps in the nursing process. To do that, you must be able to analyze a wide variety of situations and data. Thus, the great majority of NCLEX questions are written at the level of either application or analysis (NCSBN, 2007b).

WHAT YOU WILL BE EXPECTED TO KNOW: THE NCLEX TEST PLAN

The NCLEX Test Plan is not organized around medical–surgical nursing, maternal–child nursing, community health nursing, etc. in the same way the curricula of many nursing programs are. Instead, it is organized around four client need categories and four integrated processes that are fundamental to and integrated throughout nursing practice. Taken as a whole, the client need categories encompass virtually all the client needs nurses must be able to meet, and the integrated processes describe the means by which nurses go about meeting them. The NCLEX Test Plan mandates that a certain percentage of the questions on each RN licensing examination be allocated to each client need category or subcategory. For example, 13–19% of the questions on every candidate's exam must address the client need subcategory management of care, and 13–19% may be thought of as the weight allotted to that subcategory. The client need categories and subcategories (where applicable) and the relative weights assigned to them for the current test plan are shown in the following list (NCSBN, 2007a) (it is likely that these weights will be modified somewhat as of April 2010):

- Safe, effective care environment (21–33%)
  - Management of care (13–19%)
  - Safety and infection control (8–14%)
- Health promotion and maintenance (6–12%)
- Psychosocial integrity (6–12%)
- Physiological integrity (43–67%)
  - Basic care and comfort (6–12%)
  - Pharmacology and parenteral therapies (13–19%)
  - Reduction of risk potential (13–19%)
  - Physiological adaptation (11–17%)

The specific content (what you will need to know) associated with each client need category is listed on the NCSBN's Web site (www.ncsbn.org). Click on NCLEX Examinations and then on Test Plans.

As suggested by their title, the integrated processes are woven throughout the exam, and the test plan does not mandate a specific weight for any of them. The integrated processes are as follows:

- The nursing process (assessment, analysis, planning, implementation, and evaluation)
- Caring
- Communication and documentation
- Teaching and learning

The following scenarios illustrate how NCLEX items combine integrated processes and client need categories.

A. **The charge nurse is making assignments on a medical–surgical unit. Which of the following clients should be assigned to an RN?**

In this scenario, the client need category is management of care (a subcategory of safe, effective care environment), and the integrated process is the nursing process.

B. A client requests instructions about how to use a home blood pressure monitor. The nurse should tell her:

In this scenario, the client need category is health promotion and maintenance and the integrated process is teaching and learning.

Note that the first scenario involves a specific setting, a medical–surgical unit, but the second does not. Questions related to a given client need category may or may not be written in terms of various types of settings (psych–mental health units, obstetrical units, etc.) or patients of a certain age (elderly, middle-aged, or young). There is no requirement that a certain percentage of questions be related to any setting or age group. Thus, it is possible that your examination will contain anywhere from zero to quite a few scenarios concerning, say, elderly patients, and it is possible you may encounter zero or many questions set in a specific setting, such as a pediatric unit (NCSBN, 2007a).

REFERENCES

National Council of State Boards of Nursing. (2007a). *2007 NCLEX-RN detailed test plan, candidate version*. Retrieved June 3, 2009, from https://www.ncsbn.org/2007_NCLEX_RN_Detailed_Test_Plan_Candidate.pdf

National Council of State Boards of Nursing. (2007b). *2007 NCLEX-RN detailed test plan, item writer/item reviewer/nurse educator version*. Retrieved June 1, 2009, from https://www.ncsbn.org/2007_NCLEX_RN_Detailed_Test_Plan_Educator.pdf

National Council of State Boards of Nursing. (2009). *2009 detailed NCLEX process*. Retrieved June 3, 2009, from https://www.ncsbn.org/2009_Detailed_NCLEX_Process.pdf

Chapter 4

CAT-Anatomy:
How Computer-Adaptive Testing Works

Marian C. Condon

WHAT YOU WILL LEARN IN THIS CHAPTER

- What computer-adaptive testing is
- How NCLEX is scored
- Which test-taking strategies you should *never* use on NCLEX

WHAT COMPUTER-ADAPTIVE TESTING IS

As you no doubt already know, the NCLEX is not a paper-and-pencil test; it is what is known as a *computer-adaptive test* (CAT). This type of test is currently the most efficient and accurate method of ascertaining whether a candidate possesses the minimum level of knowledge and competency necessary for safe and effective practice as an entry-level registered nurse. Prior to the advent of CAT in 1994, NCLEX was a pencil-and-paper test, and every candidate in a given year was presented with the exact same questions. The old tests took many hours to complete, and candidates had to wait much longer for their results than they do now. CAT is a vast improvement over pencil-and-paper testing because CAT allows each candidate to be presented with a unique exam that will reveal his or her level of competence as efficiently as possible.

HOW NCLEX IS SCORED

When you take the NCLEX, you will be presented with a unique examination tailored specifically for you; each time the computer selects a new question from the test bank, it will base its selection on your answer to the previous question. Here's how that works: when you begin your licensing exam, you will be presented with an initial question related to one of the client need categories or subcategories. The difficulty level of that question will be moderately low. If you answer that initial question correctly, the computer will choose as your next question a similar but somewhat more difficult test bank item. If you answer that question correctly, the computer will upgrade its estimate of your competence, which is known as your ability level, and present you with an even more difficult question. The process will continue until you finally answer a question incorrectly. At that point, your ability level regarding that particular client need category or subcategory will have become established, and the computer will then present you with another moderately difficult question related to a different client need category. It will keep selecting more and more difficult questions on that topic until you finally answer one of them incorrectly. The process will continue until all client need categories and subcategories have been covered and the computer has determined with 95% accuracy that you do or do not possess the minimal level of nursing competency required for licensure. If you are either very well prepared or very poorly prepared for the NCLEX, the computer may need your answers to only 75 questions to decide whether you passed or failed. If you are somewhere in the middle range of preparedness, it may need you to answer more questions, up to a maximum of 265, to arrive at a pass–fail decision (National Council of State Boards of Nursing [NCSBN], 2009a).

TEST-TAKING STRATEGIES YOU SHOULD *NEVER* USE ON NCLEX

The tests used as evaluation criteria in nursing courses are almost always administered in a paper-and-pencil format or a computerized equivalent in which everyone answers the same questions. Therefore, NCLEX will likely be the very first computer-adaptive test you will take, and it is essential that you use only test-taking strategies that are appropriate for it. Some of the strategies that may have served you well on the paper-and-pencil tests you took in school will be disastrous if you use them during a CAT.

One of the big differences between the NCLEX and the exams you took in school has to do with time. When faced with a nursing school examination, you knew how many questions you had to answer and how much time you had to answer them. Because most nursing program exams contain 50–60 items and must be completed within an hour, you may be accustomed to allowing yourself only a minute or two to ponder the best answer to each question. On the NCLEX, however, you will have a maximum of 6 hours to complete between 75 and 265 questions, and you will not know at any point in time how many more questions await you. Even though the minutes you spend completing the online tutorial at the test center (see Chapter 5) will count toward the 6 hours, as will any time you spend taking breaks, you are still likely to have more time than you are accustomed to having, especially if you are presented with fewer than 265 questions. Very few NCLEX candidates run out of time; more than half complete the examination in less than 2.5 hours (NCSBN, 2005). My advice related to the time you should allot to each question is as follows: for each of the first 75 questions, take all the time you need to feel pretty certain about the answer you choose because if you do very well on the first 75 items, the computer will shut off and you will have passed the NCLEX. However, if the computer presents you with a 76th question, allow for the possibility that you may be presented with as many as 189 more questions ($265 - 76 = 189$) and begin to move through the test a bit more quickly. Allow yourself enough time to consider each question carefully—you will not be able to go back and change your answer to any question you've already answered—but do not waste time. On average, candidates spend between 60 and 70 seconds on standard multiple-choice NCLEX questions (NCSBN, 2009b).

Another time-related strategy you may have used on exams in school but should *not* use on NCLEX is random guessing. By random guessing, I mean choosing answers haphazardly, without having thought about the question or the answer choices. Random guessing is a strategy you may have used while taking nursing school exams if you knew you were running out of time and wanted to avoid having an item marked incorrect because it was not completed. If you used random guessing, you likely reasoned that if you left a given item blank, you would have no chance of getting credit for it, but if you guessed randomly, you had at least a one in four chance of getting credit. Using random guessing on the NCLEX, however, will not increase your chances of passing. What random guessing on the NCLEX will do is increase your chances of failing because each random guess that is incorrect (which will be most of them) will trigger the computer to select your next question at a lower level of difficulty. If you keep guessing randomly, you will soon display a pattern of answering even low-level questions incorrectly, and the computer will decide you lack the requisite level of knowledge to pass the exam.

In the unlikely event that you do run out of time, it will still be possible for you to pass your licensing exam because the computer will base its pass–fail decision on the ability level you demonstrated while answering *the last 60 questions* (NCSBN, 2009a). Thus, even if the 6 hours allowed for the examination is almost up and the computer is still presenting you with questions, you should not start hurrying through them or guessing randomly.

REFERENCES

National Council of State Boards of Nursing. (2005). *Is how fast I respond to items an important factor for passing the NCLEX?* Retrieved March 3, 2009, from https://www.ncsbn.org/06_07_05_NCLEX_Speed_Fact.pdf

National Council of State Boards of Nursing. (2009a). *2009 detailed NCLEX process.* Retrieved June 18, 2009, from https://www.ncsbn.org/2009_Detailed_NCLEX_Process.pdf

National Council of State Boards of Nursing. (2009b). *Frequently asked questions about NCLEX alternate item formats.* Retrieved June 18, 2009, from https://www.ncsbn.org/Alt_Item_FAQ.pdf

Chapter 5

Registration, Results, and Test-Center Smarts

Marian C. Condon

WHAT YOU WILL LEARN IN THIS CHAPTER

- How to register to take NCLEX
- What fees are involved
- How to avoid pretest disasters
- What to expect at the test center
- What to not worry about
- How to get your results

HOW TO REGISTER TO TAKE NCLEX

To be eligible to take the NCLEX, you must be a graduate of an accredited diploma, associate degree, or baccalaureate nursing program. Toward the end of your senior year, your program will provide you with information regarding time lines and the forms that must be submitted to Pearson VUE (the company that administers the NCLEX) and your state board so you can register to take the licensing examination and apply for a temporary practice permit, which some states require graduate nurses to hold if they wish to practice before their NCLEX results are known. As of 2009, the Pearson VUE registration fee is currently $200. Your state board may levy license application and practice permit application fees as well. Pearson VUE will confirm your registration to test and inform your state board of your intention to test. You will not, however, be allowed to actually take the NCLEX until your school has notified your state board that you have successfully met the school's graduation requirements. After the state board has been notified of your eligibility to take NCLEX, it will issue you an Authorization to Test (ATT) document, and you will be able to make an appointment to take the exam at a Pearson Professional Center. The current version of the *NCLEX Examination Candidate Bulletin* contains detailed information about rules and policies related to NCLEX registration along with sample NCLEX registration forms. The bulletin can be accessed online at http://www.vue.com/nclex/. The process that must be followed by candidates who wish to take the NCLEX at a Pearson VUE test center located outside the United States is essentially the same, but additional fees and taxes may apply. Additional information about international test sites may be found at https://www.ncsbn.org/Internatl_FAQ.pdf.

AVOIDING PRETEST DISASTERS

If you follow the guidelines presented in later chapters of this book, you should be fully prepared for the NCLEX and confident of a positive result. After all your hard work, you owe it to yourself to avoid any last-minute problems that could impair your performance, stress you, or cause you to miss your appointment to take the NCLEX. The two problems discussed in the following sections are easily avoided by a bit of forethought and preparation.

Not Getting Enough Sleep

Getting a good night's sleep before you take the NCLEX is very important. If you are tired when you arrive at the test center, you won't be at your sharpest when you address the questions on your exam. Cramming into the wee hours and allowing yourself to become sleep deprived is not a good idea. If you think preexam jitters are likely to keep you awake, consider asking your nurse practitioner or physician to suggest a medication that will ensure a good night's rest. Do not, however, wait until NCLEX-eve to find out how your sleep aid will affect you. You need to know for sure what time you need to go to bed so you will wake up refreshed, as opposed to suffering from a drug hangover. Sleep-promoting medications vary as to how long their effects last. If you take one that lasts for 8 hours and then get only 6 hours of sleep, you will awaken feeling dull and lethargic instead of well rested and alert. Remember that various cold remedies can make you feel drowsy, too; be very cautious about taking any medication with which you are not familiar before or during the NCLEX.

Arriving Late for Your Test

There are only about 200 Pearson VUE test centers in the continental United States, so unless you live in or near a fairly large city, you may have to travel a considerable distance to reach the test center nearest you. I strongly suggest that if you plan to drive to the test center, you should make sure ahead of time that you know where it is, how long it will take you to get there, and where you will be able to park. A practice drive, preferably at the same time of day you will make the real one, will be well worth your investment in time. If you are more than 20 minutes late for your appointment or miss the appointment entirely, you will have to reschedule—and pay your $200 registration fee all over again. If the location in which you will be taking the NCLEX is more than an hour away from your home, you may wish to consider arriving there the afternoon or evening before the exam and staying in a nearby hotel or motel. By doing so, you will avoid a long commute and the possibility that an unanticipated traffic jam or flat tire will derail your plans.

WHAT TO EXPECT AT THE TEST CENTER

When you arrive at a Pearson Professional Center to take the NCLEX, you must have your ATT and picture ID with you or you will not be allowed to sit for the exam. Security around the NCLEX examination is stringent, and you will not be permitted to bring any study materials with you to the test center. You cannot bring any hats, scarves, coats, watches, cell phones, PDAs, or scratch paper into your computer cubicle; lockers are provided at most test centers. (A dry eraser tablet and marker will also be provided for you.) Your picture and a fingerprint will be taken when you arrive at the test center (National Council of State Boards of Nursing [NCSBN], 2009).

You (and other candidates who test at the same time) will be directed to an individual computer station and provided with a brief online orientation to the computer—how to go about choosing and submitting answers to test questions and how to use the optional on-screen calculator. You should review the NCLEX tutorial online at www.pearsonvue.com/nclex before your test day so you can skip the tutorial and get right to the exam. You must take care to avoid any behavior that might lead the test center staff to think you are attempting to cheat on the exam; do not talk to other test takers or leave your cubicle without a staff member's permission. Make sure you do not have an overlooked cell phone or any other sort of electronic device in your pocket.

WHAT YOU DON'T HAVE TO WORRY ABOUT

Some clients have told me that while taking the NCLEX, they just knew they had gotten certain questions wrong because the computer presented them with those same questions a second time. My clients, however, were incorrect. What they noticed was that they had been presented with some of the same *scenarios* more than once. NCLEX item writers are permitted to use the same scenario in more than one test item, but the questions asked about the scenario and the answer choices must be different. If a question looks really familiar to you, do not assume that you are being presented with it again because you got it wrong; you are merely noticing similarities in the question's stem.

Another thing about which you need not be concerned is how long the computer takes to generate new questions. Any delay the computer seems to be experiencing has nothing to do with your performance; it simply means that several candidates have submitted answers at nearly the same moment, and the computer needs a bit of extra time to process them.

GETTING YOUR RESULTS

When a candidate passes the NCLEX, his or her results are conveyed by Pearson VUE to the NCSBN, which in turn makes that information available to the nursing board in the jurisdiction (state) in which the candidate took the examination. The nursing board then posts on its Web site that an RN license has been issued to the individual. Candidates can visit their board's Web site to see whether a license has been issued in their name. As of January 2009, many boards provide licensure information by linking their Web sites to the NCSBN's new paperless licensure verification system, Nursys. This computer system contains information about nurse licensure (and disciplinary action) provided by participating boards of nursing in the United States and its territories. You can access Nursys directly at https://www.nursys.com, via links on the NCSBN's Web site (www.ncsbn.org), or from a link on your state board's Web site if it participates in Nursys. Do not call your state board to inquire about your license; none of the state boards releases NCLEX results over the phone (NCSBN, 2009).

REFERENCE

National Council of State Boards of Nursing. (2009). *2009 detailed NCLEX process.* Retrieved June 3, 2009, from https://www.ncsbn.org/2009_Detailed_NCLEX_Process.pdf

Chapter 6

Test Yourself: How Good Are You at Doping Out Test Questions?

Marian C. Condon

WHAT YOU WILL LEARN IN THIS CHAPTER

- How effective your current approach is
- The best way to systematically analyze a test question
- Why noticing key words is vitally important
- How to respond to specific key word categories
- How to evaluate answer choices
- The importance of congruency

HOW WELL DO YOU ANALYZE TEST QUESTIONS?

If you want to pass the NCLEX, it is absolutely essential that you become an expert test-question analyzer. To do that, you must first identify weaknesses in your current approach to test questions and then eradicate them. You can evaluate your current level of expertise by carrying out the following exercise.

Exercise

Address the following practice question and attempt to answer it correctly. As you do that, use the numbered blank lines to record each step you take in the order in which you took it. For example, if you began by reading the entire question, write "read entire question" on the first line. Also record the cognitive steps you took, such as "tried to recall everything I know about renal failure." When you have finished the question and chosen your answer, compare the steps you took with the recommended ones outlined in the next section of this chapter.

When evaluating a nursing intervention designed to treat a patient's pain, the nurse does which of the following?
A. Uses suggestion to enhance drug action
B. Asks the patient to rate the pain on a 1–10 scale
C. Verifies the dose and the route of administration
D. Checks the patient's chart for drug allergies

Record the steps in your process here:

1. _____
2. _____
3. _____

4. _____

5. _____

6. _____

7. _____

8. _____

THE OPTIMAL QUESTION-ANALYZING PROCESS

The following question-analyzing process is the one I teach to all my NCLEX clients. They get the hang of it quite quickly and are pleased to find that using it becomes almost automatic with time.

Step 1: Cover the answer choices and read only the stem (scenario).

When you first address a test question, your initial cognitive activity should be to read through the stem without looking at the answer choices. You should not look at the answer choices right away because if you lean a bit toward the global cognitive style discussed in Chapter 1 and you read the answer choices right away, you may decide prematurely (and without realizing you are doing it) that one of them is the key (correct answer). Then, when you start to focus on the scenario, you will be in danger of zeroing in on the elements that seem to support your favored answer choice and glossing right over the ones that do not.

Remember: When you actually take NCLEX, cover the answer choices with your hand or your dry erase tablet before you start to read the scenario.

Step 2: Make sure you know what the question really is.

After you have read through the scenario, your second step should be to focus on the question that is embedded in the scenario and rephrase that question in your own words. Here's the sample scenario with the embedded question underlined:

When evaluating a nursing intervention designed to treat a patient's pain, <u>the nurse does which of the following?</u>

Note that rephrasing the question clarifies its meaning a bit:

What does the nurse do to determine whether a treatment for pain has been effective?

Here's another underlined embedded question you can use to practice rephrasing:

The nurse is administering the drug alteplase (recombinant tissue plasminogen activator) to a client who was admitted with severe chest pain. <u>Which of the following would the nurse recognize as a side effect of the drug?</u>

Your rephrased question should look like this:

What negative sign or symptom might a patient display that was caused by alteplase?

Step 3: Underline the key words in the scenario.

The key words, or in some cases, key phrases, in a test question's scenario provide information that you must take into consideration to answer the question correctly;

think of key words as the clues you need to solve the mystery of which answer choice is correct. Failing to consider even one of the key words in a scenario can cause you to answer the question incorrectly because each key word counts; item writers are not allowed to include irrelevant information in scenarios. Each key word in a given scenario prompts you to consider the implications of one of the following:

- The illness, condition, or problem
- The stage or phase of the illness
- Signs and/or symptoms
- A pertinent characteristic of the patient
- A drug, treatment, or device
- The step in the nursing process that has been stipulated
- The level of priority or likelihood
- The relative merits of one course of action over another

Here are some examples of key words that should alert you to consider the implications of a particular illness, condition, or problem:

- Diabetic ketoacidosis, myocardial infarction, pancreatitis, renal failure, cancer, dementia, pregnancy
- Fracture, burn, head injury, laceration, bleeding
- Pain, discomfort, distress, anxiety, fear, confusion

Here are some examples of key words that should alert you to consider the implications of a particular stage or phase of an illness or hospital stay:

- Onset, acute, early
- Chronic, late, advanced
- End stage, terminal, palliative
- Newly admitted, preop, postop, prior to discharge

Here are some examples of key words that should alert you to consider the implications of a particular physical sign, symptom, or state:

- Moaning, groaning, distress, short of breath
- Comatose, unresponsive, unconscious, confused
- Hungry, thirsty, constipated, nauseated, vomiting
- Paralyzed, weak, numb, aphasic, light headed
- Red, warm, oozing, cool, blue, dusky, cyanotic, swollen, pitting, febrile

Here are some examples of key words that should alert you to consider the implications of a particular age, psychological state, or circumstance:

- Neonate, 2-year-old, adolescent, 80-year-old
- Widowed, lonely, grieving, blind, deaf
- Psychotic, disoriented, forgetful, withdrawn, suicidal
- Fearful, anxious, irritated, dissatisfied, angry, abusive, assaultive
- Allergic
- NPO, DNR

Remember: If the patient's age is stipulated, that information is there for a reason. Make sure the answer you choose is age appropriate or makes sense in terms of the patient's age.

Here are some examples of key words that should alert you to consider the implications of a particular drug, treatment, procedure, or device:

- Heparin, Lasix, Ativan, alteplase, neomycin, potassium, morphine
- Blood, transfusion, packed cells, albumin
- D5W, NSS, D5NSS, Ringer's lactate, TPN
- Hemodialysis, peritoneal dialysis
- Central line, arterial line, continuous infusion, IV push
- Intramuscular, subcutaneous
- Cast, traction, crutches, walker, wheelchair
- Nasogastric tube, tube feeding

Remember: When considering questions concerning procedures, never confuse a nursing action with an action performed by a different member of the healthcare team. For example, if a question concerns the nurse's role in central line insertion, the answer may be gathering equipment or monitoring the patient, but it will not be inserting the catheter.

Here are some examples of key words that should alert you to consider a particular step in the nursing process:

- Assessment
- Analysis
- Planning
- Intervention
- Evaluation

Remember: If a particular step in the nursing process is stipulated in the question, always be sure your answer choice is congruent with the stipulated process. For example, if the question asks which nursing intervention would be most appropriate, make sure the answer you choose is an intervention and does not involve assessing or evaluating.

Here are some examples of key words that should alert you to recognize and consider the level of priority or likelihood inherent in a situation:

- First, initially, priority, immediately
- Most likely, least likely

The key words *first, initially, priority,* and *immediately* are typically found in two types of questions: (1) those that are designed to test your knowledge of the steps in which a procedure should be carried out, and (2) scenarios in which the patient is at risk for some negative development and you are being asked to decide what you should do first to minimize or abolish the risk. Questions that ask you to indicate the order in which you would carry out the steps of a procedure in a nonemergency situation are more likely to contain the words *first* and *initially* and are fairly straightforward; if you see hand washing as an answer choice, you should consider it carefully.

Questions that include the words *immediately* or *priority* (and sometimes *first* or *initially*) are often about safety. When faced with such scenarios, you may assume that you have a physician's order and all the resources you need to deal with the situation. Although in the real world of nursing practice it is possible to delegate or do two things simultaneously, in the world of NCLEX it is not. Thus, when answering prioritization questions, it is usually best to choose as the answer the action it would be best for the nurse to personally carry out first. The following question requires you to choose the best initial action.

The nurse answers a call light and finds the patient, who is lying flat in bed, pale and breathing rapidly and with difficulty. The nurse's first action should be to do which of the following:
A. Call the rapid response team.
B. Elevate the head of the bed.
C. Start oxygen at 2 L/min via nasal cannula.
D. Take the patient's vital signs.

Did you choose B, elevate the head of the bed? That is the best choice because the patient's oxygenation status must be improved as rapidly as possible, and people take in more air when their upper body is raised so their lungs can expand downward easily. If this question were a Drag-and-Drop or Ordered Response question in which you had to list the answer choices in the order in which you would carry them out, you would indicate that choice C, starting oxygen, would be your next nursing action because doing that would further increase oxygenation status. When you read a question such as this one, you might initially recognize oxygen administration as your second-best move but then start thinking to yourself, "but what if there is no oxygen available at the bedside?" You might then decide that the second-best thing for the nurse to do would be to summon the rapid response team, in which case you would get the question wrong. When answering questions on the NCLEX, you may assume that any device listed as an answer choice is available at the bedside.

Remember: When analyzing test-question scenarios and answer choices, do not base your answers on "but what if" speculation; base them only on the information provided in the scenario.

Key phrases such as *most likely* and *least likely* alert you that you are being asked to differentiate between symptoms, side effects, or responses of some kind that are common and expected and those that are less so or that don't apply at all.

A male patient who has recently been started on Tenormin (atenolol) to control his hypertension is most likely to complain of which of the following symptoms:
A. Racing pulse
B. Sexual dysfunction
C. Headache
D. Cough

Did you choose B, sexual dysfunction? That is a common side effect of beta-blocker therapy. A racing pulse is unlikely because beta blockers slow the heart rate, headache is not listed as a side effect, and cough is associated with ACE inhibitors.

Remember: Questions in which you are asked to prioritize are often about safety.

Some key words or phrases alert you to consider the relative merits of one course of action over another. Usually more than one of the answer choices will represent a reasonable and desirable action, but one of those is more important than the others. The following key words or phrases should cue you that you are being asked to decide relative merit:

- Best action
- Best course of action
- Best practice

A nurse who is preparing to administer digoxin (Lanoxin) discovers that the patient, who previously had a regular heart rate, now has an irregular heart rate of 48. Which of the following actions would represent best practice?
A. Reassessing the apical heart rate for a full minute
B. Withholding the ordered dose of medication
C. Administering the dose to regulate the heart rate
D. Assessing for signs of hypovolemia

Both choice A and choice B make sense in the context of this question, but one absolutely *must* be carried out, and the other *could* be carried out. Although it is feasible that a nurse might decide to recheck the heart rate to ensure accuracy, the critical action is withholding the dose of digoxin.

Remember: On standard NCLEX questions, you may choose only one answer. Choose the critical behavior, not one that is merely desirable.

Exercise
See if you can underline all the key words or phrases in the following question:

When evaluating a nursing intervention designed to treat a patient's pain, the nurse does which of the following?

How did you do? Did you identify all the key words as illustrated in the following answer?

When <u>evaluating</u> a <u>nursing intervention designed to treat a patient's pain</u>, the nurse does which of the following?
The key word *evaluating* signals that the nurse should be carrying out a particular step in the nursing process—evaluation. The key phrase *nursing intervention designed to treat a patient's pain* cues you that the nurse's goal is to evaluate the degree to which a pain medication, or some other intervention related to pain management, has been effective.

Exercise
Here's another question you can use to practice underlining key words:

When assessing a patient in diabetic ketoacidosis, the nurse's priority is to:

How did you do with that one? Did you underline all the key words as illustrated in the following answer?

When <u>assessing</u> a patient in diabetic <u>ketoacidosis</u>, the nurse's <u>priority</u> is to:

The key word *assessing* signals that you are addressing a particular phase of the nursing process—assessment. The key word *ketoacidosis* refers to a particular illness, and the key word *priority* indicates that you are being asked to identify an assessment procedure that the nurse must carry out to ensure the patient's safety.

Step 4: Consider the implications of each key word or phrase.

In this step, focus on each key word or phrase and reflect on what you know about it and how it may relate to other key words before you start reading the answer choices. As previously mentioned, if your learning style is more global than analytical, it is absolutely essential that you discipline yourself to focus on individual parts (key words in the scenario) before you consider the question as a whole (key words plus answer choices).

Exercise

Each key word (assessing, ketoacidosis, and priority) from the previous scenario is listed below with lines after it. Use those lines to record all the knowledge and understanding you have about the word and how it may relate to the other key words. Let's call each bit of knowledge and understanding a *nugget*. You will read more about nuggets in Chapter 8.

Key words:

Assessing

_____

_____

_____

_____

Ketoacidosis

_____

_____

_____

_____

Priority

_____

_____

_____

_____

I have listed the key words and some related nuggets in the following list. I started with ketoacidosis because knowledge about its pathophysiology and treatment determines which assessments the nurse will perform.

Key words:

Ketoacidosis
- Patients with ketoacidosis are usually Type 1 diabetics with very high serum glucose levels.
- They are in metabolic acidosis because, due to their lack of insulin, they must metabolize protein instead of glucose, and acidic ketone bodies are a by-product of protein metabolism.
- They are severely dehydrated and may have electrolyte imbalances and hypotension.
- They are treated with intravenous normal saline and short-acting insulin.
- Rapid fluid replacement plus insulin puts them at risk for hypertension and hypoglycemia.
- They may have an altered level of consciousness due to the acidosis.
- Their serum potassium levels can shift dramatically during treatment and may cause cardiac dysrhythmia.

Assessing: Based on the previous information, the nurse must assess the following:
- Glucose levels
- Electrolyte levels
- Blood gas levels
- Level of consciousness
- Urinary output
- Vital signs
- Cardiac rhythm

Priority: Although all the previously listed assessments are important, the nurse's priority is to monitor cardiac rhythm because certain dysrhythmias can be life threatening.

Step 5: Think about what the correct answer might be.

Before you look at the answer choices, try to anticipate what the correct answer is. Consider what you know about the key words and the nature of the question that is being asked, and generate some possible correct answers. That process will require you to think about the correct answer totally in terms of the scenario and its components and may help you choose the correct answer choice instead of one that appeals to you for some reason not directly related to the scenario.

Exercise

Generate some possible answers to the following question:

The nurse finds a patient lying in bed and vomiting. The nurse's priority is to:

Write your answers *before* you look at the complete question below.

Possible answer 1: _____

Possible answer 2: _____

Possible answer 3: _____

Here's the question again, along with the answer choices:

The nurse finds a patient lying in bed and vomiting. The nurse's priority is to:
A. provide an emesis basin.
B. prevent aspiration.

C. raise the head of the bed.
D. administer a prn antiemetic drug.

Was prevent aspiration one of your answer choices? If so, congratulations!

Step 6: Consider the answer choices in light of each key word.

The answer choices should be considered one by one, in the order they are presented, and without looking at the next choice. Each successive answer choice should be considered in light of the information brought to mind by each key word and then either ruled out or retained as a possible correct answer. Here's that question concerning a patient in ketoacidosis again, followed by a demonstration of how to consider each answer choice.

When assessing a patient in ketoacidosis, the nurse's priority is to:
A. administer insulin intravenously
B. monitor level of consciousness
C. test urine for the presence of ketone bodies
D. monitor heart rhythm

Answer choice A: Administer insulin intravenously
When considered in light of the key word *assessment*, this choice would be immediately ruled out as a possible correct answer because administering insulin is a nursing intervention, not a nursing assessment. There is no need to move on to the next two key words.

Answer choice B: Monitor level of consciousness
This choice is appropriate in light of the key word *assessment* because it does represent a nursing assessment. It is also appropriate in terms of the key word *ketoacidosis* because level of consciousness is definitely a concern when a patient is in that condition. Whether monitoring level of consciousness is the priority assessment, however, depends on what the next answer choices are. Thus, you would allow answer choice B to remain in consideration as a possible correct answer.

Answer choice C: Test urine for the presence of ketone bodies
This choice is appropriate in light of the key word *assessment* but not in light of the next key word, *ketoacidosis*, because the patient has already been diagnosed as being in diabetic ketoacidosis. Testing urine for ketone bodies is a diabetic screening test and would be pointless in this scenario. Choice C would be ruled out as a possible correct answer.

Answer choice D: Monitor heart rhythm
This choice is appropriate in light of the key word *assessment* and the key word *ketoacidosis* and is indeed the priority assessment because the cardiac dysrhythmias caused by potassium imbalances are potentially life threatening. This answer choice is the key (correct answer).

Remember: One of the characteristics almost all my NCLEX clients share is not knowing how to systematically analyze a test question. Knowing how to properly dissect questions and address their components separately and in the proper order is absolutely essential to passing NCLEX because if you cannot do that, you will be prone to making one or more of the following fatal errors: (1) failing to perceive exactly what the question is asking, (2) failing to rule out answer choices that are incongruent with one of the key words in the question, (3) overlooking one or more of the key words, or (4) not recognizing the significance of certain key words. If you use the previously outlined process step by step, you will analyze every test question properly, every time.

Chapter 7

Test Yourself: How Good Is Your Knowledge Base?

Marian C. Condon and Karen S. March

WHAT YOU WILL LEARN IN THIS CHAPTER

- Whether you have a little or a lot of NCLEX prep work to do
- How the exams and practice tests in this book are constructed
- How to keep track of your progress

INTRODUCTION

Taking Comprehensive Practice Exam 1 (later in this chapter) will give you quite a good idea of where you stand right now in terms of your overall knowledge base. The exam includes questions related to all the realms and domains of nursing knowledge that you studied in school: med–surg, peds, OB, psych–mental health, community health and leadership, as well as all body systems (cardiovascular, renal, etc.) and all the steps in the nursing process. Because there is no way of foreseeing how many med–surg questions, neuro questions, assessment questions, etc. you will encounter when you take the NCLEX itself, it is essential that you be fully prepared for any and all realm–domain–nursing process combinations. All questions on this diagnostic exam are written at the same levels as the questions you will face on the NCLEX—application and analysis.

We would rather have you underestimate your current level of preparedness for NCLEX rather than overestimate it. Therefore, we suggest that you consider yourself to be very well prepared for NCLEX only if you answer 90% or more of the questions on this exam correctly. If you answer between 85 and 89% of the questions correctly, you are probably quite well prepared and just need to strengthen your knowledge in certain areas. If you answer fewer than 85% of the questions correctly, you may have significant gaps in your knowledge, but here's the good news: we wrote this book specifically for you! We have prepared 15 topic-specific Practice Tests and two more Comprehensive Practice Exams you can use to identify the information or concepts that you have not yet mastered, and, in the next chapter, you will learn a foolproof method of quickly bringing yourself up to speed. You will also be supplied with some tools you can use to keep track of the progress you are making.

COMPREHENSIVE PRACTICE EXAM 1

1. Which of the following statements made by a patient would alert the nurse that the patient may be noncompliant with treatment for hypertension?
   A. "Both my father and grandfather died of stroke."
   B. "My blood pressure normally runs about 150/100 mm Hg."
   C. "I share my blood pressure medicine with my husband."
   D. "My blood pressure medicine is very expensive."

2. A patient with heart failure is being prepared for discharge. Which of the following lunch menu choices indicates to the nurse that dietary instruction has been effective?
   A. chicken salad with cranberries on whole wheat, hot tea, orange sherbet
   B. hamburger on bun, french fries, dill pickle, cherry pie
   C. hot dog on roll, macaroni and cheese, tomato juice, white cake
   D. beef broth, saltines, hot tea, fruit ice, bottled water

3. The nurse is caring for a patient who develops this rhythm on the monitor:

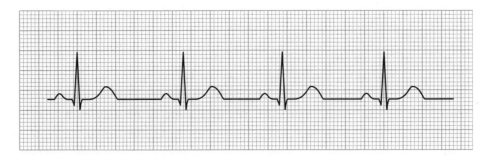

   The patient complains of dizziness and is hypotensive. Which of the following should the nurse do first?
   A. Prepare to assist with pacemaker insertion.
   B. Prepare to send the patient to surgery.
   C. Prepare for synchronized cardioversion.
   D. Administer intravenous atropine.

4. Depressed ST segments on the 12-lead EKG are indicative of which of the following?
   A. injury
   B. ischemia
   C. necrosis
   D. reperfusion

5. When a patient receives a drug with positive chronotropic effects, the nurse expects which of the following outcomes?
   A. increased sympathetic tone
   B. increased conduction velocity
   C. increased contractility
   D. increased heart rate

6. **The nurse is caring for a patient admitted with the following lab work:**

Laboratory Results	
Laboratory test	**Result**
Complete blood count	
Hematocrit (HCT)	42%
Hemoglobin (HGB)	14%
Red blood cells (RBC)	5.0 million/µL
Mean cell volume (MCV)	88 µ/m^3
Mean cell hemoglobin (MCH)	29 pg
Mean cell hemoglobin concentration (MCHC)	36.2%
White blood cells (WBC)	6000/µL
Platelets (Plt)	280,000/µL
Serum electrolytes	
Carbon dioxide	28 mEq/L
Chloride	99 mEq/L
Potassium	2.1 mEq/L
Sodium	138 mEq/L
Serum digoxin	0.8 ng/mL

Upon review, the nurse notes that the patient has which of the following abnormalities?
A. The patient is neutropenic.
B. The patient is anemic.
C. The patient is hypokalemic.
D. The patient is digoxin toxic.

7. **The nursing assistant reports a blood pressure reading to the nurse who notes that the cuff used was too small for the patient. Which effect would the size of the blood pressure cuff have on the blood pressure?**
A. The blood pressure measurement would be unaffected.
B. The blood pressure measurement would be falsely high.
C. The blood pressure measurement would be falsely low.
D. The blood pressure measurement would be 20% higher.

8. **A physician states that the patient's condition reveals a strong sympathetic influence. The nurse understands that the physician is talking about the patient's:**
A. increased blood pressure.
B. decreased blood pressure.
C. increased heart rate.
D. decreased heart rate.

9. The parents of a 4-year-old child who has been diagnosed with cystic fibrosis undergo genetic counseling. Which of the following statements by the parents indicates accurate understanding of some of the genetic implications of cystic fibrosis?
   A. "Any children we have will be born with cystic fibrosis."
   B. "The chance of having a child with cystic fibrosis is 1 in 4."
   C. "Cystic fibrosis is more commonly found in Hispanics."
   D. "All of our male children will have the disease."

ALTERNATE FORMAT

10. The nurse receives the following arterial blood gas results from the laboratory:

pH	7.46
pCO_2	48
HCO_3-	28
pO_2	89

Which of the following terms should the nurse use to properly interpret these results? SELECT ALL THAT APPLY.
A. partially compensated
B. uncompensated
C. compensated
D. respiratory
E. metabolic
F. acidosis
G. alkalosis
H. hypoxia
I. normal ABG

ALTERNATE FORMAT

11. The nurse receives the following arterial blood gas results from the laboratory:

pH	7.38
pCO_2	35
HCO_3-	19
pO_2	91

Which of the following terms should the nurse use to properly interpret these results? SELECT ALL THAT APPLY.
A. partially compensated
B. uncompensated
C. compensated
D. respiratory
E. metabolic
F. acidosis
G. alkalosis
H. hypoxia
I. normal ABG

ALTERNATE FORMAT

12. The patient is prescribed hydrocortisone sodium succinate (Solu-Cortef) 60 mg IV now. The drug is available in vials of "Solu-Cortef 125 mg/2mL." What volume of drug will the nurse withdraw from the vial to administer the correct dose?

_____

13. The nurse has provided medication teaching to the parents of a child with cystic fibrosis. Which of the following statements by the parents indicates that teaching has been effective?
    A. "I will administer the pancreatic enzymes to my child twice per day."
    B. "Pancreatic enzyme helps to decrease the viscosity of my child's mucous."
    C. "I can mix the pancreatic enzymes along with other medications in milk."
    D. "I will administer the pancreatic enzymes to my child before meals and snacks."

14. A young male patient is brought to the emergency department with a diagnosis of traumatic head injury following a motor vehicle accident. Upon admission, vital signs are unstable, pupils are equal but react sluggishly, Glasgow Coma score = 3, and ICP is 30 mm Hg. Based upon this initial assessment, the nurse understands that:
    A. further evaluation is warranted before care is provided.
    B. the patient is in a coma and has elevated ICP.
    C. the patient is unlikely to survive because of the head injury.
    D. the patient needs a head CT scan immediately.

15. Which of the following is considered to be a risk factor for cerebral aneurysms?
    A. smoking
    B. male gender
    C. diabetes
    D. age under 40

16. The patient with a spinal cord injury has had a halo vest applied. The nurse should include which of the following statements in providing discharge teaching?
    A. "You may bend over occasionally if needed."
    B. "You may drive occasionally."
    C. "You will have to turn your head very slowly."
    D. "This device will stabilize your cervical fracture."

17. The nurse is caring for a patient who begins to experience seizure activity while in bed. Which of the following actions by the nurse is indicated?
    A. Immediately call out for help.
    B. Raise the padded side rails.
    C. Restrain the patient's limbs.
    D. Insert a tongue blade in the mouth.

18. A 40-year-old patient is diagnosed with amyotrophic lateral sclerosis (ALS). In planning care for this patient, the nurse must be attentive to which of the following characteristics of the disease?
    A. rapid, acute onset of symptoms
    B. involves descending paralysis
    C. begins with bilateral upper extremity weakness
    D. cognitive function remains intact

19. Which of the following drugs is prescribed for treatment of Alzheimer's dementia?
    A. nortriptyline (Pamelor)
    B. selegiline (Eldepryl)
    C. rivastigmine (Exelon)
    D. valproic acid (Depakote)

20. The nurse is providing care for a patient who has developed neuroleptic malignant syndrome. The nurse understands that side effects of this syndrome include which of the following?
    A. flaccidity, fever, bradycardia, somnolence
    B. agitation, extrapyramidal effects, diarrhea
    C. loss of memory, severe anxiety, insomnia
    D. muscle rigidity, diaphoresis, drooling

21. The nurse is providing care for a patient who is experiencing a reaction to disulfiram (Antabuse). The nurse understands that the severe effects are likely to last:
    A. for up to 12 hours.
    B. for 6 to 8 hours.
    C. for 3 to 6 hours.
    D. for 1 to 2 hours.

22. The nurse understands that patients with renal failure are typically anemic because of which of the following factors?
    A. Kidneys in failure do not produce erythropoietin.
    B. Patients lose RBCs during hemodialysis treatments.
    C. Patients with renal failure have severe dietary restrictions.
    D. The kidneys do not manufacture normal amounts of RBCs.

ALTERNATE FORMAT

23. The nurse is caring for an elderly patient who was admitted for short-term hospitalization following elective surgery. Upon reviewing the patient's medication record, the nurse becomes concerned about administering which of the following medications to this patient? SELECT ALL THAT APPLY.
    A. furosemide (Lasix)
    B. ketorolac (Toradol)
    C. vancomycin
    D. acetaminophen (Tylenol)

24. The nurse understands that which of the following problems is a likely etiology of prerenal azotemia?
    A. glomerulonephritis
    B. hypovolemic shock
    C. intrarenal calculi
    D. pyelonephritis

25. The nurse assesses the patient for symptoms of hypocalcemia by:
    A. tapping the acromion process.
    B. inflating a blood pressure cuff on the forearm.
    C. applying a blood pressure cuff to the lower leg.
    D. monitoring the patient's blood pressure very closely.

26. The nurse is providing care for a patient who has a very low hemoglobin and hematocrit related to kidney failure. Which of the following medications is indicated to stimulate production of red blood cells?
    A. epoetin alfa (Epogen)
    B. filgrastim (Neupogen)
    C. enoxaparin (Lovenox)
    D. ondansatron (Zofran)

27. The nurse is caring for a patient who developed heparin-induced thrombocytopenia. Which of the following medications will be required for anticoagulation?
    A. heparin
    B. warfarin (Coumadin)
    C. vitamin K (AquaMEPHYTON)
    D. lepirudin (Refludan)

28. The nurse is reviewing lab work on a patient and finds the following values:

Red blood cells (RBC)	4.8 million/μL
White blood cells (WBC)	3800/μL
Platelets	168,000/μL
Hemoglobin	14.2 g/dL
Hematocrit	45.4%

    The nurse realizes that the laboratory findings are consistent with which of the following?
    A. thrombocytosis
    B. leukocytosis
    C. pernicious anemia
    D. pancytopenia

29. The nurse is providing care for a patient diagnosed with osteoporosis. The nurse understands that which of the following is a risk factor for development of osteoporosis?
    A. thin, small body frame
    B. large body frame
    C. African American ethnicity
    D. male

30. The nurse is providing discharge teaching for a patient who has had a total hip replacement. The nurse realizes that teaching has been effective when the patient makes which of the following statements?
    A. "I will be using this walker for several months to get around."
    B. "I will be sure to take antibiotics before I have dental work."
    C. "It is important for me to get as much rest as possible for healing."
    D. "I will be able to take a bath as soon as I get home from the hospital."

31. Treatment for compartment syndrome may include which of the following?
    A. elevation of the extremity
    B. acetaminophen (Tylenol)
    C. prednisone
    D. fasciotomy

32. The nurse is caring for a patient with acute diverticulitis. Prior to discharge, the nurse should instruct the patient to avoid which of the following foods in the diet?
    A. squash, potatoes, brown rice
    B. chicken, hamburger, peanut butter
    C. grapes, raspberries, popcorn
    D. salmon, grilled vegetables, pears

33. The nurse should encourage the patient with diverticulitis to increase which of the following products in the diet upon discharge?
    A. carrots, apples, oat bran
    B. wheat bread, cucumbers, popcorn
    C. peas, strawberries, corn
    D. tomatoes, peas, broccoli

34. The nurse working in a primary care office sees a patient who came in for evaluation of gastroesophageal reflux disease. When documenting the patient's history, the nurse expects the patient to report that symptoms are worse when:
    A. exercising.
    B. lying down.
    C. sitting.
    D. walking.

35. The nurse understands that which of the following is a viral pathogen that frequently causes acute diarrhea in young children?
    A. *giardia*
    B. *shigella*
    C. *rotavirus*
    D. *salmonella*

36. The nurse is caring for a 4-year-old child with celiac disease. The nurse expects to find which of the following manifestations of the disease while assessing the child and obtaining the health history from the patient's mother?
    A. malnutrition, foul-smelling stools, muscle wasting
    B. vomiting, diarrhea, abdominal pain, jaundice
    C. constipation, abdominal cramping, flatulence
    D. nausea, vomiting, diarrhea

37. The nurse is providing discharge teaching for the patient with Type II diabetes who has been ordered the following medications prior to discharge:

Medication administration record
atenolol (Tenormin) 25 mg PO daily
metformin (Glucophage) 850 mg PO T.I.D.
hydrochlorothiazide (HCTZ) 25 mg PO B.I.D.
enteric coated aspirin 81 mg PO every day
glipizide SR (Glucotrol XL) 10 mg PO B.I.D.

Which of the following statements by the patient indicates understanding of the implications of drug interactions between these medications?

A. "I need to monitor my glucose levels at home so I know if the meds are working."

B. "I may not always know if I am becoming hypoglycemic because of these meds."

C. "I need the HCTZ because the metformin and aspirin make my ankles swell."

D. "I need the atenolol because the metformin and glipizide cause my heart to race."

38. **A patient with Type I diabetes asks the nurse if it is okay to eat foods that contain sugar. The best reply by the nurse is:**

A. "You can eat some sugary foods as long as you reduce other carbs for the day."

B. "Unfortunately, you will need to eat things with a sugar substitute only."

C. "You can eat as much sugar as you want as long as you cover it with insulin."

D. "It is important to use sugar substitutes as your primary sweetening agent."

39. **If the patient's dose of NPH insulin was administered at 8 a.m., the nurse should be particularly alert to signs of hypoglycemia:**

A. between 11 a.m. and noon.

B. between 3 p.m. and 5 p.m.

C. between 11 p.m. and midnight.

D. between 3 a.m. and 5 a.m.

40. **The nurse is providing education about treatment for candidiasis. In response, the patient recognizes which of the following as a means by which the normal vaginal flora can be restored?**

A. Eat 8 ounces of yogurt daily.

B. Take daily doses of antibiotics.

C. Use vinegar douches daily.

D. Use miconazole (Monistat) as ordered.

41. **The nurse who is providing care for a patient with pelvic inflammatory disease would anticipate finding which of the following clinical manifestations upon assessing the patient?**

A. abdominal tenderness and distention

B. severe lower abdominal pain and dysuria

C. urinary tract infection and malaise

D. pain that abates with movement

42. **The nurse is caring for a patient whose last menstrual period began on October 10, 2009. Using Nägele's rule, the estimated date of birth is which of the following?**

A. January 10, 2010

B. April 17, 2010

C. June 10, 2010

D. July 17, 2010

ALTERNATE FORMAT

43. **Place in order the seven cardinal movements of labor that occur in a vertex presentation.**

A. Restitution

B. Descent

C. Flexion

D. Expulsion

E. Extension

F. External rotation

G. Internal rotation

44. The nurse is caring for a patient who has developed HELLP syndrome. The nurse knows that definitive treatment for HELLP requires which of the following?
    A. replacement of platelets and clotting factors
    B. magnesium sulfate infusion
    C. induction of labor and delivery of the infant
    D. intensive steroid therapy

45. The nurse is providing care for a pre-operative patient who normally takes enalapril (Vasotec). The nurse will verify with the physician whether or not to hold the drug prior to surgery because it is likely to cause which of the following during surgery?
    A. hypotension
    B. impaired cardiac function
    C. respiratory depression
    D. bronchospasm

46. The nurse is caring for a female patient who is concerned that she may be at higher than normal risk of breast cancer. Which of the following factors identified by the patient place her at higher than normal risk?
    A. 50 years of age
    B. works in a physician's office
    C. breast fed two children
    D. mother and sister diagnosed at 38 and 35 years of age

47. The nurse understands that all of the following are classified as warning signs of cancer by the American Cancer Society except:
    A. unintentional weight loss.
    B. indigestion or difficulty swallowing.
    C. change in bowel or bladder habits.
    D. obvious change in a wart or mole.

48. The nurse understands that a patient with colon or rectal cancer is likely to have which of the following clinical manifestations?
    A. hematuria
    B. fatigue
    C. weight gain
    D. vomiting

49. The nurse is concerned that a colleague may be diverting drugs for personal use. Which of the following provides justification for this claim?
    A. The colleague finishes every medication round expeditiously.
    B. The colleague rarely asks for a witness to waste medications.
    C. Patients do not get pain relief when medicated by the colleague.
    D. The colleague volunteers to pass medications every day.

50. The nurse has been confronted by management concerning elements of dress and personal adornment seen as inconsistent with agency guidelines. Based on a federal court ruling, it is unlawful for management to request the removal or covering of which of the following?
    A. a religious head-covering
    B. body piercings
    C. tattoos
    D. 10 earrings per ear

ANSWERS

1. **(C)**; To achieve an appropriate therapeutic effect, blood pressure medicine must be taken regularly. If the patient is sharing the drug with her husband, she is noncompliant. Having a blood pressure of 150/100 mm Hg does not necessarily imply noncompliance. It is possible that the patient does not have good control of blood pressure even with medication. The other two choices do not have anything to do with compliance.

2. **(A)**; Dietary concerns are largely related to sodium content of foods. Chicken salad with cranberries on whole wheat, hot tea, and sherbet are all foods with relatively low sodium content. In each of the other options, foods with high sodium content are included—french fries, cherry pie, dill pickle, macaroni and cheese, tomato juice, broth, and saltines.

3. **(D)**; The patient is symptomatic in a very slow sinus bradycardia, which requires administration of atropine IV.

4. **(B)**; Depressed ST segments on the 12-lead EKG are indicative of myocardial ischemia.

5. **(D)**; A drug with positive chronotropic effects increases heart rate.

6. **(C)**; The patient is hypokalemic. The serum potassium level is 2.1 mEq/L, which is considerably below normal (3.5–5.5 mEq/L) and could have serious consequences for the patient. The WBC is within normal limits, as are hemoglobin and hematocrit. The serum digoxin level is within normal limits.

7. **(B)**; Obtaining accurate results from blood pressure monitoring depends upon the use of appropriately sized equipment. The result of using a blood pressure cuff that was too small for the patient would be a falsely elevated blood pressure.

8. **(C)**; Sympathetic influences increase heart rate and speed conduction through the AV node.

9. **(B)**; Cystic fibrosis is inherited as an autosomal recessive trait with an overall incidence of 1 in 4.

ABG component	Value	What it reveals related to acid-base balance
pH	7.46	Alkalotic; partially compensated because both pCO_2 and HCO_3- are out of normal range, one causing dysfunction (HCO_3-) while the other (pCO_2) is trying to buffer
pCO_2	48	Elevated; acts to buffer alkalosis
HCO_3-	28	Elevated; contributes to alkalotic pH; primary problem
pO_2	89	

10. **(A, E, G)**; This ABG result reveals partially compensated metabolic alkalosis.

11. (**C, E, F**); This ABG result reveals compensated metabolic acidosis.

ABG component	Value	What it reveals related to acid-base balance
pH	7.38	Acidotic; compensated
pCO_2	35	Decreased; acts to buffer acidosis
HCO_3-	19	Decreased; contributes to acidotic pH; primary problem
pO_2	91	

12. (**0.96 mL**); $\dfrac{125 \text{ mg}}{2 \text{ mL}} = \dfrac{60 \text{ mg}}{x \text{ mL}}$; THEN $125x = 120$; $x = \dfrac{120}{125}$; THEN $x = 0.96$ mL

13. (**D**); Pancreatic enzymes help to improve absorption of fat, proteins, and carbohydrates. The medication should be taken just before or with meals and snacks. Pancreatic enzymes should never be mixed with other medications in any fluid.

14. (**B**); The nurse understands that the patient is in a coma and has elevated ICP. In general, it is widely accepted that a Glasgow Coma Score of less than 8 indicates coma. Any prolonged ICP of greater than 15 mm Hg is considered to be elevated ICP.

15. (**A**); Risk factors for cerebral aneurysms include smoking, hypertension, previous aneurysms, connective tissue disorders, age greater than 40 years, female gender, and blood vessel injury or dissection.

16. (**D**); Halo devices completely immobilize the cervical spine. The patient with a halo brace should be cautioned not to bend over to reduce the risk of falling because the device raises the patient's center of gravity and completely immobilizes the cervical spine. The patient may not drive. The nurse should instruct the patient to turn the entire body to scan the environment.

17. (**B**); When a patient experiences seizures, the nurse should be attentive to airway issues and try to prevent injury to the patient. In this case, raising the padded side rails is a very good idea. The nurse should not try to restrain the patient's limbs or to insert a tongue blade in the mouth.

18. (**D**); Amyotrophic lateral sclerosis (ALS) is a degenerative, progressive, incurable, and fatal disease that has a slow, subtle onset. Initially, the patient may experience weakness in the distal extremities. Over time the weakness progresses to ascending paralysis. The patient's cognitive ability remains intact, which means that the client is extremely aware of what is occurring. Anxiety is very common. Death ultimately results from aspiration, infection, and respiratory failure.

19. (**C**); Exelon patch is prescribed for treatment of Alzheimer's dementia. In clinical trials it facilitated improvement in slightly more than half of the people who took it.

20. (**D**); The patient with neuroleptic malignant syndrome has muscle rigidity, hyperpyrexia, tachypnea, diaphoresis, and drooling. The syndrome is a severe, life-threatening side effect of psychotropic therapy.

21. (**D**); Disulfiram (Antabuse) works along classical conditioning principles as it inhibits drinking because the patient tries to avoid the unpleasant physical effects that result from the alcohol-disulfiram reaction. These effects, which may be severe, include

sweating, throbbing, facial flushing, neck pain, tachycardia, respiratory distress, potentially severe hypotension, nausea, and vomiting. The effects typically last 1 to 2 hours. Usually the person becomes very drowsy and naps. Typically, when the patient wakes up, the effects are gone.

22. **(A)**; Erythropoietin is a hormone that stimulates RBC production. Erythropoietin is produced by normal, healthy kidneys, but not by kidneys in failure. Without erythropoietin, the patient develops anemia.

23. **(B, C, D)**; Individually, ketorolac (Toradol), vancomycin, and acetaminophen (Tylenol) are known nephrotoxic agents. Taken by a post-operative elderly patient, the risk of nephrotoxicity is compounded. Although the risk does not necessarily require discontinuation of the drugs , it does mandate close monitoring of renal function throughout therapy.

24. **(B)**; Prerenal azotemia is caused by factors that interfere with blood flow (perfusion) to the kidneys.

25. **(B)**; The nurse can assess for hypocalcemia by monitoring Trousseau's sign, evidence of a carpopedal spasm (of the hand) when the blood pressure cuff is left inflated over the forearm.

26. **(A)**; Epoetin alfa (Epogen) is a drug manufactured by recombinant DNA technology that stimulates red blood cell production in the same manner as endogenous erythropoietin.

27. **(D)**; Lepirudin is an anticoagulant used to treat patients with heparin-induced thrombocytopenia. Heparin is contraindicated, and vitamin K improves clotting ability, which is not desirable.

28. **(B)**; The lab results reveal decreased WBCs (leukocytosis).

29. **(A)**; Risk factors for osteoporosis include female gender, Caucasian or Asian-American ethnicity, thin or small body frame, smoking, anorexia, steroid medications, and more.

30. **(B)**; Patients who have had joint replacements are at risk for development of osteomyelitis. Therefore, it is important for them to take prophylactic antibiotics prior to any invasive procedures, including dental work, for the rest of their lives.

31. **(D)**; Fasciotomy involves a deep incision into the fascia to relieve pressure within the compartment. Timing of this treatment is crucial. Done too early, the patient will lose a lot of blood. Done too late, tissue death will occur.

32. **(C)**; The patient with acute diverticulitis should be instructed to avoid foods with small seeds; nuts and foods with skins, like raisins and grapes; raspberries; blueberries; figs; rye bread with caraway seeds; sesame seeds; poppy seeds; sunflower seeds; nuts; and okra. Avoidance of these foods will help to decrease exacerbation of diverticulitis.

33. **(A)**; The patient should be instructed to increase foods that are high in fiber when the acute inflammation has subsided. These high fiber foods include such things as wheat bran, oat bran, shredded wheat, oatmeal, whole wheat bread, multigrain bread, cooked asparagus, broccoli, squash, spinach, lettuce, carrots, peaches, apples, and oranges.

34. **(B)**; Gastroesophageal reflux symptoms are most pronounced with activities that increase intra-abdominal pressure, such as bending, straining, lifting, and lying down.

35. (**C**); Rotavirus frequently causes acute diarrhea in young children.

36. (**A**); Clinical manifestations of celiac disease include steatorrhea, foul-smelling stools, malnutrition, muscle wasting, anemia, anorexia, abdominal distention, irritability, fretfulness, uncooperativeness, and apathy.

37. (**B**); This patient may not always be aware of episodes of hypoglycemia because the atenolol (Tenormin) tends to mask the signs.

38. (**A**); Patients with diabetes can eat some amount of any food of their choice, as long as they adjust their carbohydrate intake. Therefore, if a patient eats something with sugar, the amount of carbohydrate in that food must be subtracted from the usual allotment for that particular meal and considered within the carbohydrate allowance for the entire day.

39. (**B**); If the patient received NPH insulin at 8 a.m., the nurse should be alert to signs of hypoglycemia in this patient between 3 p.m. and 5 p.m. because the effects of the insulin would peak by that time and it is not yet dinner time.

40. (**A**); The patient can help to restore the normal vaginal flora by consuming 8 ounces of yogurt with live active cultures daily.

41. (**B**); Patients with pelvic inflammatory disease have clinical manifestations that include fever, nausea, malaise, severe lower abdominal pain, dysuria, nausea and vomiting, and purulent and foul-smelling vaginal discharge.

42. (**D**); Using Nägele's rule, the calculation would occur as follows: Begin with the first day of the last menstrual period and subtract 3 months (October 10 − 3 months = July 10). Add 7 days (July 10 + 7 days = July 17, 2010).

43. (**B, C, G, E, A, F, D**); The cardinal movements of labor, in order, are descent, flexion, internal rotation, extension, restitution, external rotation, and expulsion.

44. (**C**); The nurse knows that when HELLP syndrome is diagnosed and the patient's condition is stabilized, definitive treatment requires delivery of the infant as soon as possible regardless of gestational age.

45. (**A**); Enalapril (Vasotec) is an ACE inhibitor that can cause hypotension. Unless it is prescribed to treat heart failure, the surgeon may elect to hold the drug on the morning of surgery.

46. (**D**); Hormonal risks for development of breast cancer include use of birth control pills or hormone replacement therapy; early menarche (before 12 years of age); late menopause (after 55 years of age); and first pregnancy after 30 years of age. Non-hormonal risk factors include family history, lack of regular exercise, postmenopausal obesity, increased use of alcohol, working the night shift, older than 65 years of age, no full-term pregnancies, never breast fed, higher socioeconomic status, Jewish heritage, and two or more first-degree relatives with breast cancer at an early age.

47. (**A**); The seven warning signs of cancer acknowledged by the American Cancer Society are: change in bowel or bladder habits; a sore that does not heal; unusual bleeding or discharge; thickening or lump in the breast or elsewhere; indigestion or difficulty in swallowing; obvious change in wart or mole; and nagging cough or hoarseness.

48. (**B**); Patients with colon or rectal cancer are likely to have changes in bowel habits, occult blood in the stool, flatulence, indigestion, weight loss, and fatigue.

49. (**C**); When a nurse is diverting medications for personal use, patients often notice that they achieve pain relief when medicated by other nurses but not when they are medicated by the nurse who is diverting drugs. This presumably results when the diverter "medicates" the patients with normal saline rather than medication.

50. (**A**); Religious head coverings are protected under the right to freedom of expression. Body piercings, tattoos, and excessive jewelry are not protected.

Please see Chapter 8 for information about how to use the Nugget Method (see the following template) to help you pass the NCLEX.

Nugget List

Chapter number _____ Topic _____

How to Use What You *Don't* Know to Pass the NCLEX

Marian C. Condon

WHAT YOU WILL LEARN IN THIS CHAPTER

- Why getting real about what you *don't* know is critical
- How to use the Nugget Method to identify gaps in your knowledge base
- How to master information and concepts quickly and easily
- How to make sure you will recall information when you need it
- How to evaluate your progress

In Chapter 7 you took a Comprehensive Practice Exam designed to give you a ballpark idea of the current strength of your knowledge base. In this chapter, you will learn how to use the questions you answered on that exam, and on the other Practice Tests and Comprehensive Practice Exams in this book, to identify gaps in your knowledge base—areas of nursing knowledge on which you need to bring yourself up to speed to be ready for the NCLEX. You may recall from Chapter 1 that most of my clients who fail NCLEX are not particularly good at accessing their own knowledge. They may believe, for example, that they are well informed regarding a certain topic when the reality is that all they have is the gist—the general idea. The beauty of the method you are about to learn, the *Nugget Method*, is that it forces you to focus specifically on what you don't know so it will be impossible for you to unknowingly waste your NCLEX-prep time going over facts and concepts you've already mastered. I've been refining the Nugget Method over the years during which I've been tutoring graduate nurses who failed NCLEX, and I know for an absolute fact that it works. In the latter part of this chapter, you will be introduced to memorization and recall strategies you can use to incorporate new nugget material firmly into your arsenal of nursing knowledge, and you will find out how to use the Keep Track boxes included with every Practice Test to map the progress you are making.

THE NUGGET METHOD

As you work your way through the topic-specific Practice Tests and Comprehensive Practice Exams in this book, you will use the Nugget Method to identify and commit to memory additional nursing knowledge you need to master. Here's how the Nugget Method works: When working on a specific test or exam, you will answer the first 25 or so questions and then you will look up the answers to those questions in the provided answer key. When you come to a question you answered incorrectly, you will ask yourself why you got it wrong—what nugget or nuggets of information did you lack? A

---

given nugget might consist of a fact, such as the normal CO_2 range for arterial blood, or a concept, such as a pathological process. Completing the following sentence in your mind may help you to identify nuggets:

If I'd known that _____, and that _____, and if I'd understood _____, I would have been able to answer that question correctly.

When you have identified a nugget, you will enter it into the *nugget list* that follows the Practice Test you're working on. You will write the nugget in the form of a question in the left-hand column of the nugget list and write the answer in the right-hand column. Then you will go on to the next question you answered incorrectly and do the same thing.

What is the normal pCO_2 range for arterial blood?	35–45
What are the signs and symptoms of left-sided heart failure?	Crackles; being short of breath; orthopnea; paroxysmal nocturnal dyspnea
What are the signs and symptoms of right-sided heart failure?	Peripheral edema; jugular vein distention; frequent nocturnal urination
List three complications related to calcium channel blocker drugs.	Hypotension; dysrhythmia; edema

By the time you've addressed all the questions you answered incorrectly on a given test, you may well have quite an extensive list of new information you need to add to your knowledge base. The final step in the Nugget Method is to review that information by covering the answers in the right-hand column and seeing if you can answer the questions to the left. Blank nugget list pages are provided following every Practice Test and Comprehensive Practice Exam in this book.

Because strengthening your knowledge base is one of the two critical things you must do if you want to pass NCLEX (the other is to learn to properly analyze questions), it is essential that you learn to use the Nugget Method properly.

Identifying Nuggets

Because nuggets represent information you need to add to your knowledge base, it is essential that you are able to identify them. The following exercises will help you learn to do that.

Exercise

Read the following practice question and see if you can identify all the nuggets of information you would have to have in your knowledge base to answer the question correctly. Write the nuggets you identify on the lines after the question.

QUESTION

The nurse is caring for a patient who is being weaned from a ventilator. Which of the following blood gas analysis results suggests the patient is not ready for further reduction in ventilator support?
A. PaO_2 = 50 mm Hg
B. $PaCO_2$ = 38
C. HCO_3 = 24
D. pH = 7.4

Nugget 1 _____
Nugget 2 _____
Nugget 3 _____
Nugget 4 _____
Nugget 5 _____

How did you do? Were you able to identify all the nuggets of knowledge and understanding in the following list?

Nugget 1: The term *weaning* refers to withdrawing ventilator support from patients gradually and safely.
Nugget 2: The normal range for PaO_2 is 80–100 mm Hg.
Nugget 3: The normal range for $PaCO_2$ is 35–45 mm Hg.
Nugget 4: The normal range for HCO_3 is 22–26.
Nugget 5: The normal range for pH is 7.35–7.45.

If you answered that question incorrectly because you did not know the meaning of the word *weaning* or because you did not know the normal range for any of the blood gas parameters referenced in the answer choices, you would write that information as a question and enter it into the left-hand column of your nugget list with the answer in the right-hand column. For example, if you did not know the normal range for PaO_2, your nugget question would be, What is the normal PaO_2 range?

Exercise
Read the following question and then list the nuggets of information you would need to have in your knowledge base to answer the question correctly.

QUESTION

A pregnant woman who wishes to stop smoking to protect the health of her baby has attended a smoking cessation class sponsored by the prenatal clinic. The nurse knows teaching has been effective when the client makes which of the following statements?
A. If I smoked while nursing, nicotine would get into my milk.
B. I can use as much nicotine gum as I need to stop cravings.
C. I should apply a nicotine patch whenever I feel the urge to smoke.
D. As long as I stop smoking a month before delivery, my baby will not be harmed.

Nugget 1 _____
Nugget 2 _____
Nugget 3 _____
Nugget 4 _____

How did you do? Did you identify all the nuggets of knowledge in the following list?

Nugget 1: Nicotine passes freely from the maternal blood to breast milk.

Nugget 2: A maximum of 30 pieces of nicotine gum are allowed daily.

Nugget 3: Nicotine patches are left on throughout the day and removed only at night.

Nugget 4: Smoking is harmful to the fetus throughout pregnancy. Stopping smoking during the last month does not undo earlier harm.

Exercise

Write each nugget in the previous list in the form of a question that is suitable for entry into the following nugget list:

How did you do? Does your nugget list look like this?

If a pregnant woman smokes, does the nicotine from the mother's blood pass into her breast milk?	Yes
What are the guidelines for the use of nicotine gum?	Chew each piece for 30 minutes. Use no more than 30 pieces in 24 hours.
How are nicotine patches used?	Applied to skin throughout the day and removed at night
During which months of pregnancy is smoking harmful to the fetus?	All months

Nugget List Errors

One of the reasons I ask clients to bring their nugget lists to tutoring sessions is so I can review the lists and spot and correct any misconceptions or problems. The most common errors my clients make when they first begin to use the Nugget System are described in the following discussion, along with illustrative questions and nugget list entries.

Common nugget list error 1: Writing nugget questions for some, but not all, of the information you lacked regarding a specific test question.

One of my clients, whom I'll call Sandra, chose " C. Broken water" as the answer to the following question.

QUESTION

The nurse recognizes which of the following as a sign of imminent birth?
A. Effacement
B. Bulging perineum
C. Broken water
D. Contractions

The nugget Sandra wrote for that question looked like this:

A sign that delivery is imminent is:	The perineum is bulging

When I discussed the question with Sandra, she admitted that she had not known what the word *effacement* (choice A) meant and that she was not really familiar with the usual sequence of events that occur during birth. Thus, Sandra should have written two additional nuggets based on that question, as shown in the following nugget list:

A sign that delivery is imminent is:	The perineum is bulging
What does effacement mean?	That the cervix is fully dilated
What occurs during labor and delivery and in what order?	Contractions, water breaks, cervix becomes effaced, perineum bulges, fetus is expelled

Common nugget list error 2: Writing the original test question itself in the left-hand column as the nugget question and then writing the rationale from the prep book in the right-hand column as the answer.

Because we are picking on Sandra today, let's say that she chose answer choice B instead of the correct choice, D, to the following question:

A school nurse has presented a program on preventing skin cancer. Students who understand risk factors will choose which of the following people as being at the greatest risk of developing skin cancer?
A. An office worker who is 35 years old
B. A high-school student who is 16 years old
C. A mountain biker who is 40 years old
D. A professional fisherman who is 60 years old

The rationale for the correct answer, D, is that professional fishermen are on the water and exposed to the sun all day; because sun damage is cumulative, older people are at increased risk. Outdoor hobbies, such as mountain biking, involve less sun exposure than outdoor jobs, and the mountain biker is younger than the fisherman. People who spend most of their time indoors, such as office workers and students, are at lower risk.

Sandra's incorrect nugget list entry is as follows:

Who is at highest risk for skin cancer?	Professional fishermen

By focusing only on the question itself and the rationale for the correct answer, Sandra completely missed the entire point of the Nugget System, which is to identify basic nursing knowledge that can be applied to any relevant scenario. Sandra's nugget question and answer actually make little sense because there are plenty of other occupations with high sun exposure and greater cancer risk—migrant farm work, for example.

The correct nugget list entry is as follows:

What are the risk factors for skin cancer?	Exposure to sun (warm climates; high altitude)
	High degree of cumulative exposure (older age groups)
	Fair skin
	Family or personal history
	A history of sunburn

Common nugget list error 3: Writing the answers to nugget questions without knowing what the answer actually means.

Entering information into your nugget list without really understanding what the information means is a pointless waste of your time. You'll recall from Chapter 3 that virtually all the questions on the NCLEX (and on the tests and exams in this book) are written at levels that require you to know, comprehend, and be able to apply facts and concepts related to nursing. A client I'll call Norm chose answer A instead of answer D (the correct answer) for the following question:

In taking a client's health history, the nurse notes that the client is being treated with lisinopril (Prinivil, Zestril) for essential hypertension. Which of the following assumptions would the nurse be justified in making?
A. The client smokes.
B. The client does not exercise.
C. The client requires no treatment.
D. The client should be taught to monitor his blood pressure.

When Norm looked up the answer to the question, the rationale for choice D was as follows: "Self-monitoring is an important part of hypertension management. All cases of hypertension require treatment. Assumptions about a client's lifestyle cannot be based on a diagnosis of hypertension." Norm added the following question and answer pair to his nugget list:

What should patients with essential hypertension do?	Monitor their blood pressure

When I reviewed Norm's nugget list with him, I asked him what his understanding of essential hypertension was and found that he thought the word *essential* implied that the blood pressure was so severe that it was essential that it be treated. Norm had not looked up the term *essential hypertension*; he made an assumption about what the term meant, and his assumption was incorrect.

STRATEGIES FOR ENHANCING MEMORY AND RETENTION

One of the requirements for passing the NCLEX is the ability to retain in your memory an enormous amount of information related to nursing practice and then recall it so that you can apply it to patient care scenarios. Fortunately, cognitive psychologists have identified a number of strategies that can be used to speed the memorization process, enhance retention, and facilitate recall. Some of these strategies involve cognitive processes, such as rehearsal, chunking, creating acronyms, and visualization, and others are related to study session design and timing. The specific strategies I wish to share with you are derived from some basic principles related to the memorization process.

THE BASICS OF MEMORIZATION

To say that you have learned something, let's say the actions, contraindications, and side effects of a certain drug, means that you have stored that information in your long-term memory. Short-term memory is differentiated from long-term memory by length of recall (Intelegen, 2009). When you look up a phone number and recall it long enough to dial it into the phone, you have stored the number in short-term memory. Unless you make an effort to really learn the number (store it in your long-term memory) so you will not have to look it up again, you will forget it after a few minutes.

Rehearsal

Think of some phone numbers you know by heart. You know them because you've dialed them repeatedly. In the terminology used by cognitive psychologists, you've rehearsed them sufficiently often that they became stored in your long-term memory. When you cover up the answer side of your nugget lists and challenge yourself to recall the answers to the questions from memory, you are rehearsing the nuggets of knowledge you know you need to master. Each time you review the knowledge in a given nugget list, you lodge it more and more firmly in your long-term memory.

Chunking

It is a physiological fact that most people can hold only about seven discrete bits of information in their short-term memory, which is why your phone number, xxx-xxxx, comprises only 7 digits instead of 15. If you are trying to remember multiple facts related to a central concept, for example, all the steps in a procedure or all the actions and side effects of a specific drug, you will find that dividing the bits into chunks of seven or fewer will make the memorization process easier. For example, if you wanted to memorize information regarding a specific class of drugs so you could apply that information to test question scenarios, you would quite naturally divide (chunk) the information into various categories, such as specific drugs that belong to the class, actions, side effects, contraindications, and important nursing assessments. If there was quite a bit of information in one or more of those categories, you could further chunk the information into subcategories.

Acronyms

Acronyms are formed by using the first letter of each word in the list of words to form a new word (Intelegen, 2005). You probably know and use many acronyms. Have you ever asked someone to do something ASAP? This, of course, is an acronym for *as soon as possible*. Creating acronyms to help you recall bits of information is a useful learning strategy. You may already be familiar with a common acronym used by healthcare providers to remind them how to treat sprains and some other types of soft tissue injuries; RICE means rest, immobility, compression, and elevation. Acronyms can be used along with chunking to make complex nursing information easier to retain, but they do have a downside: it is not always easy to convert the first letters of various bits of information into a recognizable and memorable word.

Suppose, for example, that you wanted to commit to long-term memory the most basic and important nursing-related facts about diuretic drugs. Although there are various subcategories within the diuretic class (loop diuretics, thiazides, potassium-sparing drugs, osmotic diuretics, and carbonic anhydrase inhibitors), and although all have some similar and dissimilar effects, you can recall the main factors you must keep in mind by using part of the alphabet as an acronym:

A = Alkalosis. Loss of chloride ions (caused by loop diuretics and thiazides) can lead to metabolic (hypochloremic) alkalosis.

B = Blood dyscrasias. The loop diuretics, the thiazides, and the carbonic anhydrase inhibitors can cause agranulocytosis and other blood abnormalities.

C = Constant urination. Patients must be taught to take diuretics early in the day so they will not have to get up frequently during the night.

D = Dehydration. All diuretics can lead to excessive water loss.

E = Electrolyte imbalances. High serum potassium levels (caused by K+-sparing diuretics) or low serum potassium levels (caused by thiazides and loop diuretics) are of particular concern.

F = Fainting. Hypotension can cause weakness and dizziness, particularly in the elderly.

G = Gout and glucose. Thiazide and loop diuretics can cause hyperuricemia and gout as well as elevated blood glucose levels.

Encoding

Before information can be stored in memory, whether short or long term, it must be encoded, which means translated into a mental representation that can be stored in memory (Weiss, 2000). Information can be encoded in several ways: semantically, as words that convey meaning; visually, as a picture; or acoustically, as a sound. Here are examples of the three ways in which you might go about encoding for storage in your brain the information that the drug Lasix (furosemide) is a potassium-wasting diuretic:

- Semantic encoding: You read and reread the information, add it to your nugget list, and then use your nugget list to quiz yourself on it.
- Visual encoding: You create a mental image of a huge syringe marked *Lasix* alongside another image of a patient draining copious amounts of urine into a Foley bag with a big K$^+$ on it for potassium.
- Acoustic encoding: You read and reread the information aloud and continue to speak it or sing it to yourself as you transpose it onto a flash card or nugget list and then quiz yourself on it.

Retrieval

Retrieval, also known as recall, is the process of accessing information stored in memory. If you've ever had the experience of encountering an acquaintance whose name you know but can't quite recall, you are aware that retrieval can sometimes be problematic. To prepare yourself adequately for the NCLEX, you must utilize learning strategies that foster both long-term storage of information and reliable retrieval. Retrieval is enhanced when encoding and storage have occurred via multiple modalities as opposed to only one. Encoding is related to another concept from the educational psychology literature, preferred learning style.

PREFERRED LEARNING STYLES

The term *preferred learning style* refers to the sensory channel via which a given individual prefers to access information that is to be learned. Although all human beings whose sensory systems (seeing, hearing, and touching) are intact constantly access sensory information from their environment using all three modalities, most have one that is preferred (easiest and most natural) and another that is secondarily preferred. Many of you are probably visual learners who grasp concepts most easily by viewing illustrations, DVDs, and demonstrations. That visual learners predominate is not surprising because 90% of the learning that occurs naturally, just as a consequence of living in the world, is visual, and 85% of the human brain is wired in a manner that facilitates visual processing (Weiss, 2000). Depending on your individual learning style profile, you may also benefit from exposing yourself to auditory learning materials. If you like to tape-record lectures so you can hear them again, or if you speak material you are reading aloud to yourself, you may have a preference for auditory learning. Finally, you may be primarily what is known as a kinesthetic learner. Kinesthetic learners like to involve their bodies in the learning process. They typically pick up psychomotor tasks, such as carrying out procedures, easily because such tasks involve using the body (particularly the hands) to touch, feel, and manipulate. Kinesthetic learners benefit from drawing conceptual relationships on paper in the form of concept maps and other kinds of diagrams.

USING VISUALIZATION TO ENHANCE MEMORY

If you are primarily a visual learner, you already know that you learn well from repeated exposure to flash cards, videos and DVDs, etc. You may, however, be unfamiliar with visualization, a powerful visual encoding–storage strategy. To visualize is to create an image in your mind's eye. For example, to avoid wandering aimlessly in convenience stores trying to recall what I want to buy, I often create in advance a mental image of the objects of my desire cavorting colorfully (and memorably) together. I might picture, say, a dozen eggs and a loaf of bread astride a roll of toilet paper that is rocking from side to side. I'll be sure to make the eggs and bread different colors and to have them pulsate or gyrate in some way; the more color and motion you can build into a visual memory, the better. Just the act of constructing such an image—conjuring the layout and applying the motion and color—relates the objects to one another and makes them very hard to forget, at least for a while. If I take the time to construct a vivid mental representation before entering the store, I absolutely never forget what I want to buy. Of course, if I wished to enter the image into my long-term memory, I would have to revisit it on the schedule suggested in the following section on designing and timing your study sessions. Memorization strategies based on visualization work well for almost all of my clients. They find their mental creations interesting to devise and fun to revisit during review sessions.

The Method of Loci

A visualization strategy that I unfailingly teach to my clients for recalling fairly large amounts of information is called the *method of loci* (Intelegen, 2005). The method of loci is an ancient memorization technique that storytellers in preliterate cultures used to pass tribal lore down to succeeding generations. To use this method, you must first visualize a location or route with which you are very familiar, such as your parents' home or the streets you traverse when you walk or drive to a specific location. Because people store new information more easily when they link it to something they already know well, you will then mentally associate specific elements of the new body of information you want to learn with specific elements of the location or route that is already firmly embedded in your memory.

Let's say you wish to link information about cardiovascular diseases, the drugs used to treat them, and nursing priorities associated with them to the familiar territory of your parents' home. You would do that by associating the various components of your topic to specific landmarks (rooms, closets, staircases, furniture) in the home in an order that makes sense in terms of how the components are related to one another. For example, you might choose to assign the cardiovascular disease hypertension to the entryway of the home because hypertension is a risk factor that can lead to more serious problems. Following that line of reasoning, you might assign angina to the next room, myocardial infarction to the next, and congestive heart failure to the next. You could address related procedures and problems, such as cardiac catheterization, angioplasty, bypass surgery, and cardiogenic shock, either by assigning each to a specific area of the home or by visualizing another locale, such as an emergency department treatment area or cardiac catheterization lab. In each room, you would create a scenario that links symbols of the relevant medications, devices, and nursing priorities to familiar objects in the room, incorporating as much color, drama, and movement as you need to make your scenario highly memorable.

The combined processes of deciding the order in which the selected conditions or problems should be accessed and how the related concepts will be grouped and symbolized in the various rooms constitutes a powerful encoding–storage strategy that will serve you well on NCLEX day. Revisiting (reviewing) the entire location frequently will further embed the information into your long-term memory. The following four examples demonstrate how the method of loci might be used to link facts and concepts related to cardiovascular nursing to the rooms and features of a home.

The Hypertension Hallway

Visualize a man standing in the entrance hallway. He has a large cartoon blood pressure cuff on his arm with the needle just past 140 on the dial. To the right is a two-shelf wooden storage rack suitable for boots and shoes. This rack contains several large medication bottles. A large bottle labeled *Thiazides* is on the first shelf. Two symbols can be seen on either side of it: ↓ K^+ for *potassium* and ↑ *glucose*. An obviously inflamed, painful big toe (symbolizing gout) sits atop the bottle.

The second shelf contains a large drug bottle labeled *Beta Blockers -olol* (as in atenolol, metoprolol, etc.). Next to it is a large picture of the television family the Brady Bunch; all are checking their heart rates via their carotid pulse. A few inches away from the beta blocker bottle sits another bottle. This one is large and white and has the words *Calcium Channel Blockers -pine* (as in nifedipine, amlodipine) emblazoned on it. Next to it is a small cartoon figure of a woman with very swollen ankles struggling to loosen (dilate as in diltiazem) the lengths of clear plastic wrap (as in verapamil) that surround her. A rhythm strip pulsates constantly in the background.

The third shelf contains a large medicine bottle painted to resemble a playing card. It is labeled *ACE Inhibitors -pril* (as in lisinopril), and dangling from it is the ↑ K^+ symbol. Sitting atop the bottle is a woman; her swollen ankles are dangling noticeably.

Room 1: The Angina Living Room

A man is lifting heavy logs into the fireplace. He is grimacing and rubbing his *chest* and *arm* because he is having pain there. Lightning bolts symbolizing pain are shooting out of his back *between his shoulder blades* because he has pain there, too. He reaches for a large *opaque* pill bottle on the mantel. It is labeled *Nitrostat* in glowing, neon colors. He puts one of the pills *under his tongue* and starts rubbing his head because he has a *headache*. Bright, gold stars appear around his head because he feels a bit *dizzy*.

Room 2: The MI Dining Room

In this room, a man is having supper while arguing heatedly with his partner. He starts to *perspire* (large water droplets are popping out on his head) and clutches his *chest* and rubs his left *arm* and *jaw–neck* area. He looks *pale*. He is also retching a bit because he is *nauseated*. On the dining room table are a bottle of *aspirin* and a phone with *911* displayed. The paramedics arrive and administer *oxygen*, start an *IV*, and attach cardiac *monitoring leads* to the man's chest. You zoom in and notice exactly where leads are placed. Using a huge syringe with a very large label, they give the man *morphine sulfate* for his pain. They load him onto a gurney and elevate his head to facilitate breathing.

You take a side trip to the emergency department with the man. You see a large IV bag very prominently labeled *Alteplase* (tissue plasminogen activator; TPA). You notice that bright red *blood* is dripping from the man's nose and is visible on his gums, and you recall that bleeding is a complication of alteplase. You notice markedly *elevated S-T segments* on the monitor and also some runs of V-tach for which a *lidocaine infusion* is started. You notice the MI-specific lab slips that are being sent: *CK-MB* and *troponin*. You make those lab slips very large and bright.

You follow the man on another side trip to the cardiac cath lab. You hear a nurse asking the man whether he is allergic to *shellfish* (she is holding a large clam in one hand) or has *renal disease* (she is holding a kidney in the other). After the procedure, you notice the man has a pressure device (huge and impossible to miss, of course) over an artery in his groin and that the nurse has driven stakes into the bed around his leg so that he cannot move it. You notice also that the leg is very *cold* and *pale* in color and that the nurse is upset about that. You hear the nurse ask the man about *back pain* and can see yellow lightning bolts of pain shooting out from under him. The nurse immediately takes the man's *blood pressure*. You notice that another nurse is holding a big, flapping lab slip marked *BUN* and *creatinine*.

Room 3: The Heart Failure Bedroom

In this room, a transparent cartoon man with a large heart that looks very weak and tired is sleeping. He is propped up on several *pillows* so he can breathe more easily. His *bladder* is very full of bright yellow liquid, and you recall that it tends to fill rapidly at night when he lies down. You see water dripping off Cartoon Man's *lungs* and you add a bit of acoustic encoding to your scene by hearing *crackles* (rales) as Cartoon Man inhales. You notice that the large, blue *jugular veins* in Cartoon Man's neck are bulging and that he has *swelling* in his feet and ankles.

You notice that on Cartoon Man's nightstand there is a cluster of two yellow bottles with a loop of twine draped over them. Propped next to them is a sign that says *Loop Diuretics*. The yellow bottles are labeled *Lasix* and *Bumex*. Dangling from the twine that surrounds all of them is a large ↓ K^+/*lytes* symbol.

There are two large medication bottles on the chair next to the bed. One is labeled *ACE Inhibitors* and the other is labeled *Beta Blockers*. You recall having seen those bottles before in the hypertension hallway. There is a smaller medication bottle labeled *Digoxin* on the dresser, and you recall that some doctors might use digoxin to help Cartoon Man's heart contract more strongly. You can see a red danger sign and a ↓ *Potassium* symbol on the bottle. You notice that tacked to the head of Cartoon Man's bed is a large lab slip requesting a *BNP level*.

Other Uses for Method of Loci

If the method of loci appeals to you, you can use it to encode and store memories of any sort. You could, for example, assign various mental health illnesses to different classrooms and then visualize your professors exhibiting the symptoms of the most appropriate disorder (you might as well have some fun with this!) as well as the side effects of the drugs used to treat them.

DESIGNING AND TIMING YOUR STUDY SESSIONS FOR MAXIMAL RETENTION

Because you are using the Nugget Method of NCLEX prep, your study sessions will consist primarily of answering the practice questions in the remaining chapters of this book, entering questions and answers into your nugget lists, and reviewing the material in the nugget lists. Occasionally, however, you may identify a concept that you just don't understand very well. When that happens, you will need to consult your class notes, a textbook or Internet source, or an actual human who may be able to shed some light on the topic that is perplexing you.

Two concepts related to memorization, primacy and recency, have implications for how you should utilize your study sessions—the time periods you set aside for adding to your nugget lists and reviewing them. According to the principles of primacy and recency, people recall the material they addressed at the beginning and end of a given study session better than the material they encountered in the middle of it (Intelegen, 2009). Thus, for purposes of retaining information in long-term memory, it is better to break long sessions into shorter minisessions. For example, if you have a 3-hour block of time set aside for study, it is best to break those 3 hours up into three 50-minute minisessions separated by 10-minute breaks so that there will be more high-retention beginnings and endings. And (good news!) your brain will encode those new memories more efficiently if you spend those 10-minutes breaks doing something enjoyable and unrelated to studying.

The frequency with which you review your nugget lists has implications for how long and how well you will retain in your memory the information you need to pass NCLEX. Consider this: according to the educational psychology literature, if you listen to a body of information presented in class and take notes but don't review them at all after that, you will have forgotten 80% of it within 1 or 2 days (Intelegen, 2009). Thus, it is absolutely essential that you conduct systematic reviews of all your nugget lists to ensure that the information you've worked so hard to retain will be available when you need it on NCLEX day. Here's what you should do: At the end of each 50-minute study minisession, just before you take your 10-minute break, quiz yourself on the nugget list questions you've made during that minisession. Then, in about 24 hours, review all the questions from the entire study session to avoid the erosion of memory that typically occurs about a day after a given session. Reviewing the material at or near the 24-hour mark should cause the information to remain encoded in your memory over the next week, after which (as you've no doubt anticipated) it will be time for yet another review. Happily, that review will stick the information in your mind for about a month, and, according to the literature on memorization, if you review it again at the 1-month mark, you should be able to access it easily over the next 6 months (Intelegen, 2009). Because you will be creating new nugget lists frequently, however, the simplest way to implement your understanding of how memory works will be to review all your nugget lists weekly. If you do that, you will gradually become a veritable font of nursing knowledge and remain so for about 6 months, within which time you will have taken NCLEX and passed.

After you become licensed and are no longer reviewing a wide spectrum of nursing knowledge regularly, you will gradually lose whatever information you don't use fairly frequently in the course of your clinical practice. You will, however, replace it with new knowledge that is more specific to the nature and demands of your job.

Remember: Stick to the following nugget list question review schedule:
- *Review the new nuggets right after each minisession.*
- *Review each study session's nuggets 24 hours after the session.*
- *Review all your nugget lists weekly.*

Remember also that memorizing facts or principles, although necessary, is not sufficient to guarantee success on the NCLEX. You must also practice considering them in the various contexts you will encounter in question scenarios, and the topic-specific Practice Tests and Comprehensive Practice Exams included in this book will provide ample opportunity for you to do that.

USING KEEP TRACK BOXES TO MONITOR YOUR PROGRESS

One of the things you absolutely do not want to do is take the NCLEX before you're really ready for it. As mentioned in Chapter 1, failing your licensing examination is a miserable experience that can harm you emotionally and financially. Ongoing self-evaluation in terms of your ability to analyze test questions and the strength of your knowledge base is a built-in feature of this book. Every chapter that consists of a topic-focused Practice Test or Comprehensive Practice Exam also contains a Keep Track box identical to the one shown here:

Keep Track

- Percent correct. (Divide the number of questions you answered correctly by the total number of questions you answered.) _____

- Number of questions you missed due to a reading error: _____

- Number of questions you missed due to errors in analysis: _____

- Number of assessment questions you missed: _____

- Number of lab value questions you missed: _____

- Number of drug/treatment questions you missed: _____

The Keep Track boxes provide space for you to record the following information that is essential to your ongoing self-evaluation: (1) your score on each test or exam, (2) the number of questions you answered incorrectly because you made a reading error, (3) the number of questions you missed because you made an analytical error, and (4) the number of questions you missed that pertained to three aspects of nursing practice that you are sure to be tested on during the NCLEX: assessment, interpretation of lab values, and appropriate administration of drugs and treatments.

Test and Exam Scores

Your score on a given test or exam tells you what percentage of the total number of questions you answered correctly. Having spent most of your life undergoing one phase or another of the educational process, you are no doubt very familiar with percentage scoring. Your scores on the topic-focused Practice Tests will tell you whether your knowledge base pertaining to a given topic (cardiovascular nursing, psych–mental health nursing, etc.) is adequate or whether you need to access additional practice questions on that topic from another source so you can extract more nuggets from them. When you have completed all the topic-focused tests, you will take the second Comprehensive Practice Exam and calculate your score. If all is going well, your score on that exam should be close to 90% or higher, particularly if you did pretty well on Comprehensive Practice Exam 1. If you did not do so well on exam 1 but scored 85% or better on Exam 2, you are making excellent progress and just need to firm up your knowledge a bit more. If you scored less than 85% on Comprehensive Practice Exam 2, however, you should gear up to do a bit more work before you take the NCLEX. You should note any content areas in which you were weak, access another source of questions in those areas, and create nugget questions based on them. When you feel that you've done sufficient work in your weak content areas, take Comprehensive Practice Exam 3. If you score 85% or higher on it, go ahead and schedule the NCLEX. If you score 84% or lower, however, you should identify your weak areas and repeat the remedial steps previously outlined. Do *not* take the NCLEX unless you have scored 90% or higher on several comprehensive exams from other books or online programs. It is much better to overprepare for the NCLEX than to fail it.

Reading Errors

You will recall from Chapter 6 that one of the keys to passing the NCLEX is making sure you understand what each test item is asking and then notice each and every key word in the scenario. When you have answered a question incorrectly because you didn't understand what the question was really asking or because you overlooked one or more key words, you made a reading error. As you hone your test item reading skills with practice, your Keep Track boxes should reflect that the number of reading errors you made on each successive Practice Test is decreasing. If, after you've completed a few Practice Tests, you find that this is not the case, reread the section of Chapter 6 that addresses question rewording and key word identification.

Analysis Errors

If you missed a question because you neglected to consider one or more of the answer choices in light of each and every key word or phrase, you've made an analysis error.

Quite a few of my clients have had to struggle to eradicate an entrenched tendency to choose answers based on hunches or hasty reasoning instead of a deliberate, step-by-step analytical process. If you find that you are continuing to answer questions incorrectly due to analysis errors, reread the relevant section of Chapter 6 and redouble your efforts to apply each step in the question-analyzing procedure to each Practice Test question you answer.

Questions on Assessment, Lab Values, and Drugs and Treatments

You will recall from Chapter 3 that the steps in the nursing process (assessment, analysis, planning, intervention, and evaluation) are woven throughout the NCLEX. I have included assessment in the Keep Track boxes because there is a specific and fairly discrete body of assessment-related information that you definitely should have in your knowledge base in case you get a lot of assessment questions on the NCLEX.

You will also recall from Chapter 3 that safe, effective care environment and physiologic integrity are two of the most heavily weighted client need categories on the NCLEX. I want you to keep track of how you are doing on questions pertaining to interpretation of lab values and questions pertaining to drug administration and treatments because both are included in those client need categories and because both tend to be challenging for my clients.

REFERENCES

Intelegen. (2005). *Mnemonic techniques and specific memory tricks to improve memory, memorization.* Retrieved June 20, 2009, from http://www.web-us.com/memory/mnemonic_techniques.htm

Intelegen. (2009). *Your memory's natural rhythms.* Retrieved June 19, 2009, from http://www.web-us.com/brain/brainmemoryrythms.htm

Weiss, R. P. (2000, July). *Brain based learning. Training and development.* Retrieved June 25, 2009, from http://findarticles.com/p/articles/mi_m4467/is_7_54/ai_64059320/?tag=content;col1

Chapter 9

Practice Test: Nursing Management of Patients with Cardiac Disorders

Karen S. March

PRACTICE TEST

General

1. Which of the following statements made by a patient would alert the nurse that the patient may be noncompliant with treatment for hypertension?
   A. "Both my father and grandfather died of an aneurysm."
   B. "My blood pressure normally runs about 140/98 mm Hg."
   C. "I take my blood pressure medicine when I have headaches."
   D. "My blood pressure medicine is very expensive."

2. The nurse has been teaching a patient about dietary modifications to help control blood pressure. Which of the following food choices by the patient indicates understanding of the instructions?
   A. French onion soup and salad
   B. vegetarian wrap with chips
   C. grilled chicken salad with fresh salsa
   D. chicken bouillon and saltine crackers

3. A patient who has been diagnosed with variant (Prinzmetal's) angina asks the nurse how this type of angina differs from stable angina. The nurse's reply should include:
   A. "Variant angina is normally triggered by exertion."
   B. "The pain of variant angina is less than that of stable angina."
   C. "Variant angina may be associated with EKG changes."
   D. "The chest discomfort of variant angina is worse."

4. The nurse articulates the difference between unstable angina and acute myocardial infarction (AMI) by which of the following explanations?
   A. "The pain of unstable angina is far less severe than the pain of AMI."
   B. "Unstable angina results from coronary artery occlusion for at least one hour."
   C. "Unstable angina and AMI can occur as a consequence of severe emotional stress."
   D. "Myocardial tissue dies as a result of acute myocardial infarction."

5. Death after myocardial infarction most frequently occurs due to which of the following complications?
   A. cardiogenic shock
   B. dysrhythmias
   C. heart failure
   D. pulmonary edema

6. A patient with heart failure is being prepared for discharge. Which of the following lunch menu choices indicates to the nurse that dietary instruction has been effective?
   A. turkey on whole wheat, mixed green salad, hot tea, orange sherbet
   B. hamburger on bun, french fries, dill pickle, cherry pie
   C. hot dog on roll, macaroni and cheese, tomato juice, white cake
   D. beef broth, saltines, hot tea, fruit ice, bottled water

ALTERNATE FORMAT

7. The nurse is preparing a patient for cardiac catheterization. Which of the following teaching points are pertinent for the nurse to include before the procedure? **SELECT ALL THAT APPLY.**
   A. "You will have to lie flat for several hours after the procedure."
   B. "You will receive medication to relax you but you will be awake."
   C. "You will feel a very cool sensation when the dye is injected."
   D. "You will be placed on a hard table that moves during the procedure."

8. The nurse understands that a patient with atrial fibrillation has lower cardiac output than a patient with normal sinus rhythm. The primary mechanism responsible for this is which of the following?
   A. loss of atrial kick
   B. rapid heart rate
   C. slow heart rate
   D. inefficient conduction

9. The nurse is caring for a patient who develops this rhythm on the monitor:

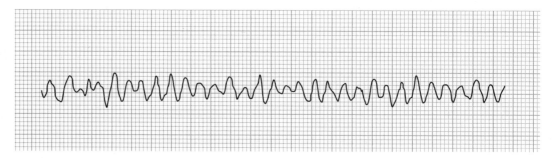

   Which of the following should the nurse do first?
   A. Prepare to assist with pacemaker insertion.
   B. Prepare to send the patient to surgery.
   C. Prepare for synchronized cardioversion.
   D. Prepare for defibrillation.

ALTERNATE FORMAT

10. The nurse must defibrillate a patient who is in ventricular tachycardia. Place an X over areas of the torso to indicate correct paddle placement.

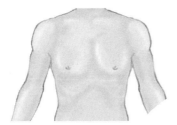

11. The nurse knows that which of the following congenital heart defects results in increased pulmonary blood flow?
    A. ventricular septal defect
    B. tetralogy of Fallot
    C. pulmonary stenosis
    D. coarctation of the aorta

12. The mechanism most commonly responsible for myocardial infarction is which of the following?
    A. coronary artery thrombosis
    B. plaque fissure or hemorrhage
    C. coronary artery spasm
    D. unstable angina

13. The most common symptom of acute myocardial infarction is which of the following?
    A. shortness of breath
    B. pain in the shoulder and left arm
    C. substernal chest pain unrelieved by rest
    D. pain relieved by nitroglycerin

14. The nurse knows that which of the following is a reliable indicator of reperfusion following thrombolytic therapy?
    A. ventricular dysrhythmia
    B. appearance of Q waves
    C. elevated ST segments
    D. reoccurrence of chest pain

15. The nurse realizes that complications commonly follow acute myocardial infarction. Which of the following complications occurs most frequently?
    A. dysrhythmias
    B. pulmonary edema
    C. cardiogenic shock
    D. sudden cardiac death

16. Elderly patients are prone to increased complications related to tissue perfusion following acute myocardial infarction because:
    A. peripheral vascular resistance increases with aging.
    B. peripheral vascular resistance decreases with aging.
    C. blood is hypercoagulable and clots more quickly.
    D. cardiac medications are less effective for this population.

17. Elevated ST segments during the early phase of an acute myocardial infarction are indicative of which of the following?
    A. injury
    B. ischemia
    C. necrosis
    D. reperfusion

18. The nurse expects which of the following EKG changes in the patient who is experiencing myocardial ischemia?
    A. elevated PR interval
    B. depressed PR interval
    C. prolonged QT interval
    D. ST segment depression

19. When caring for a patient admitted with endocarditis, the nurse must ask which of the following questions as part of the history?
    A. "Have you had any recent surgery?"
    B. "Do you have family history of heart disease?"
    C. "Have you ever used or abused IV drugs?"
    D. "Do you now or have you ever smoked?"

20. The nurse anticipates which of the following EKG changes when a patient experiences myocardial infarction?
    A. prolonged PR interval
    B. short QT interval
    C. ST segment elevation
    D. prominent U waves

21. The nurse understands that abnormal Q waves develop on the EKG following acute myocardial infarction because:
    A. necrotic tissue cannot conduct electrical current.
    B. reduced blood flow leads to reduced cardiac output.
    C. speed of impulse conduction is facilitated by infarction.
    D. they indicate that the patient needs a pacemaker.

Physical Assessment

1. A patient with a history of heart disease complains of dyspnea when ambulating in the hallway. The nurse understands that this finding is:
   A. normal for a patient with heart disease.
   B. a sign of severely impaired respiratory function.
   C. indicative of diminished cardiac reserve.
   D. a sign of impending pulmonary embolism.

2. During initial assessment of a patient with heart failure, which of the following findings should alert the nurse to monitor the patient closely?
   A. capillary refill of less than 3 seconds
   B. blood pressure of 142/88 while standing
   C. respiratory rate of 22 breaths per minute
   D. distended neck veins with HOB elevated

3. The nurse is aware that which of the following is one of the earliest signs of left ventricular failure?
   A. dyspnea
   B. cough
   C. jugular venous distention
   D. orthopnea

ALTERNATE FORMAT

4. A patient presents to an urgent care center with recurrent pressure and chest pain. The patient describes the pain as mild "pressing" or "aching," which typically is associated with diaphoresis and dizziness. Which of the following questions provide(s) important information for differential diagnosis? SELECT ALL THAT APPLY.
   A. "Where is the pain located?"
   B. "Does the pain subside with rest?"
   C. "What were you doing when the pain began?
   D. "Does anything help to relieve the pain?"

ALTERNATE FORMAT

5. A 75-year-old woman presents to the emergency department with the following symptoms: extreme nausea, dizziness, shortness of breath, and pale gray skin color. When approached by a nurse, the patient becomes very anxious. Which of the following should be priority actions taken by the nurse? SELECT ALL THAT APPLY.
   A. Provide oxygen.
   B. Attach an EKG monitor.
   C. Start an IV.
   D. Manage anxiety with lorazepam (Ativan) IV.

6. In assessing a patient who receives treatment with digoxin (Lanoxin), the nurse must be astute to cues of digoxin toxicity. Which of the following are most commonly early indicators of digoxin toxicity?
   A. abdominal discomfort and weakness
   B. ventricular tachycardia and confusion
   C. nausea and vomiting
   D. visual disturbances and headache

7. The nurse is caring for a patient admitted from the emergency department with the diagnosis "rule out myocardial infarction." The patient begins to experience chest pain. Which of the following findings would be most significant in light of the diagnosis?
   A. The pain improves when the patient sits upright in bed.
   B. The pain is relieved following two nitroglycerin tablets.
   C. The pain is described as pressure or aching in the right chest.
   D. The pain is accompanied by ST segment elevation on the monitor.

8. A 3-year-old child is diagnosed with tetralogy of Fallot. Upon assessment, the nurse expects which of the following findings?
   A. The child favors squatting.
   B. The child is growing normally.
   C. The child is acyanotic except with exertion.
   D. The child is highly active.

9. The nurse caring for a child with patent ductus arteriosus (PDA) would expect which of the following findings upon physical examination?
   A. bounding pulses and murmur
   B. vigorous activity with much energy
   C. active child without symptoms
   D. signs of increased cardiac output

10. The nurse is caring for a child with a large ventricular septal defect. Which of the following findings should the nurse anticipate upon detailed examination?
    A. symptoms of heart failure
    B. normal arterial blood gases
    C. skin is pink and warm
    D. hypoplastic right ventricle

11. A toddler has returned from cardiac catheterization. Which of the following assessment findings during the immediate postcardiac catheterization period is indicative of serious complications?
    A. capillary refill < 2 seconds and ability to wiggle toes
    B. temperature of 98.4°F with a heart rate of 114
    C. weak pedal pulse with a cool foot
    D. blood pressure of 82/50 with a dry dressing

12. The nurse should be most concerned about which of the following findings associated with chest pain?
    A. pain increases with inspiration
    B. pain lasts longer than 20 minutes
    C. pain is relieved with 1 nitroglycerin
    D. pain is relieved with rest

13. While administering nitroglycerin for chest pain, the nurse must assess which of the following parameters?
    A. heart rate
    B. blood pressure
    C. cardiac output
    D. stroke volume

14. When caring for the patient who has received thrombolytic therapy, the nurse will assess for which of the following side effects?
    A. dysrhythmias
    B. disorientation
    C. oozing at IV sites
    D. bradycardia

15. When a patient receives a drug with negative chronotropic effects, the nurse expects which of the following outcomes?
    A. loss of sympathetic tone
    B. decreased vascular tone
    C. decreased contractility
    D. decreased heart rate

16. **A patient presents with symptoms of angina while asleep or at rest. Based upon this information, the nurse is aware that a goal of therapy is which of the following?**
    A. increasing oxygen supply
    B. decreasing oxygen demand
    C. treatment with vasoconstrictors
    D. adequate control of pain

17. **Which of the following is the most important finding when the nurse assesses chest pain? The pain:**
    A. is decreased with repeated deep breathing.
    B. is not relieved by nitroglycerin
    C. improves while lying flat.
    D. is relieved following antacid.

18. **The nurse obtains a blood pressure of 62/30 on a patient who is sitting in bed and talking with family members. What should the nurse do next?**
    A. Ask the family to leave the room immediately.
    B. Reapply the cuff and repeat the blood pressure.
    C. Explain to the patient why he or she must lie supine.
    D. Prepare for imminent resuscitation procedures.

Interpretation of Lab Values

1. **The nurse is caring for a patient admitted with the following lab work:**

Laboratory Results	
Laboratory test	**Result**
Complete blood count	
Hematocrit (HCT)	42%
Hemoglobin (HGB)	14%
Red blood cells (RBC)	5.0 million/µL
Mean cell volume (MCV)	88 µ/m³
Mean cell hemoglobin (MCH)	29 pg
Mean cell hemoglobin concentration (MCHC)	36.2%
White blood cells (WBC)	6000/µL
Platelets (Plt)	280,000/µL
Serum electrolytes	
Carbon dioxide	28 mEq/L
Chloride	99 mEq/L
Potassium	2.8 mEq/L
Sodium	138 mEq/L
Serum digoxin	2.5 ng/mL

Upon review, the nurse notes that the patient suffers from which of the following conditions?

A. The patient is neutropenic.
B. The patient is anemic.
C. The patient is hyperkalemic.
D. The patient is digoxin toxic.

2. A patient has the following lab work:

Laboratory Results	
Laboratory test	**Result**
Complete blood count	
Hematocrit (HCT)	40%
Hemoglobin (HGB)	13.2%
Red blood cells (RBC)	5.0 million/µL
Mean cell volume (MCV)	88 µ/m3
Mean cell hemoglobin (MCH)	29 pg
Mean cell hemoglobin concentration (MCHC)	36.2%
White blood cells (WBC)	6120/µL
Platelets (Plt)	285,000/µL
Serum electrolytes	
Magnesium	2.2 mEq/L
Calcium	8.8 mg/dL
Potassium	2.8 mEq/L
Sodium	138 mEq/L
Serum digoxin	2.5 ng/mL

Which of the electrolyte values is most likely to precipitate changes in the serum digoxin level?

A. Mg++ 2.2 mEq/dL
B. Ca++ 8.8 mg/dL
C. K+ 2.8 mEq/dL
D. Na+ 138 mEq/L

3. The nurse is caring for a patient who survived cardiopulmonary resuscitation following ventricular dysrhythmias. A priority nursing intervention for this patient should be which of the following?

A. Review serum electrolytes.
B. Prepare to defibrillate.
C. Administer antidysrhythmic drugs.
D. Obtain a 12-lead EKG.

4. A child with congenital heart defect has an elevated hemoglobin and hematocrit. Which of the following interpretations provides a correct rationale for this occurrence?
   A. The child is not anemic because both the hemoglobin and hematocrit are elevated.
   B. Elevation of hemoglobin and hematocrit is a compensatory response to chronic hypoxia.
   C. The child is severely dehydrated, and loss of intravascular fluid has produced hemoconcentration.
   D. The child is hyperoxygenated with increased oxygen-carrying capacity of the blood.

ALTERNATE FORMAT

5. Which of the following therapeutic effects are expected as outcomes of nicotinic acid (Niacin) therapy? **SELECT ALL THAT APPLY.**
   A. reduction in LDL cholesterol
   B. raises HDL cholesterol levels
   C. hyperglycemia
   D. hypokalemia

6. Which of the following laboratory tests has been referred to as an independent risk factor for cardiovascular events?
   A. C-reactive protein (CRP)
   B. brain natriuretic peptide (BNP)
   C. phospholipids
   D. total cholesterol

7. Which of the following serum levels is indicative of severity of heart failure?
   A. serum sodium level
   B. brain natriuretic peptide (BNP)
   C. serum osmolality
   D. creatine kinase

Drugs and Treatments

1. The patient is prescribed digoxin (Lanoxin) 125 micrograms PO every day. The nurse finds digoxin (Lanoxin) 0.250 milligram tablets in the Pyxis. Which of the following is the appropriate action for the nurse?
   A. Call the pharmacy to request delivery of the correct dose.
   B. Administer 4 tablets from the Pyxis to deliver the full dose.
   C. Administer 1/2 tablet for the dose and waste the remainder.
   D. Notify the physician for a clarification of the order.

ALTERNATE FORMAT

2. The nurse is preparing to administer Lanoxin 0.125 mg IV push to the patient as ordered. The drug is available in ampules labeled "digoxin 500 mcg/2 mL." Which of the following actions will be performed by the nurse prior to and during administration of this drug? **SELECT ALL THAT APPLY.**
   A. Take an apical heart rate for a full minute prior to administration.
   B. Draw up 1 mL of drug from the ampule with a filter needle.
   C. Dilute the drug in 4 mL D5W and administer over 5 minutes.
   D. Review the patient's lab work for serum sodium levels.

3. The patient is ordered dopamine by infusion at 5 mcg/kg/min. The IV bag contains 400 mg of dopamine in 250 mL of 0.9% NaCl. The patient weighs 220 lb. Based on this information, the infusion pump must be set at what rate to ensure that the medication is infused correctly?
   A. 1.9 mL/hr
   B. 3.8 mL/hr
   C. 9.4 mL/hr
   D. 18.8 mL/hr

4. The patient is ordered dobutamine by infusion at 5 mcg/kg/min. The IV bag contains 250 mg of dobutamine in 250 mL D5W. The patient weighs 198 lb. Based on this information, the infusion pump must be set at what rate to infuse the medication correctly?
   A. 24 mL/hr
   B. 27 mL/hr
   C. 30 mL/hr
   D. 40 mL/hr

ALTERNATE FORMAT

5. The patient has an order for an IV of 1000 mL NSS with 20 mEq KCl to infuse at 2 mEq/hr by infusion pump. At what rate should the nurse set the infusion pump to ensure that the fluid is delivered as ordered?

6. An IV of 1000 mL lactated Ringer's (LR) with 20 grams magnesium sulfate arrives from the pharmacy. The nurse is to deliver a bolus of 3 grams magnesium sulfate over 30 minutes followed by a maintenance infusion of 1.5 grams/hr. The nurse knows that the correct rates for the bolus and the maintenance infusion are:
   A. 30 mL/hr for the bolus, then 15 mL/hr for the maintenance infusion.
   B. 150 mL/hr for the bolus, then 75 mL/hr for the maintenance infusion.
   C. 150 mL/hr for the bolus, then 50 mL/hr for the maintenance infusion.
   D. 300 mL/hr for the bolus, then 75 mL/hr for the maintenance infusion.

7. Morphine 10 mg IV is prescribed for the patient. The nurse finds that morphine is available in 4 mg/mL prefilled syringes. How many syringes must the nurse use to obtain the full dose?
   A. 1
   B. 2
   C. 3
   D. 4

ALTERNATE FORMAT

8. The nurse is reviewing the patient's medication administration record and laboratory results as follows:

Medication Administration Record

Medication	Dosage	Frequency
digoxin (Lanoxin)	0.125 mg PO	daily
verapamil (Calan)	240 mg PO	HS
furosemide (Lasix)	40 mg IV	daily
metoclopramide (Reglan)	10 mg PO	AC and HS
vitamin B$_{12}$	500 mcg SL	daily

Laboratory Results

Laboratory test	Result
Complete blood count	
Hematocrit (HCT)	42%
Hemoglobin (HGB)	14%
Red blood cells (RBC)	5.0 million/µL
Mean cell volume (MCV)	88 µ/m^3
Mean cell hemoglobin (MCH)	29 pg
Mean cell hemoglobin concentration (MCHC)	36.2%
White blood cells (WBC)	6000/µL
Platelets (Plt)	280,000/µL
Serum electrolytes	
Carbon dioxide	28 mEq/L
Chloride	99 mEq/L
Potassium	2.8 mEq/L
Sodium	138 mEq/L
Serum digoxin	2.5 ng/mL

The nurse notes the following rhythm on the cardiac monitor:

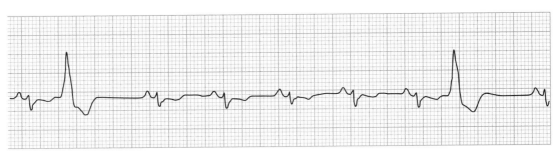

The nurse realizes that one or more of the following drugs or lab results has affected the rhythm. SELECT ALL THAT APPLY.
A. furosemide (Lasix)
B. verapamil (Calan)
C. digoxin (Lanoxin)
D. potassium
E. sodium
F. serum digoxin

9. A patient presents to an urgent care center with recurrent pressure and chest pain. The patient describes the pain as mild "squeezing" or "aching" that occurs with exertion. Which of the following drugs is most likely to provide effective relief?
A. one baby aspirin
B. intravenous morphine
C. nitroglycerin
D. oxygen

10. A 69-year-old woman is admitted to the hospital's CCU with severe anterior chest pain that radiates to her shoulders and arms. The patient is nauseous, vomiting, and diaphoretic with an apical heart rate of 100 and a blood pressure of 140/80. The drug of choice for this patient's pain is which of the following?
A. one baby aspirin
B. intravenous morphine
C. nitroglycerin
D. oxygen

11. Digoxin (Lanoxin) is used for treatment of patients with heart failure in which of the following circumstances?
A. to control heart rate in atrial fibrillation
B. to reduce myocardial oxygen consumption
C. to sustain high cardiac output states
D. to produce a positive chronotropic effect

ALTERNATE FORMAT

12. When a patient with heart failure is being treated with digoxin (Lanoxin), the nurse must be cautious about assessment for digoxin toxicity. Which of the following medications are most likely to increase serum digoxin levels? SELECT ALL THAT APPLY.
A. quinidine
B. verapamil
C. metoclopramide
D. amiodarone

13. A patient with heart failure is being prepared for discharge from the hospital. Furosemide (Lasix) has been ordered daily. The nurse should teach the patient to perform which of the following at home to assess effectiveness of this therapy?
A. check weight daily
B. check blood pressure daily
C. plan a low sodium diet
D. drink at least 2000 mL daily

14. Drugs like nitroglycerin and isosorbide dinitrate (Isordil) provide effective treatment for patients with heart failure because they work by which of the following
mechanisms?
    A. suppress the renin-angiotensin-aldosterone system
    B. inhibit the effects of the sympathetic nervous system
    C. reduce left ventricular workload
    D. decrease venous return and preload

15. Enalapril (Vasotec) can be used successfully to treat heart failure. This drug works
by which of the following mechanisms?
    A. It decreases both preload and afterload.
    B. It increases cardiac output and renal perfusion.
    C. It decreases ventricular remodeling.
    D. It relaxes the smooth muscles of the veins.

16. The nurse who is preparing to administer digoxin (Lanoxin) discovers that the
patient, who previously had a regular heart rate, now has an irregular heart rate
of 48. Which of the following actions by the nurse represents best practice?
    A. The nurse reassesses the apical heart rate for a full minute.
    B. The nurse withholds the ordered dose of medication.
    C. The nurse administers the dose to regulate the heart rate.
    D. The nurse assesses for signs of hypovolemia.

17. A medication that may be used to effectively control rapid ventricular response in
atrial fibrillation or atrial flutter is which of the following?
    A. verapamil (Calan)
    B. enalapril (Vasotec)
    C. adenosine (Adenocard)
    D. digoxin (Lanoxin)

18. Metoprolol (Lopressor) is a medication that blocks sympathetic stimulation at the
sinus node to diminish tachycardias. Although it is a relatively safe drug, it
should not be used in patients with which of the following conditions?
    A. postmyocardial infarction
    B. asthma
    C. hypertension
    D. anxiety

19. The nurse has been teaching a parent about home administration of digoxin
(Lanoxin) to a toddler upon discharge. Which of the following statements by the
parent provides assurance that teaching has been understood?
    A. "If I forget a dose, I can give it up to six hours later."
    B. "It is best to mix the drug on a teaspoon with applesauce."
    C. "If my child vomits after the dose, I can give another."
    D. "It is a good idea to brush my child's teeth after each dose."

20. The nurse is prepared to administer digoxin (Lanoxin) to a 5-year-old child. The apical pulse rate is 76. Which of the following actions by the nurse is most appropriate?
    A. Notify the physician immediately because the child is in heart block.
    B. Administer the drug because the child's pulse rate is normal.
    C. Compare the child's apical and radial pulses simultaneously.
    D. Withhold the dose of digoxin and notify the physician.

21. The patient is being prepared for administration of thrombolytic therapy for acute myocardial infarction (AMI). Which of the following conditions would constitute a contraindication for thrombolytic therapy?
    A. history of urinary tract infection
    B. hemorrhagic stroke 1 year ago
    C. history of diabetes mellitus
    D. one year postabdominal surgery

22. The rationale for administering a thrombolytic agent is which of the following?
    A. to restore blood flow through an artery via lysis of the clot
    B. anticoagulation to prevent formation of new clots
    C. to dissolve atherosclerotic plaque at the site of the blockage
    D. dilation of the blocked arterial vessel, which restores flow

23. The patient has an automated implanted cardioverter defibrillator (AICD) for control of chronic ventricular dysrhythmias. The nurse understands that which of the following should occur if the patient's rhythm deteriorates into ventricular fibrillation?
    A. External defibrillation should be initiated immediately.
    B. The AICD will defibrillate automatically at a high energy level.
    C. The nurse should initiate cardiopulmonary resuscitation immediately.
    D. The nurse should put the patient on a monitor and notify the physician.

24. The nurse knows that an intravenous dose of heparin will begin to exert anticoagulant effects within what time frame?
    A. almost immediately
    B. in 30 minutes
    C. after 2 hours
    D. within 2 to 3 days

25. When a patient develops a bleeding problem following administration of intravenous heparin, the physician is likely to prescribe which of the following drugs?
    A. Aquemephyton
    B. protamine sulfate
    C. streptokinase
    D. vitamin B$_{12}$

26. During the recovery phase following acute myocardial infarction, aspirin 325 mg PO is prescribed daily for what purpose?
    A. for treatment of nitroglycerin-induced headache
    B. to help prevent reinfarction
    C. to reduce the serum cholesterol level
    D. to lower the serum potassium level

27. Captopril (Capoten) and enalapril (Vasotec) decrease peripheral resistance and lower blood pressure by which of the following mechanisms?
    A. direct arterial and venous dilation
    B. block conversion of angiotensin I to angiotensin II
    C. increase fluid excretion at the Loop of Henle
    D. peripheral vasoconstriction and central vasodilation

28. **The nurse should be certain to mention which of the following teaching points about adverse effects of nicotinic acid (Niacin) therapy?**
    A. Take 325 mg of aspirin one half hour before each dose to reduce flushing.
    B. Take with a full glass of water and keep your head elevated for 30 minutes.
    C. Take the drug on an empty stomach to ensure the full therapeutic effect.
    D. Monitor blood glucose levels at least monthly from the onset of therapy.

29. **The nurse knows that the patient understands the rationale for administering low-dose aspirin following acute myocardial infarction when the patient makes which of the following statements?**
    A. "Aspirin will keep my fever down."
    B. "Aspirin keeps my platelets from clumping."
    C. "Aspirin helps to manage my pain."
    D. "Aspirin will help me sleep at night."

30. **A patient is admitted to the intensive care unit with symptomatic bradycardia and severe hypotension. Orders are received to start an epinephrine drip at 2.1 mcg/minute. The nurse expects the epinephrine to exert what effect?**
    A. increase cardiac output
    B. increase vascular congestion
    C. decrease ventricular workload
    D. decrease stroke volume

ANSWERS

General

1. (**C**); Blood pressure meds must be taken regularly; if the patient is taking the drug only when he or she has headaches, the patient is noncompliant. Options A and D do not suggest noncompliance. Option B may indicate poor control of hypertension but does not necessarily imply noncompliance with medications.

2. (**C**); Grilled chicken salad and fresh salsa are both made from fresh (preservative-free) materials and therefore are likely to be of lower sodium content than French onion soup, chips, chicken bouillon, or saltines.

3. (**C**); Variant (Prinzmetal's) angina is characteristically associated with EKG changes related to coronary artery spasm, which results in decreased oxygen supply to the myocardium. Variant angina may occur at rest, and is similar to pain experienced with other types of angina.

4. (**D**); Myocardial cell death occurs as a consequence of myocardial infarction. With unstable angina, cell death does not occur. The pain of angina is typically less severe than AMI but not always. AMI results from coronary artery occlusion with pain that is not relieved by nitroglycerin for at least 20 minutes.

5. (**B**); Although any of the four complications can occur, the major cause of death after AMI is dysrhythmia.

6. **(A)**; Dietary concerns are largely related to sodium content of foods. Turkey, green salad, hot tea, and sherbet are all foods with relatively low sodium content. In each of the other options, foods with high sodium content are included—french fries, cherry pie, dill pickle, macaroni and cheese, tomato juice, broth, and saltines.

7. **(A, B, D)**; The patient will be placed on a hard table during the test. The table will move automatically as needed during the procedure. Although the patient will receive some medication to assist with relaxation (usually diazepam or midazolam), the patient can be aroused and can answer questions throughout the procedure. The patient will feel a very *warm* sensation with dye injection. Following the procedure, the patient will be required to lie flat for several hours with a sandbag to the groin to decrease the chance of hematoma formation or vessel rupture.

8. **(A)**; When a patient is in atrial fibrillation, there is no atrial kick. This means that the patient has approximately 30% less cardiac output than if the patient is in normal sinus rhythm with the benefit of atrial contraction.

9. **(D)**; The patient is in coarse ventricular fibrillation, which requires immediate defibrillation.

10.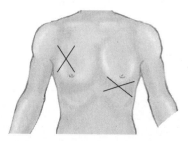

11. **(A)**; In ventricular septal defect, higher pressure on the left side of the heart means that blood flows from left to right and then into the pulmonary artery, which delivers increased pulmonary blood flow. This results in increased pulmonary vascular resistance and, eventually, right ventricular hypertrophy.

12. **(A)**; AMI is commonly due to the development of a coronary artery thrombus that completely occludes blood flow through the vessel, causing myocardial necrosis if left untreated. Hemorrhage is not a common cause of myocardial infarction (MI). Coronary artery spasm may produce angina. Unstable angina can be a warning sign of impending MI, but angina does not cause MI.

13. **(C)**; A hallmark symptom of AMI, which distinguishes it from angina, is that chest pain is unrelieved by rest (or nitroglycerin).

14. **(A)**; The occurrence of ventricular dysrhythmias following thrombolytic therapy is generally considered to be a sign of reperfusion of the coronary artery. Q waves and elevated ST segments indicate infarction. Recurrence of chest pain may indicate extension of the AMI.

15. **(A)**; Although there are a number of possible complications associated with myocardial infarction, the most common is dysrhythmia.

16. **(A)**; Elderly patients are more prone to complications related to tissue perfusion following AMI because peripheral vascular resistance increases with aging.

17. (**A**); Elevated ST segments during the early phase of AMI indicate injury. ST depression indicates ischemia; Q waves reveal necrosis; and ventricular dysrhythmia can indicate hypoxemia, hypokalemia, or reperfusion following thrombolytic therapy.

18. (**D**); ST depression indicates the occurrence of myocardial ischemia.

19. (**C**); The nurse must inquire about IV drug use because that is one of the major precipitating factors of endocarditis in the United States.

20. (**C**); The nurse anticipates ST segment elevation on the EKG when a patient experiences myocardial infarction. Prolongation of PR interval, short QT interval, and prominent U waves are not present during AMI.

21. (**A**); The nurse understands that abnormal Q waves develop on the EKG following acute myocardial infarction because necrotic tissue cannot conduct electric current.

Physical Assessment

1. (**C**); This finding is not normal. It indicates diminished cardiac reserve in a patient with known heart disease.

2. (**D**); Distended neck veins with the HOB elevated indicates significant fluid overload. Therefore, the patient should be monitored closely. The respiratory rate and blood pressure are mildly elevated, but capillary refill is normal.

3. (**B**); Cough is one of the earliest signs of LV failure. It is prompted by congestion within the pulmonary system and may be accompanied by bilateral crackles. Dyspnea is a subjective term that does not always correlate to degree of fluid accumulation. Orthopnea occurs when the patient is recumbent because increased volume return from the lower extremities prompts extreme breathing difficulty when the patient is flat. Many patients sleep in a recliner when they are prone to orthopnea.

4. (**A, B, C, D**); Each of the questions, if answered, provides important information that will lead to the differential diagnosis.

5. (**A, B, C**); This patient presents with signs and symptoms that would make one suspicious of AMI. Therefore, it is important for the nurse to provide oxygen to the patient, attach an EKG monitor, and start an IV. The anxiety is most likely related to the shortness of breath, nausea, and feeling bad. It should begin to subside as treatment begins to take effect.

6. (**C**); Although there are many signs and symptoms of digoxin toxicity, nausea and vomiting are two of the earliest.

7. (**D**); In the patient with a diagnosis of "rule out myocardial infarction," pain accompanied by ST segment elevation on the monitor would increase the suspicion of infarction.

8. (**A**); These children are typically cyanotic at birth and will favor squatting as oxygen saturation worsens. These children typically have poor growth patterns and are limited in activity because of low energy.

9. (**A**); Clinical manifestations include a significant murmur, signs of heart failure, and bounding pulses.

10. (**A**); These patients have symptoms of heart failure. They do not have normal ABGs, and their skin color is dusky as a consequence of pulmonary congestion.

11. **(C)**; Weak pedal pulse and a cool foot are indications of significant problems with perfusion, which require immediate attention.

12. **(B)**; In adults older than 35 years of age, suspicion of acute myocardial infarction is raised when chest pain lasts for more than 20 minutes. Pain relieved by one nitroglycerin tablet or rest is attributed to angina.

13. **(B)**; Nitroglycerin produces vasodilation, which can reduce blood pressure. The goal is to decrease pain while maintaining systolic blood pressure above 100 mm Hg.

14. **(C)**; Bleeding is the most common side effect associated with thrombolytic therapy.

15. **(D)**; A drug with negative chronotropic effects would be expected to decrease heart rate.

16. **(A)**; The most desirable treatment would be to increase O_2 supply because angina at rest is caused by decreased O_2 supply, not increased oxygen demand. Vasoconstrictors would worsen the problem.

17. **(B)**; The most important finding in chest pain assessment is pain that is not relieved with nitroglycerin. This pain is often associated with myocardial infarction.

18. **(B)**; The nurse should reapply the cuff and repeat the blood pressure without panic. The patient is not symptomatic.

Interpretation of Lab Values

1. **(D)**; The serum digoxin level is 2.5 ng/mL, and a normal digoxin level should be 0.8–2.0 ng/mL. Serum digoxin level is the only abnormal lab result.

2. **(C)**; Hypokalemia is known to potentiate digoxin toxicity. Magnesium, calcium, and sodium are all normal.

3. **(A)**; The nurse should review serum electrolyte results, particularly the serum potassium level. Hypokalemia and hypoxemia are two of the most common causes of ventricular dysrhythmias.

4. **(B)**; The elevated H/H represents a compensatory response to chronic hypoxia.

5. **(A, B)**; Niacin therapy helps to reduce LDL cholesterol and to raise HDL cholesterol levels. Hyperglycemia occurs as an adverse effect, not a therapeutic effect.

6. **(A)**; C-reactive protein is a marker for inflammatory changes in the vasculature. Clinical studies have demonstrated its association with increased cardiovascular risk.

7. **(B)**; Plasma concentration of BNP is used to gauge severity of heart failure and response to therapy.

Drugs and Treatments

1. **(C)**; The nurse must translate micrograms into milligrams to find that 125 micrograms equals 0.125 milligrams. Then, mathematically, the nurse can easily find that the required dose is 1/2 tablet.

2. **(A, C)**; Digoxin (Lanoxin) may be given undiluted or diluted in 4 mL NSS. There is more risk of precipitation with undiluted administration. Digoxin must be administered over a minimum of 5 minutes. Low serum potassium levels may potentiate digoxin toxicity. The required volume of drug to be drawn up in the syringe is 0.5 mL.

3. **(D)**; First, convert the patient's weight to kg by dividing 220 by 2.2, which equals 100 kg. Next, figure out how many mLs = 1 mcg by dividing the total volume (250 mL) by the number of micrograms of dopamine (400,000) to equal 0.000625 mL/mcg. Then apply the information to the following equation:

$$\frac{5 \text{ mcg} \times 100 \text{ kg}}{\text{minute}} \times \frac{60 \text{ minutes}}{\text{hour}} \times 0.000625 \frac{\text{mL}}{\text{mcg}} = 18.75 \frac{\text{mL}}{\text{hr}}$$

Because most IV pumps will infuse fractional doses expressed in tenths of a mL, you would round this to 18.8 mL/hr.

4. **(B)**; First, convert the patient's weight to kg by dividing 198 by 2.2, which equals 90 kg. Next, figure out how many mLs = 1 mcg by dividing the total volume (250 mL) by the number of micrograms of dobutamine (250,000) to equal 0.001 mL/mcg. Then apply the information to the following equation:

$$\frac{5 \text{ mcg} \times 90 \text{ kg}}{\text{minute}} \times \frac{60 \text{ minutes}}{\text{hour}} \times 0.001 \frac{\text{mL}}{\text{mcg}} = 27 \frac{\text{mL}}{\text{hr}}$$

5. 100 mL/hr; Using the ratio method, the infusion pump should be set to 100 mL/hr.

$$\frac{1000 \text{ mL}}{20 \text{ mEq}} = \frac{x \text{ mL}}{2 \text{ mEq}}$$

$$20\,x = 2000$$

$$x = 100 \frac{\text{mL}}{\text{hr}}$$

6. **(D)**; First, calculate the bolus using the ratio method:

$$\frac{1000 \text{ mL}}{20 \text{ g}} = \frac{x \text{ mL}}{3 \text{ g}}$$

$$3000 = 20\,x$$

Therefore, $x = 150$ mL to infuse over 30 minutes (0.5 hr). To determine the infusion rate per hour, divide the volume (150 mL) by the infusion time (in hours).

$$150 \text{ mL} \times 0.5 \text{ hr} = 300 \frac{\text{mL}}{\text{hr}} \text{ (BOLUS)}$$

Next, calculate the maintenance infusion using the same ratio technique:

$$\frac{1000 \text{ mL}}{20 \text{ g}} = \frac{x \text{ mL}}{1.5 \text{ g}}$$

$$1500 = 20\,x$$

Therefore, $x = 75$ mL to infuse each hour or 75 mL/hr (MAINTENANCE).

7. **(C)**; Divide the full dose (10 mg) by the number of mg/syringe (4) to find out how many syringes are needed.

$$\frac{10 \text{ mg}}{4 \dfrac{\text{mg}}{\text{syringe}}} = 2.5 \text{ syringes}$$

Therefore, the nurse must use three syringes to obtain the full dose of medication.

8. (**A, D**); The rhythm strip reveals two premature ventricular complexes (PVCs). The two most likely causes of premature ventricular contractions are hypoxia and hypokalemia. This patient's potassium level is 2.8 mEq/L, which is well below normal. The furosemide (Lasix) may have played a role in the development of hypokalemia.

9. (**C**); The patient is likely experiencing angina, which is treated with nitroglycerin.

10. (**B**); This patient's symptoms are indicative of acute myocardial infarction because of the type of pain described, as well as the accompanying nausea and vomiting. Pain medication of choice for treatment of AMI is intravenous morphine.

11. (**A**); Digoxin is useful for treatment of patients with heart failure who remain symptomatic with beta blockers and ACE inhibitors. It is also useful to control the ventricular response to atrial fibrillation.

12. (**A, B, D**); Quinidine, verapamil, and amiodarone tend to increase serum digoxin concentration, making the patient prone to development of digoxin toxicity. Metoclopramide tends to decrease the serum digoxin level.

13. (**A**); When patients with heart failure go home, it is critically important that they weigh themselves daily because weight is the most important indicator of fluid status at home.

14. (**D**); Nitroglycerin and isosorbide (Isordil) are both nitrates that decrease venous return and preload, thereby reducing symptoms of heart failure.

15. (**C**); ACE inhibitors like Vasotec decrease ventricular remodeling, which would result in less than optimal ventricular function.

16. (**B**); The dose of digoxin should be withheld if the heart rate is less than 60 or irregular. Bradycardia and dysrhythmias may indicate digoxin toxicity, so the physician should be consulted.

17. (**A**); Verapamil, a calcium channel blocker, is used to control rapid ventricular response to either atrial fibrillation or atrial flutter.

18. (**B**); Metoprolol should not be administered to patients with asthma because it can produce bronchospasm as an adverse effect.

19. (**D**); Whenever possible, the patient's teeth should be brushed after administration of digoxin to prevent tooth decay from exposure to the sweet liquid.

20. (**B**); A normal pulse rate for a 5-year-old child is 70–110. Therefore, the dose should be administered.

21. (**B**); A history of intracranial hemorrhage is a contraindication for administration of thrombolytics.

22. (**A**); Thrombolytic agents lyse clots to reestablish blood flow through coronary arteries.

23. (**B**); In response to ventricular fibrillation, the AICD will automatically defibrillate the patient.

24. (**A**); Heparin begins to take effect almost immediately when administered via intravenous push.

25. (**B**); Protamine sulfate is the antidote for heparin.

26. (**B**); Aspirin therapy is prescribed for post-MI patients to help prevent reinfarction by decreasing platelet aggregation.

27. (**B**); ACE inhibitors work by blocking the conversion of angiotensin I to angiotensin II.

28. (**A**); Niacin therapy can cause extreme flushing of the face, neck, and ears. Taking 325 mg of aspirin 30 minutes prior to the niacin helps to reduce the unpleasant flushing.

29. (**B**); The nurse knows that the patient understands the reason he or she is taking low-dose aspirin following acute myocardial infarction when the patient says, "Aspirin keeps my platelets from clumping."

30. (**A**); The nurse expects the epinephrine to increase cardiac output.

Keep Track

- Percent correct. (Divide the number of questions you answered correctly by the total number of questions you answered.) _____

- Number of questions you missed due to a reading error: _____

- Number of questions you missed due to errors in analysis: _____

- Number of assessment questions you missed: _____

- Number of lab value questions you missed: _____

- Number of drug/treatment questions you missed: _____

Nugget List

Chapter number _____ Topic _____

Practice Test: Nursing Management of Patients with Vascular Disorders

Karen S. March

PRACTICE TEST

General

1. The nursing assistant reports a blood pressure reading to the nurse, who notes that the cuff used was too large for the patient. Which effect would the size of the blood pressure cuff have on the blood pressure?
   A. The blood pressure measurement would be unaffected.
   B. The blood pressure measurement would be falsely high.
   C. The blood pressure measurement would be falsely low.
   D. The blood pressure measurement would be 20% higher.

2. A physician states that the patient's condition reveals strong parasympathetic influence. The nurse understands that the physician is talking about the patient's:
   A. increased myocardial contractility.
   B. decreased blood pressure.
   C. increased cardiac output.
   D. decreased heart rate.

3. The nurse is providing teaching to a patient about reducing modifiable risk factors for peripheral vascular disease. Which of the following would be an appropriate statement by the nurse?
   A. "Aspirin significantly increases the viscosity of the blood."
   B. "Cigarette smoking produces peripheral vasoconstriction."
   C. "Vigorous exercise increases blood viscosity."
   D. "Weight loss yields negligible peripheral vascular improvement."

4. The nurse is providing education about atherosclerosis to the patient. Which of the following statements by the patient indicates understanding of the teaching?
   A. "My arteries are narrowing and cannot carry as much blood."
   B. "The walls of my arteries are weak and bulge outward due to pressure."
   C. "I can completely reverse the effects of atherosclerosis by walking."
   D. "Atherosclerosis is due to chronic inflammation in my arteries."

5. The nurse is caring for a patient with hypertension who has been prescribed atenolol (Tenormin) 25 mg PO daily and enalapril (Vasotec) 5 mg PO twice daily. Which of the following comments by the patient might indicate noncompliance with the treatment regimen?
   A. "My mother and father died of old age."
   B. "My medicine is so expensive."
   C. "I take my medicine when I get a headache."
   D. "My blood pressure is 128/76 mm Hg."

6. The nurse is providing education to a patient who is newly diagnosed with Raynaud's disease. Which of the following statements by the patient indicates understanding of instructions for managing this disease?
   A. "I need to learn stress and relaxation techniques."
   B. "If I have a few beers, my fingers and toes will be warm."
   C. "If I drink coffee each day, I will have fewer symptoms."
   D. "Beta blockers might help decrease my symptoms."

7. Which of the following jobs would potentially be the best "fit" for a person with Raynaud's?
   A. postal carrier on a walking route
   B. downhill ski instructor
   C. personal fitness trainer
   D. school bus driver

8. The nurse is assigned to care for a patient who was admitted with Buerger's disease. Based on knowledge about this disease, the nurse anticipates which of the following information about the patient?
   A. The patient is likely to be a young male.
   B. The patient is likely to be a young female.
   C. The patient is likely to be an elderly female.
   D. The patient is likely to be an elderly male.

ALTERNATE FORMAT

9. The nurse will be receiving a patient admitted with a diagnosis of "stroke." The nurse is aware that which of the following are considered to be risk factors for stroke? SELECT ALL THAT APPLY.
   A. diabetes
   B. obesity
   C. cocaine use
   D. female
   E. male
   F. hypertension

10. The nurse is providing education to the patient about clinical manifestations of a transient ischemic attack (TIA). Which of the following statements by the patient indicates a need for further education?
    A. "TIA is like a warning when blood supply to part of the brain is interrupted."
    B. "TIA is nothing to worry about because the effects are only temporary."
    C. "Symptoms might include numbness or weakness on one side of my body."
    D. "If I have a TIA, I might lose my vision and have difficulty talking."

ALTERNATE FORMAT

11. The nurse is discussing medical management of carotid disease with a patient. Which of the following medical treatment options is available to the patient with carotid artery disease? SELECT ALL THAT APPLY.
    A. aspirin
    B. balloon angioplasty
    C. carotid stenting
    D. MRI
    E. CT

12. The nurse is providing teaching to a patient about carotid endarterectomy. Which of the following statements by the patient indicates understanding of the teaching?
    A. "This procedure can be done after a stroke to clean out my arteries."
    B. "My neurosurgeon can reduce my chance of stroke by surgically removing plaque."
    C. "If I have this procedure, I will not have a stroke and don't have to worry about it."
    D. "This is a relatively simple procedure that can be done just about anywhere."

13. The nurse caring for a patient following a transient ischemic attack (TIA) realizes that the priority nursing diagnosis for the patient is which of the following?
    A. ineffective peripheral tissue perfusion
    B. risk for infection
    C. impaired gas exchange
    D. risk for impaired mobility

14. The nurse is providing care for a patient who was admitted via the emergency department with a diagnosis of abdominal aortic aneurysm. A CT scan revealed that the aneurysm is 6.5 cm in diameter. Which of the following findings would alert the nurse to the possibility of impending rupture?
    A. anxiety, tearfulness, and verbal expression of concern
    B. chest pain, diaphoresis, and nausea
    C. restlessness, lower back pain, and hypotension
    D. biphasic pulses bilaterally by doppler

15. The nurse is assigned to care for a patient with abdominal aortic aneurysm. Which of the following findings should alert the nurse to the fact that the patient is suffering an aortic dissection?
    A. anxiety, restlessness, diaphoresis
    B. abrupt onset of severe, tearing chest pain
    C. gradual onset of severe, radiating chest pain
    D. inability to concentrate, fever, hypotension

ALTERNATE FORMAT

16. The nurse is assigned to care for a 60-year-old patient in the ICU who underwent surgical repair of an abdominal aortic aneurysm 5 days ago. The patient remains on a mechanical ventilator because of failed extubation attempts. The nurse understands that this patient is at risk for development of venous thromboembolism because of which of the following factors? SELECT ALL THAT APPLY.
    A. age
    B. abdominal surgery
    C. admission to the ICU
    D. prolonged immobility > 3 days

17. The nurse is providing education to the patient about prophylaxis for DVT. Which of the following statements by the patient indicate understanding of the education points?
    A. "I will wear my compression stockings all day long."
    B. "I do not have to use the sequential compression devices if I have TEDS on."
    C. "I have to wear thigh-high compression stockings for the best effect."
    D. "Because I have a DVT, I need to stay in bed as much as possible."

Physical Assessment

1. The nurse is assessing a patient with Raynaud's disease. Based on the patient's diagnosis, the nurse would focus history taking on assessment of:
    A. characteristics of pain, color changes of extremities, and frequency of attacks.
    B. whether or not the patient is compliant with nonpharmacologic therapy.
    C. whether or not the patient is compliant with pharmacologic treatment.
    D. full health background, including any autoimmune disorders.

2. Upon assessment of the patient with Buerger's disease, the nurse expects which of the following physical findings?
    A. paralysis of fingers and toes
    B. toe and finger ulceration
    C. pale lower extremities
    D. cool, pulseless extremities

ALTERNATE FORMAT

3. Postoperatively, the nurse caring for a carotid endarterectomy patient must include which of the following priority assessments? SELECT ALL THAT APPLY.
    A. speech
    B. airway
    C. urine output
    D. facial symmetry
    E. abdominal sounds

4. Which of the following findings would the nurse anticipate during assessment of a patient with subclavian steal syndrome?
    A. thrombosis of the subclavian vein
    B. femoral artery bruit
    C. blood pressure difference of 40 mm Hg from right to left arm
    D. unilateral pale, cool extremities with fleeting pulses

5. The nurse is providing care for a patient in the intensive care unit. Which of the following physical assessment findings would suggest the presence of a thoracic aneurysm?
    A. headache, fever, non-radiating chest pain
    B. tearing lower back pain with radiation to the abdomen
    C. substernal chest pain, dyspnea, stridor
    D. fleeting pulses, cool upper extremities

6. The nurse is assigned to care for a patient who has just returned from the operating suite following repair of an abdominal aortic aneurysm. Which of the following assessment findings would be of most concern to the nurse?
    A. The patient is groggy and hypothermic upon arrival from the OR.
    B. The patient is unable to feel the tip of a pin on the sole of the right foot.
    C. The patient is able to feel pressure from a blunt object bilaterally above the knees.
    D. The patient can push weakly on both of the nurse's hands with the feet.

Interpretation of Lab Values

1. The nurse is teaching a patient about warfarin (Coumadin) therapy. As part of the instruction, the nurse informs the patient that a treatment goal is an international normalized ratio (INR) between:
   A. 2–3.
   B. 3–4.
   C. 4–5.
   D. 5–6.

Drugs and Treatments

1. The nurse is providing care for a patient with Raynaud's disease and asks the patient for a complete list of medications. The rationale for this action is:
   A. that it is always a good idea to know what medications the patient is on.
   B. some medications, including beta blockers and hormones, precipitate vasospasm.
   C. that the patient must begin to understand the ramifications of medication therapy.
   D. to alert the patient that pharmacologic therapy may impact the treatment plan.

2. The nurse is providing discharge teaching for the patient with Buerger's disease. Which of the following instructions must be included?
   A. "You will need to attend physical therapy twice per week."
   B. "You will need to have a surgical revascularization procedure."
   C. "If you continue to smoke, you will probably require amputation."
   D. "If you maintain a cool environment, you will have fewer symptoms."

3. The nurse is providing education for follow-up of a patient diagnosed with abdominal aortic aneurysm. Which of the following comments by the patient indicates a need for reinforcement of follow-up instructions?
   A. "The main thing to remember is to notify my doctor if I have abdominal pain."
   B. "I can attend smoking cessation classes to help me stop smoking."
   C. "I will need to periodically have the size of my aneurysm checked by ultrasound."
   D. "It is important for me to have my blood pressure checked at least occasionally."

4. The nurse is aware that surgical treatment of abdominal aortic aneurysm depends upon a number of factors. Which of the following is the most likely treatment for an abdominal aortic aneurysm of 4 cm?
   A. endovascular repair
   B. open surgical repair
   C. reassess by ultrasound in 6 months
   D. reassess by ultrasound in 2 years

5. The nurse is caring for an ICU patient following carotid endarterectomy. The patient's blood pressure is 188/116 mm Hg according to an arterial line. The nurse has the following treatment options available. Which should be employed first?
   A. Zero and recalibrate the arterial line.
   B. Obtain a cuff BP for correlation with the arterial line.
   C. Initiate and titrate IV nitroprusside (Nipride) to maintain BP < 150/85.
   D. Initiate and titrate IV nitroprusside (Nipride) to maintain BP < 130/80.

6. The nurse is caring for a postoperative carotid endarterectomy patient who has required IV nitroprusside (Nipride) to maintain blood pressure within the parameters set by the surgeon. The nurse understands that:
   A. the patient's blood pressure will gradually decline to normal.
   B. the patient will gradually transition to oral antihypertensive medication.
   C. the patient must remain in intensive care until the blood pressure stabilizes.
   D. the patient will be transferred to a step down unit with the nitroprusside drip.

ALTERNATE FORMAT

7. The patient at high risk for development of DVT is likely to receive which of the following medications for prophylaxis? SELECT ALL THAT APPLY.
   A. subcutaneous heparin
   B. subcutaneous unfractionated heparin
   C. aspirin
   D. warfarin (Coumadin)

ALTERNATE FORMAT

8. According to evidence-based guidelines, which of the following are recommendations for care of the patient with confirmed DVT? SELECT ALL THAT APPLY.
   A. maintain strict bedrest
   B. ambulate as tolerated
   C. elevate the affected extremity above the heart
   D. massage the affected extremity
   E. apply dry heat directly over the area
   F. administer warfarin (Coumadin) for 3 months

ALTERNATE FORMAT

9. The nurse understands that inferior vena cava filters are used for which of the following reasons? SELECT ALL THAT APPLY.
   A. as prophylaxis for deep vein thrombosis
   B. for patients at risk for pulmonary embolism
   C. in patients who develop a clot during anticoagulation
   D. as evidence-based care for patients with DVT

10. The nurse is providing education for a patient who will be discharged with a prescription for enoxaparin (Lovenox). It will be a priority for the nurse to teach the patient:
    A. how to administer subcutaneous injections.
    B. to take the medicine with meals.
    C. to take the medicine with a full glass of water.
    D. about potential side effects of this drug.

ANSWERS

General

1. **(C)**; Obtaining accurate results from blood pressure monitoring depends upon use of appropriately sized equipment. The result of using a blood pressure cuff that is too large for the patient would be a *falsely low blood pressure*.

2. **(D)**; Parasympathetic influences decrease heart rate and slow conduction through the AV node.

3. **(B)**; Nicotine is a potent vasoconstrictor that reduces blood flow to the extremities and puts the patient at risk for peripheral vascular disease. Smoking is a modifiable risk factor. Individuals may choose to stop smoking to reduce the strong vasoconstrictive effects of nicotine.

4. **(A)**; In atherosclerosis, accumulations of lipid and fibrous tissue line the lumen of the artery, which results in narrowing of the lumen and inability to accommodate normal blood flow. Significant reduction in blood flow to tissues results in ischemic pain related to inadequate delivery of oxygen to the tissues.

5. **(C)**; When the patient admits to taking medicine when he or she gets a headache, the implication is that if there is no headache, then there will be no medicine.

6. **(A)**; Raynaud's is characterized by vasospasms that decrease blood flow to the fingers, toes, and earlobes. Vasospasms may be triggered by stress, exposure to cold, smoking, alcohol use, caffeine intake, cocaine, and amphetamines. Management of the disease depends upon the patient's specific triggers.

7. **(C)**; The best job "fit" for the person with Raynaud's would be one in which there would be control over exposure to cold. Therefore, the best fit would be personal fitness trainer, a position that is typically indoors with some environmental temperature control. Each of the other options has a significant component of exposure to extremes in the weather.

8. **(A)**; Buerger's disease, a nonatherosclerotic inflammatory vascular disorder, typically occurs in young men who are cigarette smokers.

9. **(A, B, C, D, F)**; Women are at higher risk for stroke than men. Other risk factors include hypertension, diabetes, obesity, use of illicit drugs (such as cocaine), physical inactivity, hyperlipidemia, and atrial fibrillation.

10. **(B)**; Although it is true that the effects of TIA are temporary, TIA is a warning that there is a problem with perfusion to part of the brain. As such, the occurrence of TIA should initiate investigation into the cause of the disruption in perfusion.

11. **(A, B, C)**; Medical therapy for patients with carotid disease includes aspirin for its antiplatelet properties and may include endovascular procedures that are performed by percutaneous access to the vessel. These include balloon angioplasty with carotid stenting, which can be performed in an interventional radiology laboratory or cardiac catheterization laboratory. MRI and CT are both diagnostic tools used to help identify areas in which lesions occur. Neither is considered to be part of medical management.

12. (**B**); The patient has gained some understanding of the procedure and purpose of endarterectomy if he or she is able to mention that plaque will be surgically removed from the carotid artery to reduce the chance of stroke. The procedure is not done after stroke.

13. (**A**); The priority diagnosis for the patient with TIA is ineffective peripheral tissue perfusion. That the patient suffered a TIA is a definite indication of problems with tissue perfusion, which should prompt further investigation.

14. (**C**); The nurse should be very concerned about the possibility of impending rupture of an abdominal aneurysm if the patient develops restlessness, lower back pain, and hypotension or shocky symptoms. The surgeon must be notified immediately.

15. (**B**); Aortic dissection occurs when the innermost lining of the arterial wall separates from the other two to allow blood flow between the layers rather than through the lumen of the artery, as is normal. Eventually, this can completely obstruct the true lumen of the vessel. If not addressed in a timely manner, the situation is life threatening. The most classic sign of aortic dissection is pain, often described by the patient as "ripping" or "tearing" with an abrupt onset.

16. (**A, B, C, D**); The patient is at risk for development of venous thromboembolism because of age greater than 40 years, having had major abdominal surgery, having been admitted to the ICU, and because of prolonged immobility of more than three days.

17. (**A**); The patient should wear compression stockings all day long except during bathing. The stockings should be off for no more than 30 minutes per day. There is no demonstrated added benefit to thigh-high stockings over knee-high stockings. Knee highs cost less and are easier to apply.

Physical Assessment

1. (**A**); The nurse should perform careful history taking, which includes a full description of characteristics of pain, numbness, and color changes on the hands and feet during attacks, as well as the frequency of attacks.

2. (**B**); Patients with Buerger's disease typically have symptoms associated with toe and finger ischemia. If the condition is advanced, patients frequently have ulcerations on both the fingers and toes. Complications include progressive ischemia leading to gangrene and amputation.

3. (**A, B, D**); Priority assessments include ABCs—ensuring an open airway, breathing, and circulation. Additionally, it is critical that the nurse assess cranial nerve function by assessing for speech difficulty, facial symmetry, ability to show one's teeth, determine smells, shrug the shoulders, swallow, etc.

4. (**C**); Subclavian steal syndrome can occur if the subclavian artery is obstructed, particularly if the internal mammary is then used for bypass grafting in a coronary artery bypass patient. This condition may not be apparent until after the bypass because the patient is not symptomatic until the internal mammary is used for bypass. Signs and symptoms include dizziness, syncope, and vertigo. Blood pressure difference of > 20

mm Hg between arms suggests the presence of the syndrome. Blood pressure will be lower on the affected side than on the unaffected side.

5. **(C)**; Clinical manifestations of thoracic aortic aneurysm include substernal chest pain, back and neck pain, dyspnea, cough, and stridor. Respiratory symptoms are due to pressure on the trachea.

6. **(B)**; The nurse should be concerned if the patient is unable to feel the tip of a sharp object on the sole of the foot postoperatively. This could indicate ischemic injury related to prolonged cross-clamping of the aorta. The surgeon must be notified. It is not unusual for postop abdominal aneurysm patients to return to the ICU when they are still groggy and hypothermic. That the patient can feel pressure from a blunt object above the knees is a positive indicator. Also positive is the patient's ability to push bilaterally with the feet. This indicates intact motor function.

Interpretation of Lab Values

1. **(A)**; The goal for INR during treatment with warfarin (Coumadin) is 2–3.

Drugs and Treatments

1. **(B)**; The medication history is an important component of a full assessment. This is particularly the case for patients with Raynaud's because some fairly common medications, including beta blockers and hormones, tend to cause vasospasm, which precipitates specific symptoms of Raynaud's.

2. **(C)**; Primary treatment for Buerger's focuses on smoking cessation and avoidance of secondhand smoke. Smoking cessation counseling is essential because continued smoking will enhance progression of the disease.

3. **(A)**; It is neither safe nor effective for the patient to do nothing beyond notifying the doctor if he or she experiences abdominal pain. Follow-up for the patient with abdominal aortic aneurysm includes monitoring the growth of the aneurysm at least once or twice per year because elective surgical repair is recommended when the size exceeds 5 cm. Patients should be encouraged to stop smoking, lose weight if not at optimal weight, and to maintain optimal control of blood pressure.

4. **(C)**; An abdominal aortic aneurysm measuring 4 cm is not at high risk for rupture. The patient should have repeat ultrasound for measurement of size every 6 to 12 months. When the aneurysm measures more than 5 cm in diameter, the patient should be referred for elective surgical repair. Some sources indicate that elective repair is indicated when the size exceeds 5.5 cm.

5. **(A)**; The nurse should first zero and recalibrate the arterial line. Given that there is a good waveform, the nurse should then initiate and titrate IV nitroprusside (Nipride) to maintain BP < 150/85. Carotid endarterectomy patients frequently return from the operating room with significant hypertension, but lowering the BP too dramatically all at once could lead to ischemic injury. Therefore, the higher BP parameters would be more appropriate for this patient.

6. **(B)**; The nurse understands that IV nitroprusside is used during the immediate postop period for blood pressure control. However, it is desirable to begin transitioning the

patient to oral antihypertensive medication as soon as the patient tolerates oral fluids. This will allow gradual weaning of the nitroprusside. Patients should not be moved from the intensive care unit if IV nitroprusside continues to infuse because it is an extremely potent drug that requires close monitoring by nursing staff.

7. (**A, B, D**); Pharmacological agents that can be utilized for DVT prophylaxis include subcutaneous heparin, subcutaneous unfractionated heparin, and warfarin (Coumadin). Evidence has not supported the effectiveness of aspirin in preventing DVT. Therefore, aspirin is not recommended for prophylaxis.

8. (**B, C, F**); The most recent evidence-based guidelines indicate that strict bed rest is not required for the patient with confirmed DVT. Ambulation as tolerated is appropriate. The affected extremity should be elevated 10–20 degrees above the heart when lying down. The patient should be placed on oral warfarin (Coumadin) therapy for 3–6 months.

9. (**B, C**); Inferior vena cava filters are devices that can be introduced percutaneously to capture clots and to decrease the risk of pulmonary embolism.

10. (**A**); Although it is important to teach the patient about all aspects of this drug, including side effects, the priority for the nurse is to teach the patient about proper injection technique. Enoxaparin (Lovenox) is administered subcutaneously. It would be desirable for the nurse to first teach the patient the proper injection technique and then to have the patient perform return demonstrations a few times prior to discharge.

Keep Track

- Percent correct. (Divide the number of questions you answered correctly by the total number of questions you answered.) _____

- Number of questions you missed due to a reading error: _____

- Number of questions you missed due to errors in analysis: _____

- Number of assessment questions you missed: _____

- Number of lab value questions you missed: _____

- Number of drug/treatment questions you missed: _____

Nugget List

Chapter number _____ Topic _____

Practice Test: Nursing Management of Patients with Respiratory Disorders

Karen S. March

PRACTICE TEST

General

ALTERNATE FORMAT

1. Preoperative nursing care for the patient who will undergo bronchoscopy includes which of the following measures? SELECT ALL THAT APPLY.
    A. obtaining informed consent
    B. teaching about what to expect during the procedure
    C. providing clear liquids until 1 hour before the test
    D. obtaining a preprocedural sputum specimen

ALTERNATE FORMAT

2. The nurse is providing care for a patient following bronchoscopy. Which of the following assessments should be part of early postprocedure care for this patient? SELECT ALL THAT APPLY.
    A. check for gag reflex
    B. monitor vital signs
    C. assess for dyspnea
    D. evaluate voice quality

ALTERNATE FORMAT

3. The nurse who is caring for a patient postpneumonectomy demonstrates good clinical judgment by placing the patient in which of the following positions? SELECT ALL THAT APPLY.
    A. supine
    B. prone
    C. lying on the operative side
    D. lying on the nonoperative side

4. The nurse is providing care for a 40-year-old nonsmoker who is tachycardic, has diminished breath sounds with wheezes, and has exertional dyspnea. Based on physical assessment findings, the nurse realizes the most likely etiology of this patient's problem is which of the following?
    A. emphysema
    B. chronic bronchitis
    C. alpha1-antitrypsin deficiency
    D. brain natriuretic peptide deficiency

5. The nurse is preparing to provide discharge teaching to a patient with emphysema. Which of the following instructions should the nurse include for this patient?
   A. "You may use your oxygen at 4 L/min by nasal cannula."
   B. "You should try to drink at least two liters of fluid per day."
   C. "You should try to reduce your smoking to two cigarettes per day."
   D. "You should be sure to weigh yourself daily and notify the doctor."

6. The patient with emphysema is taught about pursed-lip breathing. Which of the following statements by the patient indicates understanding of the mechanics behind this technique?
   A. "I get more oxygen with a breath if I inhale long and hard through my nose."
   B. "When I puff out my cheeks with each breath, I don't work as hard to breathe."
   C. "When I breathe through pursed lips, my airways don't collapse between breaths."
   D. "When I inhale through pursed lips, my oxygen exchange is more effective."

7. The patient with COPD should receive oxygen therapy by nasal cannula at which of the following flow rates?
   A. 1–2 L/min
   B. 3–5 L/min
   C. 6–8 L/min
   D. 10 L/min

8. The nurse is assigned to care for a patient who has had a left lower lobectomy for cancer. Which of the following issues will have a significant impact on plans for care of this patient?
   A. Most patients with lung cancer have been smokers.
   B. Public education about smoking cessation is largely inadequate.
   C. Most lung cancers are well established before symptoms are apparent.
   D. A rich oxygen supply promotes growth of cancer cells in lung tissue.

9. The nurse is caring for a postoperative patient who underwent a thoracic lobectomy. The nurse notes that the patient has two chest tubes in place—one is located toward the lower portion of the thorax, and the other is located higher up on the chest wall. When the family asks why the patient has two chest tubes, the best response by the nurse is which of the following?
   A. "Two tubes were necessary due to the amount of bleeding from the operative site."
   B. "Both tubes were required in order to drain blood from two different lung areas."
   C. "The lower tube will drain blood, and the higher tube is intended to drain air."
   D. "The primary drainage tube is lower on the thorax, and the other is for overflow."

10. The nurse provides preoperative teaching for a patient who will undergo a total laryngectomy. Upon completion of the teaching, which statement by the patient confirms full comprehension of the long-term effect of surgery on the airway?
    A. "I expect to have some difficulty breathing through my mouth after surgery."
    B. "I expect to have difficulty breathing through my nose following surgery."
    C. "I understand that I will have a temporary tracheostomy tube after surgery."
    D. "I understand that I will have a permanent tracheostomy following surgery."

ALTERNATE FORMAT

11. The nurse is caring for a patient who will undergo a radical neck dissection for cancer of the larynx. The nurse must include which of the following topics within the educational plan of care during hospitalization? SELECT ALL THAT APPLY.
    A. maintenance of airway
    B. alternate methods of communication
    C. endotracheal intubation
    D. changes in body image

12. While providing discharge instructions to the patient with a laryngectomy, the nurse cautions the patient to be careful while bathing for which of the following reasons?
    A. to prevent aspiration of water
    B. to prevent infection of the stoma
    C. a special device must cover the stoma
    D. water is not permitted around the stoma

13. The nurse is caring for a patient with chronic pulmonary disease. Which of the following signs or symptoms should the nurse recognize as signs of early onset of respiratory failure?
    A. hypotension and wheezing
    B. dyspnea and bradycardia
    C. restlessness and confusion
    D. cyanosis and pallor

14. Which of the following conditions is likely to predispose a patient to hypoxia?
    A. chronic renal failure
    B. chronic hepatic failure
    C. pancreatic failure
    D. acute adrenal insufficiency

15. The nurse is providing preoperative teaching for a patient who will undergo thoracic surgery. Which of the following teaching points are important to include for this patient? SELECT ALL THAT APPLY.
    A. "You may have chest tubes and drainage apparatus after surgery."
    B. "You will be assisted to turn, cough, and deep breathe frequently after surgery."
    C. "You will be in the intensive care unit for at least one week following surgery."
    D. "Oxygen will be administered to support your breathing if needed."

16. The nurse is caring for a patient with a 20-year history of chronic pulmonary disease. The patient is on O_2 at 2 L via nasal cannula and is dyspneic. Oxygen saturation by finger probe is 85%. When asked by the patient to increase the oxygen, the nurse's best response is to:
    A. place a nonrebreather mask on the patient and increase O_2 flow to 3 L.
    B. notify the physician of the patient's request for increased oxygen.
    C. increase the oxygen and monitor the patient's respiratory status closely.
    D. explain to the patient that too much O_2 will reduce his or her desire to breathe.

ALTERNATE FORMAT

17. The charge nurse receives notification that a patient who is coughing frequently and whose sputum is pink, frothy, and copious is about to be admitted to the unit. The patient has a history of night sweats, anorexia, and weight loss. Based on this information, the nurse should: SELECT ALL THAT APPLY.
    A. place this patient in a private room with negative air pressure.
    B. place this patient in standard and airborne precautions.
    C. wear a respirator, gown, and gloves when entering the patient's room.
    D. place the patient in a private room with positive ventilation.

18. The nurse is providing discharge teaching for the patient who was hospitalized with pulmonary embolism. Which of the following statements by the patient indicates a need for further review of information?
    A. "I should be as active as possible every day at home."
    B. "I will need to change my vena cava filter once per week."
    C. "I should notify my doctor if I develop warmth or swelling in my legs."
    D. "I will need to be on anticoagulant therapy for awhile."

19. The nurse is caring for a patient with a positive tuberculin skin test. Which of the following assessment findings is most suggestive of active disease?
    A. crackles
    B. cough with productive sputum
    C. night sweats
    D. weight gain

20. The nurse is caring for a patient who is intubated with a cuffed endotracheal tube. Which of the following statements by the nurse indicates a proper understanding of the purpose of inflating the cuff?
    A. "The inflated cuff increases oxygen delivery to the lungs."
    B. "The inflated cuff provides protection for the trachea during suctioning."
    C. "The inflated cuff helps prevent aspiration of gastric contents."
    D. "The inflated cuff prevents intubation of the right mainstem bronchus."

21. The parents of a 2-year-old child who has been diagnosed with cystic fibrosis decide to undergo genetic counseling. Which of the following statements by the parents indicates accurate understanding of the genetic implications of cystic fibrosis?
    A. "Any children we have will have cystic fibrosis."
    B. "Both of us are carriers of the gene."
    C. "Cystic fibrosis is common in Hispanics."
    D. "All of our male children will have the disease."

22. The pathophysiological mechanism responsible for respiratory distress among children with cystic fibrosis is:
    A. decreased ciliary action leading to stasis of mucous in the lungs.
    B. supralaryngeal strictures leading to severe acute bronchospasm.
    C. edema of the epiglottis causing upper airway occlusion.
    D. excessive production of thick mucous leading to obstruction.

23. A young adult male and a young adult female, both diagnosed with cystic fibrosis, become romantically involved. At a routine visit with a healthcare provider, the male patient asks the nurse about the chances of having an affected child. The most appropriate response by the nurse would be:
    A. "You probably will not be able to father a child because of your disease."
    B. "You should always use condoms to protect against unwanted pregnancy."
    C. "Young women with cystic fibrosis are not fertile."
    D. "All of your children will be carriers of the disease."

24. A patient on a telemetry floor is intubated and on a mechanical ventilator. When the ventilator alarm sounds, the nurse begins to troubleshoot the ventilator but fails to provide supplemental oxygen to the patient until the situation can be corrected. The patient becomes hypoxemic and suffers a myocardial infarction. This situation provides an example of:
    A. negligence.
    B. abandonment.
    C. injury.
    D. assault.

25. Early respiratory failure is initially demonstrated by:
    A. cyanosis and pallor.
    B. restlessness and irritability.
    C. hypotension and tachycardia.
    D. dyspnea and nasal flaring.

26. The patient with acute respiratory failure may require bronchodilator therapy if which of the following occurs?
    A. bronchospasms
    B. excessive secretions
    C. viscous secretions
    D. acute pharyngitis

27. Which of the following chest X-ray findings is consistent with left tension pneumothorax?
    A. flattening of the diaphragm
    B. shifting of the mediastinum to the right
    C. presence of gastric air bubble
    D. increased translucency of the right lung

28. Water-seal chest drainage is used to maintain:
    A. positive chest wall pressure.
    B. negative chest wall pressure.
    C. positive intrathoracic pressure.
    D. negative intrathoracic pressure.

29. Adult respiratory distress syndrome (ARDS) is suspected when:
    A. hypoxemia exists despite increases in supplemental oxygen.
    B. the patient complains of dyspnea and exhibits shortness of breath.
    C. the PaO_2 level falls into the range of 60–70 mm Hg.
    D. the SaO_2 level falls into the range of 82–86%.

30. **Major respiratory problems related to pathophysiology of ARDS include:**
    A. decreased lung compliance caused by increased membrane permeability.
    B. decreased airway resistance secondary to overdistended alveoli.
    C. overproduction of surfactant, which causes increased surface tension.
    D. bronchodilation, which decreases the amount of air flow into the lungs.

31. **The majority of pulmonary emboli originate in the:**
    A. deep leg veins.
    B. lung tissue.
    C. pelvic area.
    D. right atrium.

32. **Currently the most widely used test for diagnosing pulmonary embolus is:**
    A. arterial blood gas.
    B. bronchoscopy.
    C. spiral CT.
    D. pulmonary angiogram.

33. **The major hemodynamic consequence of massive pulmonary embolus is:**
    A. increased systemic vascular resistance leading to left heart failure.
    B. pulmonary hypertension, which ultimately leads to right heart failure.
    C. obstruction of the portal vein, which leads to ascites.
    D. embolism to the internal carotids, which results in stroke.

34. **The most effective means of preventing development of pulmonary embolism is:**
    A. encouraging frequent coughing and deep breathing.
    B. forcing fluids to at least 3000 mL/day.
    C. limiting ambulation to no more than once per day.
    D. preventing development of deep vein thrombosis.

35. **Which of the following is most likely to cause respiratory alkalosis in a patient?**
    A. airway obstruction from biting on the endotracheal tube
    B. pulmonary edema from receiving too much IV fluid too quickly
    C. excess tidal volume in a mechanically ventilated patient
    D. overuse of antacids, especially those containing aluminum hydroxide

36. **While the nurse is providing care for a mechanically ventilated patient, the low pressure alarm sounds. The first action by the nurse should be to:**
    A. auscultate the patient's lung sounds to assess for air exchange.
    B. check all connections between the patient and the ventilator.
    C. administer intravenous sedation and analgesia.
    D. instruct the patient to stop biting on the endotracheal tube.

Physical Assessment

1. **The nurse is caring for a patient who received medications about an hour ago and is now experiencing chest pain, tachycardia, and tremors. Which of the following medications is most likely to blame for these effects?**
    A. furosemide (Lasix)
    B. albuterol (Proventil)
    C. digoxin (Lanoxin)
    D. propranolol (Inderal)

2. The nurse is performing an assessment on a patient who recently returned from the operating room following sinus surgery. Which of the following findings would alert the nurse to excessive postoperative bleeding?
    A. bright red stools
    B. frequent swallowing
    C. discoloration around the eyes
    D. inability to breathe through the nose

3. The nurse is caring for a patient who is severely short of breath and able to speak only one or two words at a time. The patient has a ruddy complexion and a productive cough. Which of the following assessment parameters provides the best indication of the patient's level of oxygenation?
    A. pale nail beds
    B. sputum color
    C. ruddy complexion
    D. dusky mucous membranes

ALTERNATE FORMAT

4. The nurse is caring for a patient who was intubated because of acute respiratory failure. Immediately following the intubation, the nurse performs an assessment to determine placement of the endotracheal tube (ETT). Place an X over the area(s) where the nurse should place the stethoscope to determine ETT placement.

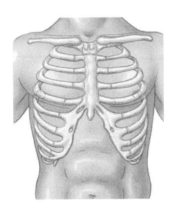

5. The nurse is caring for a patient who is postoperative. Upon entering the patient's room, the nurse notes that the patient is restless and agitated. Vital signs are T 100.9°F; P 104; R 28; BP 78/50. Further assessment reveals that the patient is complaining of chest pain, is cyanotic, and has crackles over the lung fields. Based upon assessment of this patient, the priority nursing diagnosis is:
    A. impaired gas exchange.
    B. anxiety.
    C. pain.
    D. impaired mobility.

6. The nurse is caring for a patient in the emergency department who suffered chest injuries in a motor vehicle accident. The nurse quickly assesses the patient and discovers that there are no breath sounds over the right side of the chest and that the trachea is deviated toward the left. Based on this assessment, the nurse prepares to:
   A. obtain vital signs and order stat lab work.
   B. begin CPR and have someone notify the physician.
   C. assist with chest needle decompression.
   D. perform an arterial stick for blood gases.

7. An emergency department nurse is assessing a patient who suffered blunt chest trauma in a bar fight. The patient is restless and cyanotic. Based on baseline data, it would be most important for the nurse to:
   A. apply O_2 at 2 L via nasal cannula.
   B. percuss the chest wall for resonance.
   C. observe for symmetry of chest movement.
   D. roll the patient to assess the posterior thorax.

8. The nurse is caring for a patient who received a liter of IV fluid over the past hour for treatment of hypovolemic shock. Although the patient's vital signs are normal, the patient has begun to cough. Upon hearing the cough, the nurse assesses the patient for which of the following consequences of the fluid bolus?
   A. pulmonary edema
   B. atelectasis
   C. pneumonia
   D. pneumothorax

9. The nurse is assigned to care for a 5-year-old child with suspected epiglottitis. Based on the diagnosis, the nurse would expect which of the following findings upon assessment?
   A. fever, bradycardia, and inspiratory stridor
   B. respiratory distress, tachycardia, and wheezing
   C. elevated temperature, severe sore throat, drooling, and a muffled voice
   D. flaring of the nostrils and expiratory stridor with wheezing and grunting

10. The nurse is caring for an 18-month-old child admitted to the hospital with acute laryngotracheobronchitis. Upon assessing the child's respiratory status, the nurse should anticipate which of the following findings?
    A. inspiratory stridor and brassy cough
    B. prolonged expiration and wet, productive cough
    C. nasal flaring and severe retractions
    D. nocturnal paroxysmal cough and bradypnea

Interpretation of Lab Values

ALTERNATE FORMAT

1. The nurse receives the following arterial blood gas results from the laboratory:

pH	7.31
pCO_2	54
HCO_3^-	27
pO_2	86

Which of the following terms should the nurse use to properly interpret these results? SELECT ALL THAT APPLY.
A. partially compensated
B. uncompensated
C. compensated
D. respiratory
E. metabolic
F. acidosis
G. alkalosis
H. hypoxia
I. normal ABG

ALTERNATE FORMAT

2. The nurse receives the following arterial blood gas results from the laboratory:

pH	7.34
pCO_2	46
HCO_3^-	28
pO_2	90

Which of the following terms should the nurse use to properly interpret these results? SELECT ALL THAT APPLY.
A. partially compensated
B. uncompensated
C. compensated
D. respiratory
E. metabolic
F. acidosis
G. alkalosis
H. hypoxia
I. normal ABG

ALTERNATE FORMAT

3. The nurse receives the following arterial blood gas results from the laboratory:

pH	7.41
pCO$_2$	46
HCO$_3^-$	28
pO$_2$	89

Which of the following terms should the nurse use to properly interpret these results? SELECT ALL THAT APPLY.
A. partially compensated
B. uncompensated
C. compensated
D. respiratory
E. metabolic
F. acidosis
G. alkalosis
H. hypoxia
I. normal ABG

ALTERNATE FORMAT

4. The nurse receives the following arterial blood gas results from the laboratory:

pH	7.44
pCO$_2$	42
HCO$_3^-$	23
pO$_2$	92

Which of the following terms should the nurse use to properly interpret these results? SELECT ALL THAT APPLY.
A. partially compensated
B. uncompensated
C. compensated
D. respiratory
E. metabolic
F. acidosis
G. alkalosis
H. hypoxia
I. normal ABG

ALTERNATE FORMAT

5. The nurse receives the following arterial blood gas results from the laboratory:

pH	6.99
pCO_2	34
HCO_3^-	18
pO_2	68

Which of the following terms should the nurse use to properly interpret these results? SELECT ALL THAT APPLY.
A. partially compensated
B. uncompensated
C. compensated
D. respiratory
E. metabolic
F. acidosis
G. alkalosis
H. hypoxia
I. normal ABG

ALTERNATE FORMAT

6. The nurse receives the following arterial blood gas results from the laboratory:

pH	7.25
pCO_2	48
HCO_3^-	20
pO_2	78

Which of the following terms should the nurse use to properly interpret these results? SELECT ALL THAT APPLY.
A. partially compensated
B. uncompensated
C. compensated
D. respiratory
E. metabolic
F. acidosis
G. alkalosis
H. hypoxia
I. normal ABG

ALTERNATE FORMAT

7. The nurse receives the following arterial blood gas results from the laboratory:

pH	7.35
pCO$_2$	38
HCO$_3^-$	22
pO$_2$	90

Which of the following terms should the nurse use to properly interpret these results? SELECT ALL THAT APPLY.
A. partially compensated
B. uncompensated
C. compensated
D. respiratory
E. metabolic
F. acidosis
G. alkalosis
H. hypoxia
I. normal ABG

ALTERNATE FORMAT

8. The nurse receives the following arterial blood gas results from the laboratory:

pH	7.38
pCO$_2$	35
HCO$_3^-$	20
pO$_2$	89

Which of the following terms should the nurse use to properly interpret these results? SELECT ALL THAT APPLY.
A. partially compensated
B. uncompensated
C. compensated
D. respiratory
E. metabolic
F. acidosis
G. alkalosis
H. hypoxia
I. normal ABG

ALTERNATE FORMAT

9. The nurse receives the following arterial blood gas results from the laboratory:

pH	7.48
pCO_2	48
HCO_3^-	27
pO_2	86

Which of the following terms should the nurse use to properly interpret these results? SELECT ALL THAT APPLY.
A. partially compensated
B. uncompensated
C. compensated
D. respiratory
E. metabolic
F. acidosis
G. alkalosis
H. hypoxia
I. normal ABG

ALTERNATE FORMAT

10. The nurse receives the following arterial blood gas results from the laboratory:

pH	7.52
pCO_2	34
HCO_3^-	28
pO_2	87

Which of the following terms should the nurse use to properly interpret these results? SELECT ALL THAT APPLY.
A. partially compensated
B. uncompensated
C. compensated
D. respiratory
E. metabolic
F. acidosis
G. alkalosis
H. hypoxia
I. normal ABG

ALTERNATE FORMAT

11. **The nurse receives the following arterial blood gas results from the laboratory:**

pH	7.21
pCO_2	48
HCO_3^-	18
pO_2	69

Which of the following terms should the nurse use to properly interpret these results? SELECT ALL THAT APPLY.
A. partially compensated
B. uncompensated
C. compensated
D. respiratory
E. metabolic
F. acidosis
G. alkalosis
H. hypoxia
I. normal ABG

ALTERNATE FORMAT

12. **The nurse receives the following arterial blood gas results from the laboratory:**

pH	7.39
pCO_2	42
HCO_3^-	24
pO_2	94

Which of the following terms should the nurse use to properly interpret these results? SELECT ALL THAT APPLY.
A. partially compensated
B. uncompensated
C. compensated
D. respiratory
E. metabolic
F. acidosis
G. alkalosis
H. hypoxia
I. normal ABG

13. **Which of the following arterial blood gas values would indicate a need for oxygen therapy?**
A. $PaO_2 = 80$ mm Hg
B. $PaCO_2 = 35$ mm Hg
C. $HCO_3^- = 24$ mEq
D. $SaO_2 = 87\%$

14. **Which of the following patients would be considered hypoxemic?**
    A. a 70-year-old patient with a PaO_2 of 80
    B. a 50-year-old patient with a PaO_2 of 65
    C. an 84-year-old patient with a PaO_2 of 96
    D. a 68-year-old patient with a PaO_2 of 84

Drugs and Treatments

1. **The nurse knows that the patient has a good understanding about a newly pre-scribed medication, montelukast sodium (Singulair), when the patient makes which of the following statements?**
    A. "I should always keep this medication with me in case I have an acute asthma attack."
    B. "I can take up to four tablets per day to help control my asthma symptoms."
    C. "This medication reverses acute bronchospasm during an asthma attack."
    D. "This medication works prophylactically to control my exercise-induced asthma."

ALTERNATE FORMAT

2. **The process by which a primary care provider decides the appropriate antibiotic therapy for a patient with signs and symptoms of a serious infection involves a series of decisions. Please indicate the order in which these decisions normally occur.**
    1. The primary care provider selects an antibiotic known to kill common organisms.
    2. Upon identification of the causative organism, susceptibility testing is done.
    3. A narrow spectrum antibiotic is ordered.
    4. The area of infection is cultured.
        A. 1, 2, 3, 4
        B. 2, 3, 1, 4
        C. 4, 1, 2, 3
        D. 4, 2, 1, 3

3. **A patient has an order for Ancef 1 gm IV q 8 hours. A note on the patient's medication administration record (MAR) states that the patient is allergic to penicillin. Which of the following rationales or actions is appropriate?**
    A. Administer the drug as ordered even if the patient had a severe reaction to penicillin.
    B. Administer the Ancef with caution if the patient had only mild hives with penicillin.
    C. Do not administer the Ancef because the patient will have a life-threatening reaction.
    D. Do not administer the Ancef because it is a penicillin derivative.

4. **The nurse realizes that which of the following medications should not be administered to the patient with a documented severe allergic reaction to penicillin?**
    A. amoxicillin + clavulanic acid (Augmentin)
    B. sulfamethoxazole (Bactrim)
    C. indomethacin (Indocin)
    D. gentamicin

5. **Which of the following statements by a 26-year-old female patient indicates understanding of medication side effects for the prescribed drug, piperacillin + tazobactam (Zosyn)?**
    A. "It is important for me to take the medication for at least two days after I feel better."
    B. "I should report any problems with breathing to my physician immediately."
    C. "It is safe for me to take this drug even though I have a penicillin allergy."
    D. "I should use an alternate form of birth control while I take this medication."

ALTERNATE FORMAT

6. The patient is prescribed hydrocortisone sodium succinate (Solu-Cortef) 100 mg IV. The drug is available in vials of "Solu-Cortef 125 mg/2 mL." What volume of drug will the nurse withdraw from the vial to administer the correct dose?

_____

ALTERNATE FORMAT

7. The COPD patient is ordered ipratropium (Atrovent) 1 puff and triamcinolone acetonide (Azmacort) 2 puffs at 6 p.m. Place in order the sequence that should be used for proper administration of these drugs.
   1. Administer 2 puffs of Azmacort.
   2. Identify the patient by two identifiers.
   3. Administer 1 puff of Atrovent.
   4. Verify that both drugs are correct as ordered.
   5. Encourage the patient to gargle.
      A. 2, 4, 1, 3, 5
      B. 3, 1, 2, 4, 5
      C. 4, 2, 3, 1, 5
      D. 5, 4, 2, 1, 3

8. The nurse is assigned a postoperative patient. Which of the following actions by the nurse is likely to result in more effective coughing by the patient?
   A. instructing the patient to cough while supine
   B. offering pain medication prior to coughing
   C. encouraging the patient to ambulate after coughing
   D. offering incentive spirometry after the patient coughs

9. The nurse is caring for a patient with respiratory failure who has been admitted to a telemetry floor for monitoring. The nurse knows that the sigh mechanism on the ventilator helps to prevent which of the following adverse effects of mechanical ventilation?
   A. pneumothorax
   B. pulmonary embolism
   C. pneumonia
   D. atelectasis

10. The nurse is providing education about medications to the patient with tuberculosis. Which of the following statements by the patient indicates adequate understanding related to medications for this disease?
    A. "I need to notify my healthcare provider if my skin turns yellow."
    B. "I will need to take intravenous antibiotics for at least six weeks."
    C. "I need to notify my healthcare provider if my ankles swell."
    D. "If my urine turns orange, I should notify my healthcare provider."

11. The nurse is caring for a patient diagnosed with pulmonary embolus. Which of the following treatments should the nurse anticipate for this patient?
    A. bronchoscopy to remove retained pulmonary secretions
    B. bronchodilators to improve ventilation-to-perfusion matching
    C. administration of a heparin drip to prevent clot extension
    D. antibiotic therapy to eradicate persistent microorganisms

12. Which of the following interventions should the nurse implement to most effectively enhance coughing in the postthoracotomy patient?
    A. Allow at least 8 hours of rest between deep breathing and coughing.
    B. Premedicate the patient with a narcotic at least 2 hours before coughing.
    C. Have the patient drink two 8-ounce glasses of water before coughing.
    D. Place the patient in semi-Fowler's position and provide splinting before coughing.

13. The nurse expects a child with laryngotracheobronchitis to receive treatment with corticosteroids to:
    A. treat the infectious process.
    B. reduce subglottic edema.
    C. accelerate healing.
    D. mask signs of infection.

14. The nurse has provided medication teaching to the parents of a child with cystic fibrosis. Which of the following statements by a parent indicates that teaching has been effective?
    A. "I will administer the pancreatic enzymes to my child twice per day."
    B. "Pancreatic enzyme helps to decrease the viscosity of my child's mucous."
    C. "I can mix the pancreatic enzymes along with other medications in milk."
    D. "Pancreatic enzyme improves absorption and digestion of fat and proteins."

15. A patient has been mechanically ventilated because of an exacerbation of COPD. Which of the following statements by the nurse is correct regarding readiness for ventilator weaning based on the patient's most recent arterial blood gas values?

pH	7.40
pCO_2	42
HCO_3^-	24
pO_2	80

    A. "Weaning is indicated. The arterial blood gas values are normal."
    B. "Weaning is not indicated. Respiratory acidosis must be corrected."
    C. "Weaning is indicated. Respiratory acidosis stimulates breathing."
    D. "Weaning is not indicated. Normal PaO_2 and $PaCO_2$ will stunt respirations."

ALTERNATE FORMAT

16. The nurse is caring for a postoperative patient following thoracotomy with left lower lobectomy. The patient has one chest tube. The nurse must ensure that which of the following supplies are available at the bedside? **SELECT ALL THAT APPLY.**
    A. sterile gauze
    B. suture material
    C. thoracotomy tray
    D. sterile petrolatum gauze
    E. sterile gloves

ANSWERS

General

1. **(A, B)**; Informed consent should be obtained, and the patient should be taught what to expect during the procedure. The patient should remain NPO for a minimum of 6 hours prior to the procedure. If a sputum specimen is required, it can easily be obtained during the procedure.

2. **(A, B, C, D)**; After the procedure the nurse must check for return of the gag reflex before administering any ice or fluids. Vital signs should be monitored. The patient should also be monitored for signs of laryngeal edema, including dyspnea, stridor, and hoarseness.

3. **(A, C)**; Postoperative pneumonectomy patients should be positioned either supine or on the operative side to facilitate ventilation and perfusion. This position also allows fluid drainage to consolidate in the pleural space on the operative side rather than in the patient's remaining lung.

4. **(C)**; The patient has classic symptoms associated with emphysema but is a young non-smoker. Therefore, the most likely etiology is alpha1-antitrypsin deficiency.

5. **(B)**; The patient should be encouraged to drink 2 liters per day to help to liquefy secretions. The patient should have only low-flow oxygen (1–2 L/min) to prevent respiratory depression. Respiratory drive is dependent upon high CO_2 and low O_2 levels. Higher O_2 levels can result in loss of respiratory drive.

6. **(C)**; Breathing through pursed lips slows exhalation and maintains inflation of the distal airways, which enhances respiration.

7. **(A)**; COPD patients should receive oxygen at flow rates of 1–2 L/min to prevent respiratory depression. Higher rates of flow can cause respiratory depression, resulting in the need for intubation.

8. **(C)**; The nurse should be aware that most lung cancers are in advanced stages before the patient becomes symptomatic. This has implications for both short-term and long-term care options for the patient. Although most patients with lung cancer have been smokers, this is not a certainty because many patients have been unwittingly exposed to secondhand smoke or radon over their lifetimes. Public education about smoking cessation has improved considerably over the past 10 years. Oxygen supply to the lungs has not been implicated in supporting this type of cancer.

9. **(C)**; The nurse should explain that the tube placed lower on the thorax will drain blood while the tube placed higher on the thorax will allow for removal of air.

10. **(D)**; The patient will have a permanent tracheostomy.

11. **(A, B, D)**; Education for the patient who will undergo radical neck dissection must include discussion of how to maintain a patent airway, alternate methods of communication related to removal of the larynx, and changes in body image related to extensive surgical dissection of the neck.

12. **(A)**; The nurse cautions the patient to be careful while bathing to avoid aspiration of water through the tracheal stoma.

13. **(C)**; Restlessness and altered level of consciousness are early signs of respiratory failure. Although hypotension may be associated with respiratory failure, wheezing is not considered to be a hallmark sign or symptom. Dyspnea and bradycardia represent late signs of respiratory failure, as do cyanosis and pallor.

14. **(A)**; Chronic renal failure is likely to predispose a patient to hypoxia because of an associated decrease in production of erythropoietin, which is required for red blood cell (RBC) production. Patients lacking RBCs have reduced oxygen-carrying capacity.

15. **(A, B, D)**; A patient undergoing thoracic surgery should be taught preoperatively about treatment expectations during the postoperative period. It is important for the patient to be aware that chest tubes will be inserted during surgery and that he or she will be required to turn, cough, and deep breathe frequently following surgery. The patient should be aware that supplemental oxygen may be required following surgery. Patients who undergo thoracic surgery are not necessarily admitted to an intensive care unit postoperatively.

16. **(C)**; This patient has an oxygen saturation of 85%, which is inadequate. Therefore, the nurse should increase the oxygen to achieve a saturation of 90% while closely monitoring the patient's respiratory status. If the nurse were to apply a nonrebreather mask, it would be essential to set the flow rate between 10 and 15 L per minute to achieve an appropriate response. Research has not demonstrated that increasing oxygen results in decreased respiratory effort.

17. **(A, B, C)**; This patient's history and present status suggests that the patient may have tuberculosis. The charge nurse should place the patient in a private room with negative air pressure with standard and airborne precautions. When entering the patient's room, the nurse should wear a respirator, gown, and gloves as personal protective equipment.

18. **(B)**; The vena cava filter, which is placed intravascularly, will remain in place indefinitely. The patient will not change the device at home. The patient should be encouraged to be as active as possible and to limit immobility. The patient will be on anticoagulant therapy following discharge and should notify the doctor if any signs of deep venous thrombosis develop.

19. **(C)**; Clinical manifestations of active tuberculosis include cough with frothy pink sputum, night sweats, anorexia, and weight loss.

20. **(C)**; The inflated cuff prevents aspiration of gastric contents. It does not protect the trachea, increase oxygen delivery to the lungs, or prevent intubation of the right mainstem bronchus.

21. **(B)**; For a child to inherit the gene for cystic fibrosis, both parents must be carriers of the gene. It is inherited as an autosomal recessive trait with an overall incidence of 1 in 4.

22. **(D)**; The pathophysiological mechanism responsible for respiratory distress among children with cystic fibrosis is excessive production of thick mucous leading to obstruction.

23. **(A)**; The most appropriate response by the nurse would be that the young male will probably not be able to father a child because males with cystic fibrosis are sterile. Young women with the disease generally have difficulty becoming pregnant because of excessively viscous cervical mucus. Additionally, there is a high incidence of fetal loss with pregnancy.

24. **(A)**; When the nurse fails to provide oxygen to the patient during a ventilator malfunction that results in patient suffering, the nurse has been negligent.

25. **(B)**; Restlessness and irritability are among the early signs of respiratory failure. Cyanosis, pallor, hypotension, dyspnea, and nasal flaring are later signs.

26. **(A)**; The patient with acute respiratory failure may require bronchodilator therapy if bronchospasms occur.

27. **(B)**; In tension pneumothorax, there is mediastinal shift to the opposite side of the chest.

28. **(D)**; Water-seal chest drainage is used to maintain negative intrathoracic pressure.

29. **(A)**; A hallmark of ARDS is hypoxemia despite administration of increasing levels of oxygen.

30. **(A)**; During ARDS, increased membrane permeability allows an influx of fluids and other large molecules into the lung tissues, which results in decreased lung compliance.

31. **(A)**; The majority of pulmonary emboli originate in the deep leg veins.

32. **(C)**; Currently the most widely used test for diagnosing pulmonary embolus is spiral CT.

33. **(B)**; The major hemodynamic consequence of massive pulmonary embolus is pulmonary hypertension, which ultimately leads to right heart failure.

34. **(D)**; The most effective means of preventing development of pulmonary embolism is by preventing development of deep vein thrombosis.

35. **(C)**; When a ventilated patient receives excess tidal volume, too much CO_2 is blown off. This results in production of respiratory alkalosis.

36. **(B)**; The first thing the nurse should do under the circumstances is to check that all connections between the patient and the ventilator are secure.

Physical Assessment

1. **(B)**; Albuterol (Proventil) is a beta$_2$ agonist used to control bronchospasm associated with asthma. Adverse effects associated with beta$_2$ agonists include tremors, chest pain, tachycardia, and dysrhythmia.

2. **(B)**; Excessive swallowing in the patient after sinus surgery should prompt the nurse to investigate why the patient is swallowing frequently. This is most likely due to drainage of blood into the posterior pharynx.

3. **(D)**; Dusky mucous membranes provide significant insight into the patient's oxygenation status. The patient's complexion, sputum color, and pale nail beds do not provide any definitive information about oxygenation.

4. The nurse should place a stethoscope systematically over the *right chest*, the *left chest*, and then over the *stomach*. In each case, the nurse must listen for air exchange. Even if air flow is heard over the chest area, it is essential to listen over the stomach to ensure that no air flow is heard there. The presence of air flow over the stomach area would indicate gastric intubation.

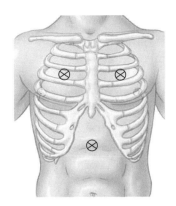

5. **(A)**; This patient has hallmark signs of pulmonary embolism. The priority nursing diagnosis must be *impaired gas exchange*. Although *anxiety* and *pain* are also issues, the airway issue must be the priority.

6. **(C)**; Based on the patient's history and presenting symptoms, the nurse must suspect tension pneumothorax, a life-threatening emergency situation. Treatment involves insertion of a needle into the second or third intercostal space on the affected side. This will allow air under pressure to escape. As soon as possible, a chest tube must be inserted to allow for lung reexpansion.

7. **(C)**; Based on the patient's history, it is most important for the nurse to assess for chest symmetry with respirations. This patient may have tension pneumothorax, which is a life-threatening emergency.

8. **(A)**; The onset of cough is most likely related to pulmonary congestion as a consequence of fluid overload. The nurse should recognize this as an early sign of pulmonary edema.

9. **(C)**; Based on the diagnosis, the nurse would expect to find that the child has a fever, severe sore throat, drooling, and a muffled voice.

10. **(C)**; The nurse should expect to assess nasal flaring and severe retractions in this child. The cough should be croupy or barking, and respirations are tachypnic.

Interpretation of Lab Values

1. **(A, D, F)**; This arterial blood gas (ABG) result reveals partially compensated respiratory acidosis.

ABG component	Value	What it reveals related to acid-base balance
pH	7.31	*Acidotic; partially compensated* because both pCO_2 and HCO_3^- are out of normal range—one is causing dysfunction (pCO_2) while the other (HCO_3^-) is trying to buffer.
pCO_2	54	Elevated; contributes to acidosis; *primary problem*
HCO_3^-	27	Elevated; acts as bicarbonate buffer
pO_2	86	

2. **(A, D, F)**; This ABG result reveals partially compensated respiratory acidosis.

ABG component	Value	What it reveals related to acid-base balance
pH	7.34	*Acidotic; partially compensated* because both pCO_2 and HCO_3^- are out of normal range—one is causing dysfunction (pCO_2) while the other (HCO_3^-) is trying to buffer.
pCO_2	46	Elevated; contributes to acidosis; *primary problem*
HCO_3^-	28	Elevated; acts as bicarbonate buffer
pO_2	90	

3. **(C, E, G)**; This ABG result reveals compensated metabolic alkalosis.

ABG component	Value	What it reveals related to acid-base balance
pH	7.41	*Alkalotic;* within normal limits; *compensated*
pCO_2	46	Elevated; acting as buffer for alkalosis
HCO_3^-	28	Elevated; contributes to alkalotic pH; *primary problem*
pO_2	89	

4. **(I)**; This is a normal ABG. All component values are within normal limits.

5. **(B, E, F, H)**; This ABG result reveals uncompensated metabolic acidosis with hypoxia.

ABG component	Value	What it reveals related to acid-base balance
pH	6.99	*Acidotic; uncompensated*
pCO_2	34	Decreased; acting as buffer for acidosis
HCO_3^-	18	Decreased; contributes to acidotic pH; *primary problem*
pO_2	68	< 80 mm Hg indicates *hypoxia*

6. **(B, D, E, F, H)**; This ABG result reveals uncompensated respiratory and metabolic acidosis with hypoxia.

ABG component	Value	What it reveals related to acid-base balance
pH	7.25	*Acidotic; uncompensated*
pCO_2	48	Elevated; contributes to acidosis; *primary problem*
HCO_3^-	20	Decreased; contributes to acidotic pH; *primary problem*
pO_2	78	< 80 mm Hg indicates *hypoxia*

7. **(I)**; All components are within normal limits. This is a normal ABG.

8. **(C, E, F)**; This ABG result reveals compensated metabolic acidosis.

ABG component	Value	What it reveals related to acid-base balance
pH	7.38	*Acidotic; compensated*
pCO$_2$	35	Decreased; acts to buffer acidosis
HCO$_3^-$	20	Decreased; contributes to acidotic pH; *primary problem*
pO$_2$	89	

9. **(A, E, G)**; This ABG result reveals partially compensated metabolic alkalosis.

ABG component	Value	What it reveals related to acid-base balance
pH	7.48	*Alkalotic; partially compensated* because both pCO$_2$ and HCO$_3^-$ are out of normal range—one is causing dysfunction (HCO$_3^-$) while the other (pCO$_2$) is trying to buffer.
pCO$_2$	48	Elevated; acts to buffer alkalosis
HCO$_3^-$	27	Elevated; contributes to alkalotic pH; *primary problem*
pO$_2$	86	

10. **(B, D, E, G)**; This ABG result reveals uncompensated respiratory and metabolic alkalosis.

ABG component	Value	What it reveals related to acid-base balance
pH	7.52	*Alkalotic; uncompensated*
pCO$_2$	34	Decreased; contributes to alkalosis; *primary problem*
HCO$_3^-$	28	Elevated; contributes to alkalosis; *primary problem*
pO$_2$	87	

11. **(B, D, E, F, H)**; This ABG result reveals uncompensated respiratory and metabolic acidosis with hypoxia.

ABG component	Value	What it reveals related to acid-base balance
pH	7.21	*Acidotic; uncompensated*
pCO$_2$	48	Elevated; contributes to acidosis; *primary problem*
HCO$_3^-$	18	Decreased; contributes to acidosis; *primary problem*
pO$_2$	69	< 80 mm Hg indicates *hypoxia*

12. **(I)**; All components are within normal limits. This is a normal ABG.

13. **(D)**; SaO_2 represents the amount of oxygen bound to hemoglobin and available for transport throughout the body. Normally, SaO_2 should be 96–100%. A value less than 90% indicates the need for supplemental oxygen therapy.

14. **(B)**; The 50-year-old patient with a PaO_2 of 65 is hypoxemic.

Drugs and Treatments

1. **(D)**; Montelukast sodium (Singulair) is a leukotriene receptor antagonist drug that is used for prophylaxis and chronic treatment of asthma. Singulair is not effective for treatment of acute bronchospasm, and it should not be used alone for treatment of exercise-induced asthma. The usual dosage is one tablet per day.

2. **(C)**; Normally, the first step is to culture the suspected infected site. While waiting for culture results, the healthcare provider selects an antibiotic known to effectively treat common organisms. When the causative organism is identified, susceptibility testing is done so that the most effective drug for treatment can be chosen. Finally, a narrow spectrum antibiotic is ordered.

3. **(B)**; Cefazolin sodium (Ancef) is a cephalosporin drug. Cephalosporins can be administered with caution to patients who are penicillin sensitive; however, it is important to monitor the patient closely because cross-sensitivity exists in about 10% of patients. This means that the patient may have an allergic reaction to the cephalosporin, too.

4. **(A)**; Amoxicillin + clavulanic acid (Augmentin) is a penicillin-derivative drug. Therefore, a patient who has demonstrated allergy to penicillin should not receive this drug.

5. **(D)**; Antibiotic drugs can decrease the effectiveness of oral contraceptives. Therefore, it is important for female patients of child-bearing age to be aware that they should use an alternate form of birth control while on the antibiotic medication.

6. **1.6 mL**; Use the ratio method of calculation: $\frac{125 \text{ mg}}{2 \text{ mL}} = \frac{60 \text{ mg}}{x \text{ mL}}$. Solving for x, you will find that $125x = 200$. Therefore, $x = 1.6$ mL.

7. **(C)**; The nurse must first verify that the drugs are correct as ordered and then identify the patient by at least two means. Next, the Atrovent (bronchodilator) should be administered followed in a few minutes by the Azmacort (glucocorticoid). Finally, the patient should gargle to decrease the chances of developing oral *candidiasis*.

8. **(B)**; Offering pain medicine about 30 minutes before asking the patient to perform coughing and deep breathing is likely to promote effective coughing. Patients experiencing significant pain will not cough deeply because it hurts. If pain is controlled, more effective coughing and deep breathing will result. Patients will not cough effectively when supine.

9. **(D)**; The sigh mechanism on a mechanical ventilator delivers a prescribed number of sighs per hour to mimic normal respiration. Use of this feature helps to prevent atelectasis.

10. **(A)**; The patient should notify the healthcare provider if the skin becomes jaundiced because it is indicative of the onset of hepatotoxicity, a major adverse effect of several medications that are used to treat tuberculosis. Patients will be on one or more oral medications for 6 to 9 months. An expected side effect of rifampin therapy is orange discoloration of body fluids.

11. **(C)**; The nurse should anticipate that the patient will have a heparin drip to prevent extension of the existing clot.

12. **(D)**; The nurse should place the patient in semi-Fowler's position and provide a pillow for splinting any incision before encouraging the patient to cough. Coughing and deep breathing should be done at least every 4 hours, if not more frequently.

13. **(B)**; Corticosteroids are used to treat children with laryngotracheobronchitis because they help to reduce subglottic edema, which helps to ease respirations.

14. **(D)**; Pancreatic enzymes help to improve absorption of fat, proteins, and carbohydrates. The medication should be taken just before or with meals and snacks. Pancreatic enzymes should never be mixed with other medications in any fluid.

15. **(D)**; The nurse is correct to predict that a patient with COPD is not ready to wean with textbook perfect blood gas results. The normal PaO_2 and $PaCO_2$ values will result in stunted respiratory effort because respiratory drive in COPD patients is stimulated by elevated $PaCO_2$ values.

16. **(A, D, E)**; Postoperatively, the nurse should have sterile gauze, sterile petrolatum gauze, and sterile gloves available in the room in case the chest tube should become dislodged or require reinforcement of the dressing.

Keep Track

- Percent correct. (Divide the number of questions you answered correctly by the total number of questions you answered.) _____

- Number of questions you missed due to a reading error: _____

- Number of questions you missed due to errors in analysis: _____

- Number of assessment questions you missed: _____

- Number of lab value questions you missed: _____

- Number of drug/treatment questions you missed: _____

Nugget List

Chapter number _____ Topic _____

Practice Test: Nursing Management of Patients with Neurologic Disorders

Karen S. March

PRACTICE TEST

General

1. The nurse is aware that which of the following is a sensitive indicator of cortical function?
   A. level of consciousness
   B. arousal
   C. orientation
   D. concentration

2. The nurse is caring for a sedated patient in the intensive care unit. When the nurse applies nail bed pressure, the patient withdraws the hand. The response by the patient indicates which of the following?
   A. confusion
   B. arousal
   C. orientation
   D. attention

3. The nurse must assess a patient's level of orientation. Which of the following patient responses indicates severe cerebral dysfunction?
   A. The patient identifies the state, city, and location of the hospital.
   B. The patient reports uncertainty about his or her location.
   C. An ICU patient reports uncertainty about the time of day.
   D. The patient does not recognize an immediate family member.

4. Which of the following provides an early indication of neurological change?
   A. impaired orientation to time
   B. confusion
   C. delirium
   D. impaired recent memory

5. To assess the patient's level of attention and concentration, the nurse should:
   A. tell the patient a story and then ask detailed questions.
   B. ask the patient to name the months of the year in reverse order.
   C. ask the patient to name the contenders in the last presidential election.
   D. ask the names, ages, and birth dates of the patient's children.

6. During assessment, the nurse asks the patient to name all of his or her children, their ages, and birth dates. Which of the following was the nurse testing?
   A. remote memory
   B. intermediate memory
   C. recent memory
   D. long-term memory

7. During assessment, an office nurse asks how the patient arrived at the appointment and with whom. The nurse also asks the patient to recall what he or she ate at breakfast. Which of the following was the nurse testing?
   A. remote memory
   B. intermediate memory
   C. recent memory
   D. long-term memory

8. The nurse names three objects for the patient to remember (for example: dog, ball, apple) and asks the patient to repeat them. The nurse informs the patient that he or she will be asked to name the objects a little later and then proceeds through other aspects of the assessment for a few minutes. After about 5 minutes, the nurse asks the patient to name the objects. The nurse has performed an assessment of which type of memory with this strategy?
   A. remote memory
   B. intermediate memory
   C. recent memory
   D. long-term memory

9. When describing the affect of a patient who seems depressed or very sad, the nurse should use which of the following descriptive terminology?
   A. euphoric
   B. flat affect
   C. apathetic
   D. dysphoric

10. The nurse is caring for a patient who suffered a cerebrovascular accident (CVA). Consequently, the patient, who seems bright and engaged in a visit, is unable to respond verbally to questions. The nurse recognizes this as:
    A. expressive speaking aphasia.
    B. expressive writing aphasia.
    C. visual receptive aphasia.
    D. auditory receptive aphasia.

11. A female patient is admitted for a full neurological work-up. A consent has been signed, and the nurse is preparing the patient for a lumbar puncture when the patient says that she does not understand the procedure or remember what to expect. The nurse's best response would be to:
    A. stat page the physician to come to explain the procedure to the patient.
    B. remind the patient that a needle will be inserted to withdraw spinal fluid for analysis.
    C. explain the proper position for the procedure and insist the patient lie down.
    D. tell the patient that someone will explain the procedure when it is time.

12. **A patient has known impairment of cranial nerve II. Based on this knowledge, the nurse should do which of the following to ensure client safety?**
    A. Provide directions by mouth and in writing.
    B. Check the temperature of food on the dinner tray.
    C. Provide an obstacle-free path for ambulation.
    D. Check the temperature of shower water.

13. **The patient has been diagnosed with a cerebellar lesion. The nurse evaluates successful adaptation to this impairment when the patient is able to demonstrate proper use of which of the following items?**
    A. raised toilet seat
    B. a reacher
    C. a walker
    D. adaptive utensils

14. **The nurse is preparing to assess function of the patient's trigeminal (CN V) nerve. Which of the following items would the nurse gather to test the nerve?**
    A. flashlight, pupil size chart, and newspaper
    B. tuning fork, otoscope, and audiometer
    C. safety pin, cold and hot items, and cotton wisp
    D. Snellen chart, opthalmoscope, reading charts

15. **The nurse is testing the function of the glossopharyngeal (CN IX) nerve and the vagus (CN X) nerve. To perform the test correctly, the nurse must:**
    A. have the patient open the mouth and say, "aaah."
    B. place warm and hot objects on each side of the face.
    C. perform both air and bone conduction tests.
    D. have the patient smile and raise the eyebrows.

16. **The nurse is assigned to care for a patient with arteriovenous malformation (AVM) prior to treatment. The patient asks the nurse what the physician will be able to do to fix the problem. The best response by the nurse is:**
    A. "You will have to ask the physician about that directly."
    B. "The treatment will depend upon the extent of your AVM."
    C. "The only treatment for an AVM is a frontal craniotomy."
    D. "I don't know. We will have to ask the physician about it."

17. **The nurse is caring for a patient who is scheduled for an electroencephalogram (EEG). When the patient asks the nurse why the test is needed, the best reply by the nurse is:**
    A. "An EEG can help to identify and locate brain tumors."
    B. "The EEG will measure the electrical activity in your muscles."
    C. "An EEG will help to measure brain response to microshocks."
    D. "The EEG will record the electrical activity of your brain cells."

ALTERNATE FORMAT

18. **In preparing a patient for an electroencephalogram (EEG), the nurse should do which of the following? SELECT ALL THAT APPLY.**
    A. Tell the patient that there will be no electrical shock.
    B. Shampoo the patient's hair before the procedure.
    C. Shampoo the patient's hair after the procedure.
    D. Sedate the patient with phenobarbital before the test.

19. The nurse is caring for a patient with a brain tumor who is scheduled for a CT scan. Which of the following factors, if present in the patient's history, would affect the manner in which the nurse prepares the patient for the scan?
    A. The patient takes anticonvulsant medication.
    B. The patient has difficulty recalling recent events.
    C. The patient developed hives when eating shrimp.
    D. The patient has paresthesias in the hands.

20. The nurse is providing teaching about brain CT scanning to a patient. Which of the following teaching points should the nurse be certain to include?
    A. "You will have to lie very still on a long, narrow table during the test."
    B. "You will be able to sit up during the test if you need to have a break."
    C. "You will have many tiny electrodes placed on your scalp during the test."
    D. "You will have contrast injected in your IV and then return for pictures."

21. A young male patient is brought to the emergency department with a diagnosis of traumatic head injury following a motor vehicle accident. Upon admission, vital signs are within normal limits, pupils are equal but react sluggishly, Glasgow Coma score = 5, and intracranial pressure (ICP) is 30 mm Hg. Based upon this initial assessment, the nurse understands that:
    A. further evaluation is warranted before care is provided.
    B. the patient is in a coma and has elevated ICP.
    C. the patient is unlikely to survive because of the head injury.
    D. the patient needs a head CT scan immediately.

22. A patient is brought to the emergency department with a diagnosis of traumatic head injury following a motorcycle accident. Upon admission, vital signs are within normal limits, pupils are equal but react sluggishly, Glasgow Coma score = 6, and ICP is 35 mm Hg. Based upon this initial assessment, the priority intervention by the nurse should be to:
    A. administer medications to reduce the increased ICP.
    B. start two large bore IVs at 100 mL per hour.
    C. monitor and record vital signs and pupillary responses.
    D. maintain a patent airway and administer oxygen.

23. Which of the following nursing interventions is indicated for a patient with elevated ICP?
    A. Encourage oral intake of 2 liters of fluid per day.
    B. Elevate the head of the bed 30 degrees.
    C. Turn and reposition the patient every hour.
    D. Maintain the patient in the prone position.

24. Which of the following is contraindicated in the patient with increased ICP?
    A. Maintain the head and neck in neutral position.
    B. Provide for a quiet environment.
    C. Maintain fluid restriction.
    D. Cluster care to provide for periods of rest.

25. An 8-year-old child is admitted with a diagnosis of epilepsy. The patient exhibits brief lapses of consciousness and vacant stares. The nurse suspects that the patient is experiencing what type of seizures?
   A. grand mal
   B. petit mal
   C. Jacksonian
   D. psychomotor

26. The nurse is caring for a patient with a history of seizures who falls to the floor and becomes cyanotic and then experiences erratic muscular contractions over the entire body. The patient's eyes are rolled back during this episode. The nurse knows that the priority nursing intervention for this patient is to:
   A. monitor the vital signs during the episode.
   B. ensure and maintain a patent airway.
   C. hold the patient's head firmly to prevent injury.
   D. administer intravenous Solu-Medrol immediately.

27. The nurse is providing postoperative teaching to a patient with transient ischemic attack (TIA). Which of the following teaching points should the nurse be certain to include in teaching?
   A. Rehabilitative therapy may be required for up to 2 months.
   B. TIAs are a significant warning sign of impending stroke.
   C. The patient will need to have assistance at home for a while.
   D. The patient may need to move to an assisted living facility.

28. The emergency department nurse is assigned to provide care for a patient diagnosed with ischemic stroke. Which of the following questions is particularly important for the nurse to ask of the patient or family member?
   A. "How long ago did you first notice the symptoms of your stroke?"
   B. "Do you live alone at home or is there someone else with you?"
   C. "Do you have a preference for a rehabilitation facility?"
   D. "Have you ever experienced symptoms like this previously?"

29. The nurse understands that mild hypothermia is a neuroprotective strategy that is useful for treatment of patients with stroke in that it:
   A. decreases metabolic action in the brain.
   B. inhibits environmental stimulation.
   C. promotes rest for the brain.
   D. decreases inflammatory responses.

30. Which of the following patients is a good candidate for carotid endarterectomy (CEA)?
   A. a patient with 45% stenosis of the internal carotid
   B. a patient with 85% stenosis of the internal carotid
   C. a patient with 45% stenosis of the internal jugular
   D. a patient with 85% stenosis of the internal jugular

ALTERNATE FORMAT

31. Which of the following are considered to be risk factors for cerebral aneurysms? **SELECT ALL THAT APPLY.**
    A. smoking
    B. male sex
    C. female sex
    D. age over 40
    E. diabetes
    F. hypertension

32. Which of the following is an important factor that influences signs and symptoms manifested by patients with cerebral aneurysms?
    A. the patient's blood pressure
    B. preexisting comorbidities
    C. location of the aneurysm
    D. availability of emergency treatment

33. The nurse observes a patient fall to the floor and begin to seize. The best response by the nurse is to:
    A. protect the patient's head from injury.
    B. restrain the patient to prevent injury.
    C. place a bite block in the patient's mouth.
    D. summon assistance to hold the patient down.

34. The nurse in the emergency department is caring for a patient who experienced a head injury with loss of consciousness. Shortly afterward, the patient regained consciousness for a period of time before experiencing a rapidly declining level of consciousness. The nurse takes quick action, realizing that the patient has developed:
    A. skull fracture.
    B. concussion.
    C. subdural hematoma.
    D. epidural hematoma.

35. The nurse is caring for a patient who has returned from the operating room having undergone a craniotomy. The nurse should position the patient in which of the following positions?
    A. supine with head of bed flat; head and neck in neutral midline position
    B. supine with head of bed flat; head turned toward operative side
    C. head of bed elevated 30 degrees; head and neck in midline position
    D. head of bed elevated 30 degrees; head turned toward operative side

36. The nurse is caring for a patient who experienced basilar skull fractures as a result of a motor vehicle accident. The nurse is concerned that the client will develop meningitis. Which of the following clinical manifestations would indicate meningitis?
    A. negative Kernig's sign
    B. positive Brudzinski's sign
    C. elevated WBCs
    D. temperature = 100.4°F

37. The nurse is providing education to a patient and other family members after the patient sustained a spinal cord injury that resulted in paraplegia. Teaching for this patient and family should focus on:
    A. selection of the most appropriate rehabilitation facility.
    B. possible surgical intervention to re-establish nerve pathways.
    C. promoting patient independence in self-care activities.
    D. discussion of alternative vocations for the patient.

38. The patient with a spinal cord injury has had a halo vest applied. The nurse should include which of the following statements in providing discharge teaching?
    A. "You should avoid bending over."
    B. "You may drive occasionally."
    C. "You will have to turn your head very slowly."
    D. "This device will stabilize your thoracic fracture."

39. Treatment for unruptured cerebral aneurysms may include:
    A. craniotomy for surgical resection.
    B. endovascular coiling.
    C. medical management.
    D. thrombolytic therapy.

40. The most common type of cerebral aneurysm is:
    A. saccular.
    B. fusiform.
    C. dissecting.
    D. supratentorial.

41. The patient with a C5 spinal cord injury has weak respiratory effort, ineffective cough, and uses accessory muscles to breathe. The priority nursing diagnosis for this patient is:
    A. impaired gas exchange.
    B. ineffective breathing pattern.
    C. risk for aspiration.
    D. risk for injury.

42. The nurse is caring for a patient who begins to experience seizure activity while in bed. Which of the following actions by the nurse is contraindicated?
    A. loosening restrictive clothing
    B. raising padded side rails
    C. restraining the patient's limbs
    D. positioning the patient on the side

43. The nurse is caring for a patient who experienced a CVA. The patient has residual dysphagia, so the nurse must avoid which of the following when feeding?
    A. giving coffee, tea, or water
    B. thickening liquids on the meal tray
    C. placing food in the unaffected side of the mouth
    D. allowing ample time for chewing and swallowing

44. A patient is admitted to the hospital with a diagnosis of Guillain-Barré syndrome. During the admission interview, the nurse asks if the patient has a history of which of the following?
    A. recent *staphylococcus* infection
    B. recent GI or respiratory infection
    C. air travel to another country
    D. seizures or brain trauma

45. An elderly female patient is admitted with Alzheimer's disease. The nurse understands that pathological changes in the patient's brain are related to:
    A. damage to the myelin sheath.
    B. abnormal accumulation of protein.
    C. destruction of neurons.
    D. increased CSF production.

46. Which of the following nursing interventions would be contraindicated for the patient with Alzheimer's?
    A. Establish a regular routine.
    B. Restrain the patient if needed.
    C. Place a clock and calendar in the room.
    D. Minimize interactions with the patient.

ALTERNATE FORMAT

47. A 40-year-old male patient is diagnosed with amyotrophic lateral sclerosis (ALS). In planning care for this patient, the nurse must be attentive to which of the following characteristics of the disease? SELECT ALL THAT APPLY.
    A. slow, subtle onset
    B. rapid, acute onset
    C. cognitive function deteriorates rapidly
    D. cognitive function remains intact
    E. respiratory failure
    F. anxiety

48. The nurse is providing education for the patient with amyotrophic lateral sclerosis (ALS). Which of the following statements by the patient indicates understanding about the disease prognosis?
    A. "I won't really know what is going on at the end."
    B. "Medical treatment has been effective for some patients."
    C. "I'll have trouble communicating my needs at some point."
    D. "This disease is curable but has exacerbations and remissions."

49. The nurse understands that emotional support is critically important for the patient with ALS because the patient:
    A. may be in the ICU for a long time.
    B. will be alert when respiratory complications develop.
    C. may not have a long-term care provider available.
    D. may be on a mechanical ventilator for a long time.

50. The nurse is admitting a patient with Guillain-Barré syndrome. The patient has ascending paralysis to the lower trunk. Based on knowledge of the progression of the disease, the nurse brings which of the following items into the patient's room?
    A. nebulizer and pulse oximeter
    B. flashlight and incentive spirometer
    C. EKG electrodes and intubation tray
    D. blood pressure cuff and glucometer

51. The nurse who cares for head-injured patients understands that which lobe of the brain controls judgment, personality, and affect?
    A. frontal
    B. parietal
    C. temporal
    D. occipital

52. The nurse understands that the most common early symptoms of myasthenia gravis are:
    A. diplopia and ptosis.
    B. anorexia and weight loss.
    C. increased susceptibility to infection.
    D. rapid, shallow respirations.

53. Plasmapheresis has been ordered for the patient with Guillain-Barré syndrome. When the patient expresses concern about what is involved, the best response by the nurse is which of the following?
    A. "It will alleviate your symptoms by removing antibodies from the blood."
    B. "You may have a mild allergic reaction with cutaneous pruritis."
    C. "It will prevent secondary bacterial infection of the nervous system."
    D. "It will reduce your need for oxygen while you are on the ventilator."

Physical Assessment

1. The nurse is caring for a head-injured male patient in the step-down unit. After performing an assessment of level of consciousness, the nurse noted the following: "The patient opened his eyes in response to hearing his spoken name, but in response to further verbal stimulation, made only incomprehensible sounds. In response to painful stimuli, the patient withdrew bilaterally." Based on these findings, the nurse would report the patient's Glasgow Coma score as which of the following?
    A. E 1; V 1; M 1 = GCS 3
    B. E 2; V 1; M 1 = GCS 4
    C. E 3; V 2; M 4 = GCS 9
    D. E 4; V 4; M 6 = GCS 14

2. The nurse is caring for a postoperative carotid endarterectomy patient and must assess cranial nerve function. To assess the function of the olfactory nerve (CN 1), the nurse should:
    A. pass a mixture of herbs under the patient's nostrils.
    B. place an ampule of ammonia under each nostril.
    C. pass a small amount of ground coffee under the nostrils.
    D. ask the patient to identify smells within the environment.

3. The nurse is caring for a postoperative carotid endarterectomy patient and must assess cranial nerve function. To assess the function of the oculomotor (CN III), trochlear (CN IV), and abducens (CN VI) nerves, the nurse should:
   A. ask the patient to follow a pencil through 6 cardinal fields of gaze.
   B. perform a funduscopic exam by using a flashlight in a dark room.
   C. ask the patient to read the smallest line possible on a Snellen chart.
   D. assess bone and air conduction tests by using a tuning fork.

4. The nurse is providing care for a patient who has been experiencing clumsiness and falls. The patient reports having a "weak" leg. The nurse realizes that the priority assessment should be targeted toward:
   A. cerebellar function.
   B. sensory function.
   C. cranial nerves.
   D. spinal nerves.

5. The nurse is caring for a patient who experienced spinal cord transection at the level of T4 in a motor vehicle accident. When assessing this patient, the nurse expects to find which of the following?
   A. fine motor movement of upper and lower extremities
   B. gross motor movement of the lower extremities
   C. paralysis of the arms, trunk, legs, and pelvis
   D. normal upper motor ability and lower paralysis

6. The nurse is assigned to a patient who was admitted with a transient ischemic attack (TIA). Which of the following manifestations would the nurse anticipate finding upon admission of this patient?
   A. confusion
   B. lethargy
   C. facial droop on the left
   D. restlessness

7. The emergency department nurse is assigned to care for a patient with suspected hemorrhagic stroke who will arrive by ambulance within 5 minutes. Based upon this brief notification, the nurse should expect to assess which of the following manifestations upon admission of the patient?
   A. loss of consciousness with severe neurologic impairment
   B. visual field impairment and sensory deficits to lower extremities
   C. cranial deficits and contralateral hemiparesis
   D. eye movement disorders and decreased visual acuity

8. The nurse is assigned to care for a patient who has experienced a cerebrovascular accident (CVA) related to thrombotic occlusion of the middle cerebral artery. Which of the following manifestations would the nurse find during assessment of this patient?
   A. drowsiness, aphasia, homonymous hemianopsia
   B. hypertension, inability to perform known tasks
   C. lethargy, confusion, restlessness, bradycardia
   D. numbness and facial weakness, difficulty walking

9. The nurse is providing care for a patient with a spinal cord injury. It would be particularly important for the nurse to assess for which of the following conditions with this patient?
   A. bladder distention
   B. impaired skin integrity
   C. fecal incontinence
   D. unrelenting pain

10. The nurse is assigned to care for a patient with Parkinson's disease. Which of the following manifestations is the nurse likely to identify in this patient?
    A. hemiplegia
    B. lethargy
    C. mask-like face
    D. cold intolerance

11. A patient is admitted to the hospital with bacterial meningitis. In addition to nuchal rigidity, the nurse should expect which of the following manifestations upon physical assessment?
    A. positive Brudzinski's and Kernig's signs
    B. positive Brudzinski's and negative Kernig's signs
    C. negative Brudzinski's and positive Kernig's signs
    D. negative Brudzinski's and Kernig's signs

12. A female patient is hospitalized with a suspected diagnosis of myasthenia gravis. During physical assessment, which of the following statements by the patient indicates the presence of a common manifestation of the disease?
    A. "I have a tough time getting up after I rest for awhile."
    B. "When I have a cold, I usually have a very strong cough."
    C. "By the end of the day, my eyelids are usually drooping."
    D. "I have a considerable amount of uncontrollable trembling."

Interpretation of Lab Values

1. The patient is prescribed phenytoin (Dilantin) for control of seizures. Which of the following serum levels indicates compliance with the medication regimen?
   A. 5 to 10 μg/mL
   B. 10 to 20 μg/mL
   C. 20 to 30 μg/mL
   D. 30 to 40 μg/mL

Drugs and Treatments

1. The nurse is caring for a patient who will undergo cerebral angiography. Following the procedure, it will be important for the nurse to encourage the patient to:
   A. ambulate as much as tolerated.
   B. lie in Trendelenburg position for 2 hours.
   C. increase fluid intake to at least 2 liters per day.
   D. remain on strict bed rest for at least 48 hours.

2. A patient is brought to the emergency department with a diagnosis of traumatic head injury following a motorcycle accident. Upon admission, vital signs are within normal limits, pupils are equal but react sluggishly, Glasgow Coma score = 6, and ICP is 35 mm Hg. The nurse is preparing to administer a dose of IV mannitol as ordered. The nurse understands that the expected outcome of this action is to:
   A. improve vital signs.
   B. reduce ICP.
   C. stabilize pupillary responses.
   D. improve renal function.

ALTERNATE FORMAT

3. Which of the following medications may be used to help to treat increased intracranial pressure? SELECT ALL THAT APPLY.
   A. osmotic diuretics
   B. loop diuretics
   C. corticosteroids
   D. thiazide diuretics

4. The nurse is teaching the parent of a pediatric patient about phenytoin (Dilantin) prior to discharge. Which of the following statements by the patient's mother indicates understanding of a common side effect of phenytoin (Dilantin)?
   A. "I will administer a glycerin suppository if my child is constipated."
   B. "If my child gets tongue lesions, I can use oral Anbesol to decrease discomfort."
   C. "I need to monitor my child's ability to detect colors in the environment."
   D. "My child should use a soft toothbrush, massage the gums, and floss daily."

5. The nurse is providing care to a patient in the emergency department who has suffered ischemic stroke. Which of the following medications provides the most advantage to the patient if administered within 3 hours of symptom onset?
   A. aspirin
   B. clopidogrel (Plavix)
   C. abciximab (ReoPro)
   D. tissue plasminogen activator (t-PA)

6. The nurse has an order to administer medication to a patient who is shivering because of treatment for hyperthermia. Which of the following medications does the nurse plan to administer?
   A. prochlorperazine (Compazine)
   B. chlorpromazine (Thorazine)
   C. thioridazine (Mellaril)
   D. fluphenazine (Prolixin)

7. The patient with a head injury has begun having very large urine output through a Foley catheter. The nurse notes that urine output for the previous shift was 3000 mL. Based on this assessment, the nurse prepares to administer which of the following drugs as ordered by the physician?
   A. desmopressin (DDAVP)
   B. furosemide (Lasix)
   C. mannitol (Osmitrol)
   D. bumetanide (Bumex)

8. Which of the following medications is likely to be used to treat status epilepticus?
   A. phenytoin (Dilantin)
   B. valproic acid (Depakene)
   C. carbamazepine (Tegretol)
   D. diazepam (Valium)

9. The nurse administers a dose of edrophonium chloride (Tensilon) to a patient intravenously. The patient demonstrates increased muscle strength for a while following the injection. The nurse interprets this finding as indicative of which of the following neurological problems?
   A. multiple sclerosis
   B. amyotropic lateral sclerosis
   C. myasthenia gravis
   D. muscular dystrophy

10. The nurse is providing teaching to a patient about taking phenytoin (Dilantin) for control of seizures. The nurse mentions that compliance with therapy will be monitored by:
    A. urine tests.
    B. blood tests.
    C. maintaining a seizure record.
    D. EEG at least once per month.

11. The patient with a history of seizures indicates understanding of discharge instructions by articulating that medication should be stopped when:
    A. side effects occur.
    B. blood levels are therapeutic.
    C. seizure activity ceases.
    D. ordered by the physician.

12. A patient with Parkinson's disease will begin treatment with levodopa (L-Dopa). Which of the following should the nurse include as a teaching point for the patient?
    A. "Rise slowly from a sitting or lying position."
    B. "Try to increase your intake of foods rich in protein."
    C. "Be sure to take supplemental pyridoxine."
    D. "Take your medication at the first sign of tremors."

13. The nurse is providing education to a young woman about phenytoin (Dilantin). During the education session, the patient indicates that she is taking birth control pills. Based on knowledge of drug interactions, which of the following teaching points must the nurse use to advise the patient?
    A. "When taking both medications, you are at risk for thrombophlebitis."
    B. "You should use an alternate form of birth control while taking Dilantin."
    C. "You can stop taking the Dilantin if you have severe GI distress."
    D. "You should not get pregnant while you are taking Dilantin."

ANSWERS

General

1. **(A)**; Consciousness is a state of awareness. Level of consciousness provides insight into the patient's level of cortical functioning.

2. **(B)**; The nurse can document that the patient exhibits some degree of arousal if, when the nurse applied nail bed pressure, the hand is withdrawn. This indicates responsiveness to sensory stimulation.

3. **(D)**; Orientation to person is generally the last orientation parameter that is lost. Lack of orientation to person occurs with severe dysfunction, such as delirium.

4. **(A)**; Impaired orientation to time often occurs early and may often be the first sign of neurological change.

5. **(B)**; The nurse can assess attention and concentration by asking the patient to count backward from 100 by 7's. The nurse could ask a less educated patient to name the months of the year or days of the week in reverse order.

6. **(A)**; Tests of remote memory may include questions such as where and when the patient was born, how old the patient is, when the patient graduated high school, and what the names, ages, and birth dates of all his or her children are. Information provided by the patient can then be validated by the family or friends.

7. **(C)**; Recent memory can be tested in a number of different ways. One way is to ask the patient to provide details about how he or she arrived at the appointment and with whom. The nurse could also ask the patient to name all of the things he or she ate at breakfast.

8. **(C)**; The nurse was testing the patient's recent memory by following the protocol as described in the scenario. A person without a cognitive deficit should be able to recall and name the three objects.

9. **(D)**; Dysphoria is an appropriate descriptor for the patient who is very depressed, despondent, or sad.

10. **(A)**; Expressive speaking aphasia is a disorder of speech and language in which the patient is unable to speak. This typically occurs as a result of a lesion at Broca's area of the frontal lobe.

11. **(B)**; A signed consent implies that the patient was informed about the procedure and, at least at the time, understood what to expect. When, during preparation for the procedure, the patient indicates that he or she does not remember what to expect, it is certainly appropriate for the nurse to remind the patient that a needle will be inserted into the spinal canal to obtain samples of cerebral spinal fluid to be sent for analysis.

12. **(C)**; Cranial nerve II is the optic nerve. Impairment of this nerve indicates that there is at least some visual challenge. Therefore, the prudent nurse would ensure that the patient has an obstacle-free path for ambulation.

13. **(C)**; Cerebellar impairment affects one's coordination and ability to ambulate. It is evident that the patient has adapted to this impairment when the patient demonstrates proper use of a walker.

14. **(C)**; The trigeminal nerve has both sensory and motor capabilities. To assess its sensory function, the nurse would use a safety pin to assess for recognition of pain; cold and hot items to identify cold and hot sensations; and a cotton wisp to evaluate recognition of touch sensations. To test motor abilities of CN V, the nurse would ask the patient to clench the jaw and close the mouth and then assess for symmetry bilaterally.

15. **(A)**; Both the glossopharyngeal and vagus nerves have both sensory and motor functions. To test the motor function, the nurse should have the patient open the mouth and say, "aaah." The palate and the uvula should move upward in response. Other testing that should be done includes checking for gag response and assessing voice quality for hoarseness.

16. **(B)**; The nurse should realize that treatment options for AVM are dependent upon a number of factors—size, location, and pattern of venous drainage. Treatment options include: (1) surgical resection at a major neurosurgical center; (2) coiling or embolization, which is performed by an interventional neuroradiologist; (3) gamma knife surgery; or (4) conservative treatment. Surgical resection involves surgical separation of the arteries and veins. Coiling or embolization involves insertion of tiny coils or glue into the arterial side of the AVM to obliterate blood flow. Gamma knife surgery can be used to treat AVMs that are not accessible for surgical resection because of their location. Conservative treatment involves symptom management and is used to treat AVMs that are unsafe for other treatment options.

17. **(D)**; The patient should be informed that an EEG is a procedure used to measure brain waves by using multiple electrodes attached to the scalp. An EEG can provide information suggestive of epilepsy, encephalitis, or dementia. It can also be used to help to determine brain death.

18. **(A, B, C)**; It is important for the nurse to let the patient know that there will be no electrical shock administered during the EEG. The EEG merely documents brain activity during the test. It is desirable for the nurse to shampoo the patient's hair both before and after the procedure—before the test for cleanliness and after the test to remove residual gel from the electrodes.

19. **(C)**; If the patient developed hives when eating shrimp, the nurse must make a notation of allergy to shellfish because this means that contrast may be contraindicated. At the very least, it will require more in-depth questioning on the part of the nurse or physician to determine if there is an absolute contraindication to contrast or whether it may be safe to administer contrast following premedication with an IV antihistamine such as Benadryl.

20. **(A)**; The nurse should mention that the test will require the patient to lie very still on a long, narrow table during the test. Movement during the test will result in interference with the quality of films.

21. **(B)**; The nurse understands that the patient is in a coma and has elevated ICP. In general, it is widely accepted that a Glasgow Coma score of less than 8 indicates coma. Any prolonged ICP of greater than 15 mm Hg is considered to be elevated ICP.

22. **(D)**; In this case, the nurse must initially think "ABC's" and maintain a patent airway and administer oxygen. Of course, it is important to rapidly begin treatment for the elevated intracranial pressure and obtain a CT of the head to document the extent of injury.

23. **(B)**; To decrease the patient's elevated intracranial pressure, it is critical for the nurse to keep the head of the patient's bed elevated 30 degrees while maintaining good body alignment.

24. **(D)**; For patients with elevated intracranial pressure, clustering care is not recommended because prolonged activity may further increase intracranial pressure.

25. **(B)**; Seizures that include brief lapses in consciousness and vacant stares would be petit mal.

26. **(B)**; The nurse should monitor the patient cautiously throughout the seizure and ensure that the patient has a patent airway. Administration of oxygen via mask or nasal cannula may be desirable depending upon the patient's status.

27. **(B)**; It is important for the nurse to let the patient know that the presence of symptoms of TIA should be viewed as a warning of impending stroke. About 1 in 10 patients who experience a TIA will subsequently experience a major stroke within a year. The biggest risk for stroke occurs within 48 hours of occurrence of the TIA.

28. **(A)**; It is particularly important for the nurse to ask how long ago the patient first began to notice symptoms of the stroke because the patient may be a candidate for thrombolytic therapy. The FDA has approved the administration of t-PA for treatment of ischemic stroke when it is administered within 3 hours of onset of symptoms.

29. **(D)**; Mild hypothermia decreases intracranial pressure and may improve mortality associated with stroke.

30. **(B)**; The patient with 85% stenosis of the internal carotid artery is a candidate for carotid endarterectomy because guidelines suggest that those with > 70% stenosis are good candidates. CEA is not indicated for patients with < 50% stenosis of the internal carotid artery. CEA is not performed for stenosis of the internal jugular vein.

31. **(A, C, D, F)**; Risk factors for cerebral aneurysms include: *smoking, hypertension,* previous aneurysms, connective tissue disorders, *age greater than 40, female gender,* and blood vessel injury or dissection.

32. **(C)**; Three major factors influence the manifestation of signs and symptoms in patients with cerebral aneurysms: location of the aneurysm, its size, and whether or not it has ruptured.

33. **(A)**; It is most important for the nurse to ensure the patient's safety. The nurse should protect the patient's head from injury. Patients who are seizing should not be restrained or held down. Placing a bite block in the patient's mouth during a seizure is not advisable because it may, in fact, occlude the airway.

34. **(D)**; The patient with a classic epidural hematoma experiences immediate loss of consciousness after traumatic injury, followed by regaining consciousness for a period of time. Later, the patient experiences a rapid decline in level of consciousness (sleepiness, confusion, obtundation, coma, and possibly death). The decline in level of consciousness after having had a period of lucidity requires immediate surgical intervention for evacuation of the hematoma.

35. **(C)**; The nurse positions the patient to maintain low intracranial pressure postoperatively by elevating the head of the bed 30 degrees and maintaining the head and neck in a neutral midline position.

36. **(B)**; Clinical manifestations of meningitis include restlessness, agitation, irritability, nausea and vomiting, severe headaches, nuchal rigidity, positive Brudzinski's sign, positive Kernig's sign, chills, high fever, confusion, altered level of consciousness, and signs and symptoms of increased cranial pressure.

37. **(C)**; During hospitalization, the nurse must teach the patient and family about promoting independence in self-care activities. This should include activities of daily living as well as self-catheterization and bowel evacuation.

38. **(A)**; The patient with a halo brace should be cautioned not to bend over to reduce the risk of falling because the device raises the patient's center of gravity and completely immobilizes the cervical spine. The patient may not drive. The nurse should instruct the patient to turn the entire body to scan the environment. Halo devices completely immobilize the cervical spine, not the thoracic spine.

39. **(B)**; Endovascular coiling is a good alternative for patients with unruptured cerebral aneurysms. The treatment, which involves placement of a coil into the aneurysm to obliterate it and significantly reduce the chances of bleeding into the brain, is performed by neurosurgeons and interventional radiologists. Research has demonstrated better than expected disability-free outcomes for patients who have had the procedure.

40. **(A)**; The most common type of cerebral aneurysm is the saccular or berry aneurysm.

41. **(B)**; The patient has an ineffective breathing pattern as defined by the weak respiratory effort, ineffective cough, and use of accessory muscles to breathe.

42. **(C)**; When a patient experiences seizures, the nurse should be attentive to airway issues and try to prevent injury to the patient. In this case, raising the padded side rails is a very good idea. The nurse should not try to restrain the patient's limbs.

43. **(A)**; The nurse will not give the patient any liquids (coffee, tea, or water) without thickening them to the consistency of oatmeal.

44. **(B)**; The nurse should inquire about recent GI or respiratory infections. Guillain-Barré is thought to be of an autoimmune nature because it often develops after viral infections of GI or respiratory origin.

45. **(B)**; Alzheimer's disease is a progressive disease in which the patient experiences irreversible deterioration of intellectual function. Nerve cells are lost, perfusion to areas of the brain is decreased, the brain atrophies, and protein accumulates in the brain tissue.

46. **(D)**; It would be desirable to establish regular routines; restrain the patient for safety if necessary; orient the patient to person, place, and time as often as necessary; and place a clock and a calendar in the patient's room. The nurse should use therapeutic communication techniques during interactions with the patient.

47. **(A, D, E, F)**; Amyotrophic lateral sclerosis (ALS) is a degenerative, progressive, incurable, and fatal disease that has a slow, subtle onset. Initially, the patient may experience weakness in the distal extremities. Over time the weakness progresses to ascending paralysis. The patient's cognitive ability remains intact, which means that the client is extremely aware of what is occurring. Anxiety is very common. Death ultimately results from aspiration, infection, and respiratory failure.

48. **(C)**; Eventually, acute dyspnea and respiratory failure occur. The patient will be placed on a mechanical ventilator, and communication will be difficult because of the inability to speak, type on a laptop, or write notes.

49. **(B)**; Emotional support is critical for the patient with ALS because the patient will remain cognitively aware throughout the progression of the devastation of the disease.

50. **(C)**; The nurse brings EKG electrodes and an intubation tray into the room in preparation for the time when the patient may require intubation and ventilatory assistance as the disease progresses.

51. **(A)**; The frontal lobe of the brain controls judgment, personality, and affect.

52. **(A)**; The most common early symptoms of myasthenia gravis are diplopia and ptosis.

53. **(A)**; Plasmapheresis can be effective to alleviate symptoms during the first 2 weeks of the disease. It involves removing plasma, separating it from the whole blood to remove antibodies that cause the disorder, and reinfusing the blood.

Physical Assessment

1. **(C)**; When documenting a Glasgow Coma score, accuracy depends upon scoring the best response in each category. For this patient, the eye response is scored at 3 because the patient responded to the spoken name. The best verbal response is scored as 2 because the patient made only incomprehensible sounds, no words. The best motor response is scored as 4 because the patient withdrew to pain bilaterally. Adding the three values together, 3 + 2 + 4 = 9, results in a Glasgow Coma score of 9.

2. **(C)**; Function of the olfactory nerve can be assessed by occluding each nostril individually while the other is tested by passing a common substance beneath it and asking the patient to identify the substance.

3. **(A)**; Cranial nerves III, IV, and VI are assessed together because they supply the muscles that move the eyes. First the nurse should assess the position of the eyes for symmetry. Extraocular movements are assessed by asking the patient to follow a pencil as the nurse moves it through the six cardinal fields of gaze. Normally, both eyes should move at the same time in the same direction.

4. **(A)**; The nurse should target the assessment toward cerebellar function because balance and coordination are under control of the cerebellum. Gait should be tested by having the patient walk normally and then on heels and toes to assess coordination.

Additionally, a Romberg's test should be done in which the patient puts the feet together and closes the eyes as the examiner stands nearby to prevent falling. To assess coordination, the nurse could have the patient touch each finger on each hand with the thumb of the hand.

5. **(D)**; When a patient suffers spinal cord trauma with transection of the cord at the T4 level, the patient will have normal upper body motor ability and paralysis of the lower portion of the body.

6. **(C)**; Manifestations of transient ischemic attack include focal neurological deficits, like inability to sense one side of the body, unilateral loss of vision, loss of speech, or facial droop. Global deficits, like restlessness, confusion, or lethargy, are not characteristic with transient ischemic attacks.

7. **(A)**; Hemorrhagic strokes occur rapidly and without significant warning signs, although some patients experience severe headache at the onset of symptoms. The nurse should anticipate that the patient with *suspected hemorrhagic stroke*, as identified by ambulance personnel, has symptoms that are significant enough to warrant the potential diagnosis from the field. Therefore, the nurse should anticipate that the patient will have loss of consciousness and severe neurologic impairment upon arrival to the emergency department.

8. **(A)**; Thrombotic strokes commonly occur in older patients with atherosclerosis. Symptoms vary according to the vessel affected. Thrombotic occlusion of the middle cerebral artery may result in drowsiness, stupor, coma, contralateral hemiplegia, sensory deficits of the arm and face, aphasia, and homonymous hemianopsia.

9. **(A)**; Patients with spinal cord injury are prone to develop autonomic dysreflexia, an exaggerated sympathetic response (and medical emergency) to specific stimuli, including bladder distention, abdominal pain, or fecal impaction. The nurse should be attentive to assessment for bladder distention or firm abdomen and fecal impaction to prevent the occurrence of this medical emergency.

10. **(C)**; Upon assessment, the nurse is likely to find any number of these clinical manifestations of Parkinson's disease: masklike face, bradykinesia, uncoordinated movements, heat intolerance, anxiety, depression, sleep disturbances, slurred speech, and short steps with propulsive gait.

11. **(A)**; Clinical manifestations of bacterial meningitis include signs of meningeal irritation, nuchal rigidity, positive Brudzinski's sign, and positive Kernig's sign.

12. **(C)**; Myasthenia gravis is a chronic progressive disorder of the peripheral nervous system in which the patient experiences muscle weakness and fatigue that worsens with exertion and improves with rest. The disease has a slow onset but can be precipitated by stress, hormonal disturbances, infections, temperature extremes, excessive exercise, etc. Manifestations include double vision and eyelid drooping.

Interpretation of Lab Values

1. **(B)**; A therapeutic drug level of phenytoin (Dilantin) indicates patient compliance with the drug regimen. The therapeutic serum level for phenytoin is 10 to 20 μg/mL.

Drugs and Treatments

1. **(C)**; Cerebral angiography depends upon the use of contrast media to define the vasculature of the brain. Following the procedure, it is desirable for the patient to increase fluid intake to facilitate excretion of the contrast.

2. **(B)**; The nurse understands that mannitol is an osmotic diuretic and that an expected outcome of treatment with this drug is a reduction in intracranial pressure.

3. **(A, B, C)**; Medications that may be used to help treat increased intracranial pressure include osmotic diuretics (mannitol), loop diuretics (furosemide), and corticosteroids (dexamethasone). Mannitol, furosemide (Lasix), and dexamethasone (Decadron) are widely used for treatment of elevated ICP. Thiazide diuretics are not indicated for treatment of elevated ICP.

4. **(D)**; A common side effect of phenytoin (Dilantin) therapy is gingival hyperplasia. This can be prevented with good oral hygiene—brushing daily with a soft toothbrush, massaging the gums, and using dental floss daily.

5. **(D)**; Tissue plasminogen activator (t-PA), approved by the FDA for treatment of ischemic stroke within 3 hours of onset of symptoms, lyses the clot and restores blood flow to the brain tissue. Clopidogrel (Plavix) is an antiplatelet agent that, when administered along with aspirin, has significantly improved clinical outcomes for patients who have experienced ischemic events. Abciximab (ReoPro) is often used in conjunction with aspirin and heparin to decrease the risk of ischemic complications of endovascular interventions.

6. **(B)**; Chlorpromazine (Thorazine) is an effective drug to interrupt shivering related to active cooling of hyperthermic patients. If shivering were allowed to continue, the temperature would likely rise rather than fall.

7. **(A)**; The patient is exhibiting signs of diabetes insipidus following the head injury. Desmopressin (DDAVP) is a synthetic form of antidiuretic hormone used for treatment of diabetes insipidus.

8. **(D)**; Status epilepticus is a life-threatening emergency that involves continuous cycles of seizure activity. Medications used to treat status epilepticus include diazepam (Valium), lorazepam (Ativan), and phenobarbital.

9. **(C)**; Patients with myasthenia gravis will demonstrate a significant increase in muscle strength for a period of time following doses of intravenous Tensilon, a cholinesterase inhibitor. The Tensilon challenge may be used in conjunction with a detailed history and physical assessment for diagnosis of myasthenia gravis.

10. **(B)**; Serum Dilantin levels will indicate level of compliance with therapy.

11. **(D)**; The patient can indicate understanding of discharge instructions by articulating that medications will continue until the physician determines that they should be discontinued.

12. **(A)**; Levodopa can cause dizziness, so patients should be cautioned to rise slowly from sitting or lying positions. The drug should be taken exactly as prescribed and the patient should be told that it may take as long as 6 months to reach the full therapeutic effect. The patient should avoid multivitamins and cereals fortified with vitamin B_6 (pyridoxine) because they may reverse the anti-Parkinson effect.

13. **(B)**; The nurse should encourage the patient to use an alternate form of birth control because Dilantin decreases the effectiveness of oral contraceptives.

Keep Track

- Percent correct. (Divide the number of questions you answered correctly by the total number of questions you answered.) _____

- Number of questions you missed due to a reading error: _____

- Number of questions you missed due to errors in analysis: _____

- Number of assessment questions you missed: _____

- Number of lab value questions you missed: _____

- Number of drug/treatment questions you missed: _____

Nugget List

Chapter number _____ Topic _____

Practice Test: Nursing Management of Patients with Psychiatric and Mental Health Disorders

Karen S. March

PRACTICE TEST

General

1. The nurse assigned to care for a patient admitted with a diagnosis of alcohol withdrawal syndrome receives a phone call from a person who identifies himself as the patient's minister. The caller asks if the patient "fell off the wagon again." The nurse's best response to the caller is which of the following?
   A. "Yes, the patient drank too much but should be fine in a few days."
   B. "We are unable to provide any information."
   C. "The patient has been admitted here but I can't say anything further."
   D. "The patient has been admitted to this facility but is not in this unit."

2. The nurse is evaluating the effectiveness of psychotropic medication on negative symptoms of psychosis in a patient by watching for a decrease in which of the following?
   A. affective flattening
   B. bizarre behavior
   C. illogicality
   D. somatic delusions

3. The nurse, who is caring for a patient with serotonin syndrome, understands that the most important nursing intervention for this patient is which of the following?
   A. administration of an anticonvulsant
   B. administration of a muscle relaxant for myoclonus
   C. discontinuation of serotonergic drugs
   D. immediately initiate body cooling procedures

4. The nurse is assigned to care for a patient who exhibits excessive emotionality, attention-seeking behaviors, and who craves novelty, stimulation, and excitement. Based on all of these factors, the nurse knows that this patient demonstrates which of the following types of personality disorder?
   A. paranoid
   B. histrionic
   C. narcissistic
   D. antisocial

ALTERNATE FORMAT

5. The nurse knows that typical characteristics seen with patients with obsessive-compulsive disorder include which of the following? SELECT ALL THAT APPLY.
A. rigid
B. perfectionistic
C. need for admiration
D. crave orderliness
E. reluctant to delegate tasks
F. manipulative

ALTERNATE FORMAT

6. The nurse is providing care for a patient who will have electroconvulsive therapy (ECT). Preparation of the patient for this therapy will involve which of the following? SELECT ALL THAT APPLY.
A. assessment of memory
B. informed consent
C. NPO after midnight prior to procedure
D. restraints during the procedure

ALTERNATE FORMAT

7. Electroconvulsive therapy (ECT) may be used for treatment of which of the following patient conditions? SELECT ALL THAT APPLY.
A. major depression
B. bipolar depressive disorder
C. mania
D. schizophrenia
E. histrionic personality disorder
F. antisocial personality disorder

8. Which of the following patients is at highest risk for suicide?
A. a 21-year-old female who lives with parents and recently broke up with a boyfriend
B. a 70-year-old widower with metastatic cancer who talks about saving his pain pills
C. a 45-year-old married female with a stressful job and significant financial stress
D. a 35-year-old religious, married man with children who has testicular cancer

9. A priority nursing intervention for the patient exhibiting psychomotor agitation would be which of the following?
A. Provide calming music or sounds as tolerated.
B. Instruct the patient on techniques to reduce anxiety.
C. Introduce the patient to diversionary activities.
D. Encourage exercise to facilitate calming of the patient.

10. The nurse providing care for a patient who has developed alcohol dependency realizes that the patient is likely to develop which of the following disorders of the liver?
A. hypercoagulability
B. hypomagnesemia
C. cirrhosis
D. pancreatic encephalopathy

11. The nurse recognizes which of the following comorbidities as being associated with eating disorders?
    A. headaches
    B. depression
    C. peripheral edema
    D. elevated B_{12} levels

12. The nurse is providing care for a patient who was recently diagnosed with major depression. The nurse realizes that which of the following is a priority for care of this patient?
    A. safety
    B. increasing participation in ADLs
    C. encouraging group therapy
    D. facilitating lengthy periods of rest

13. The nurse is approached by a friend who reports that a significant other has not left home in 3 weeks, has a very flat affect, and has lost interest in caring for the children. The nurse immediately recognizes these as symptoms of which of the following disorders?
    A. depression
    B. schizophrenia
    C. suicidal ideation
    D. bipolar manic episodes

14. The nurse is caring for a young adult patient admitted to the mental health unit with major depression and suicidal ideation. The patient has a history of cutting the wrists intermittently for more than 2 years. Upon admission, the patient stays in the room and eats only about 20% of each meal. On day three of hospitalization, the patient eats about 80% of each meal and is talking with others in group. The nurse realizes that the patient is:
    A. showing improvement.
    B. highly suicidal.
    C. exhibiting mood swings.
    D. in need of electroshock therapy.

15. The nurse is providing care for a female patient diagnosed with schizophrenia who believes that her thoughts are broadcast from her head. The nurse identifies which of the following as the most appropriate nursing diagnosis for this patient?
    A. risk for self-directed violence
    B. disturbed sensory perception
    C. impaired verbal communication
    D. disturbed thought processes

16. The nurse is providing care for a patient who is preoccupied with perfection and control, has difficulty relaxing, and cannot discard anything. The nurse knows that this patient displays symptoms of which of the following types of personality disorder?
    A. histrionic personality
    B. narcissistic personality
    C. obsessive-compulsive
    D. bipolar personality

17. The nurse is providing care for a patient with Alzheimer's dementia. Which of the following would the nurse identify as a priority nursing intervention to help orient this patient?
    A. Post a schedule of daily activities in the dining room.
    B. Use an overhead loudspeaker to announce upcoming events.
    C. Provide a daily routine and easy-to-read clocks.
    D. Place the patient alone in a private room.

18. The nurse is caring for a patient who attempted suicide and is being closely monitored for potential safety hazards. As a result of the need for close surveillance, the patient has lost the right to which of the following?
    A. social interaction
    B. decision making
    C. free time
    D. privacy

19. The nurse notices that a former patient, who is now enrolled in a community psychiatric program, is lurking outside the home of the nurse and peeping in the kitchen window. The nurse also noticed the patient at the grocery store and outside the hair salon. The nurse believes that the patient is stalking. The best response by the nurse involves:
    A. calling the local police to report the suspicion of stalking.
    B. calling the patient's spouse to discuss the behavior.
    C. inviting the patient to coffee at a cafe to discuss the behavior.
    D. waiting until the next group meeting to discuss the behavior.

20. Which of the following questions will help the nurse to identify potential stressors for a patient?
    A. Do you have a car?
    B. How do you get along with people at work?
    C. What do you want to feel like at the time of discharge?
    D. What are your goals for yourself?

ALTERNATE FORMAT

21. Which of the following experiences places a person at great risk for suicide? **SELECT ALL THAT APPLY.**
    A. hallucinations
    B. depression
    C. delusions
    D. lasting friendships

22. The nurse is caring for a patient whose goal is to focus on task performance. Which of the following types of therapy should this patient undergo?
    A. occupational therapy
    B. electroconvulsive therapy
    C. family therapy
    D. group therapy

23. A middle-aged male patient with a dual diagnosis of depression and alcohol abuse told the nurse that, upon release, he intends to kill his ex-wife with whom he has been involved in a child custody battle. The nurse shares this information with the treatment team. Which of the following is a legal duty of the team?

A. Keep the patient hospitalized indefinitely.

B. Warn the patient's ex-wife of the threat.

C. Maintain strict patient confidentiality.

D. Transfer the patient to a state hospital.

24. **The nurse is providing care for a 53-year-old man who has been taking phenytoin (Dilantin) for the past two years to control a seizure disorder. The patient has been admitted to the hospital today for new onset of seizure activity. The nurse realizes that the most likely explanation for this reoccurrence is that:**

    A. the patient is metabolizing his medication faster than normal.

    B. he has developed renal or hepatic problems that affect his drug levels.

    C. he is not being compliant with his prescribed medication regime.

    D. his serum phenytoin (Dilantin) level is ineffective because it is elevated.

25. **The nurse is providing care for a male patient who began taking paroxetine (Paxil) five days ago. When the patient states that the drug must be worthless because he doesn't feel any differently than he did without the drug, the nurse's best response is which of the following?**

    A. "You don't think the drug is working?"

    B. "Why do you feel that the drug is worthless?"

    C. "It normally takes a few weeks for the full effect."

    D. "I will report your concerns to the doctor."

26. **The nurse is providing care for a patient who has been prescribed phenelzine (Nardil) for a panic disorder. When provided with a list of foods that should not be eaten, the patient asks, "Why not?" The best response by the nurse is that:**

    A. the patient may develop severe gastrointestinal distress during consumption.

    B. the foods may precipitate life-threatening respiratory problems.

    C. the foods may precipitate a life-threatening hypertensive crisis.

    D. the patient may experience severe CNS depression following consumption.

27. **The Mini-Mental State Examination (MMSE) is used to assess which of the following?**

    A. delirium

    B. dementia

    C. orientation

    D. thinking

Physical Assessment

ALTERNATE FORMAT

1. **You are the nurse responsible for assessing a patient who has been on chlorpromazine (Thorazine) for extrapyramidal side effects (EPSEs). The nurse knows that extrapyramidal side effects include which of the following? SELECT ALL THAT APPLY.**

    A. acute dystonia

    B. akathisia

    C. amenorrhea

    D. breast secretion

    E. dyskinesia

    F. Parkinsonism

    G. sexual dysfunction

ALTERNATE FORMAT

2. The nurse is providing care for a patient with schizophrenia. Which of the following assessment questions would be appropriate for this patient? SELECT ALL THAT APPLY.
   A. "How many different voices speak to you?"
   B. "Do you recognize the voices?"
   C. "What do the voices say to you?"
   D. "What gives you relief?"

3. The emergency department nurse receives a patient who made a suicide attempt in the workplace just before being brought to the hospital. Which of the following interventions is most appropriate for the nurse to perform first?
   A. Physically search the patient for weapons and harmful materials.
   B. Place the patient in a seclusion room.
   C. Notify the employer that the patient will require extended leave.
   D. Administer an intramuscular injection of lorazepam (Ativan).

Interpretation of Lab Values

1. The nurse is caring for a patient who is prescribed lithium carbonate for control of bipolar disorder. The patient has been taking the drug for approximately 18 months. A serum lithium level drawn during this hospitalization is 2.0 mEq/L. The nurse interprets this drug level as which of the following?
   A. within normal limits
   B. borderline subtherapeutic
   C. slightly above normal
   D. within the toxic range

2. A patient has been admitted to the ICU with a diagnosis of drug overdose. The patient is lethargic, intubated, and on a mechanical ventilator. Which of the following laboratory tests should be done to provide further direction for treatment?
   A. white blood count (WBC)
   B. cardiac isoenzymes
   C. arterial blood gases (ABG)
   D. activated partial thromboplastin time (aPTT)

Drugs and Treatments

1. The nurse is providing teaching about chlorpromazine (Thorazine) to a patient who will be discharged soon. The patient demonstrates understanding of the information by making which of the following statements relative to chlorpromazine-related photosensitivity?
   A. "I will slowly build up my tolerance to bright sunshine."
   B. "I will avoid tasks that require high amounts of energy."
   C. "I will wear heavy clothing when I go outside in the sun."
   D. "I will apply sunscreen when I go outside on a sunny day."

ALTERNATE FORMAT

2. The nurse is caring for a patient who takes antipsychotic medications. The patient has developed muscle rigidity, hyperpyrexia, tachypnea, diaphoresis, and drooling. The nurse recognizes these symptoms as indicative of a severe, life-threatening side effect of psychotropic therapy which is referred to as _____.

3. The nurse is providing care for a patient who will take disulfiram (Antabuse) to support efforts toward sobriety. The nurse is confident that the patient fully understands the implications of treatment when the patient makes which of the following statements?
   A. "If I drink alcohol, I will get so sick that I will wish I could die."
   B. "If I drink alcohol, I will not be able to sleep well because I'll be hyperactive."
   C. "If I drink alcohol, I will not be able to sleep and I will be out of control."
   D. "If I drink alcohol, I will have severe mood swings and belligerent behavior."

4. The nurse is providing care for a patient who will be discharged to home within a few days. The patient has been ordered phenelzine (Nardil) for depression. The nurse understands the importance of warning the patient to avoid which of the following foods when taking this drug?
   A. pork, spinach, and fresh oysters
   B. milk, peanut butter, and yogurt
   C. cheese, bologna, and avocados
   D. orange juice, green beans, and ice cream

5. The nurse is providing education about medications to a patient who has just been started on lithium. The nurse realizes that teaching has been effective when the patient relates which of the following adverse effects that can occur and persist when lithium levels are within normal limits?
   A. fine hand tremors and polyuria
   B. tachycardia and headache
   C. tinnitus and blurred vision
   D. EKG changes and confusion

6. The nurse, who is administering antidepressant medication to a patient, understands that one major difference between the selective serotonin reuptake inhibitors (SSRIs) and the tricyclic antidepressants (TCAs) is which of the following?
   A. SSRIs are more effective than TCAs in relieving depressive symptoms.
   B. SSRIs produce a more sedative effect on patients than do the TCAs.
   C. TCAs are lethal in overdose, and SSRIs are relatively safe.
   D. TCAs have fewer cardiovascular effects than do SSRIs.

ALTERNATE FORMAT

7. The patient is being treated for depression with imipramine hydrochloride (Tofranil) 200 mg orally per day, with one half of the dose taken in the morning and one half of the dose taken in the evening. The pharmacist dispenses Tofranil 25 mg tablets. How many tablets would the nurse administer to the patient in the morning?

   _____

ALTERNATE FORMAT

8. The nurse is providing care for a patient who is prescribed olanzapine (Zyprexa) 7.5 mg daily by mouth for schizophrenia. The pharmacy dispenses the drug as 2.5 mg tablets. How many tablets must be dispensed for the ordered dose?

_____

9. The nurse is providing care for a patient prior to an electroconvulsive therapy (ECT) treatment. The nurse administers a drug to reduce secretions and protect against vagal bradycardia. Which of the following medications was administered by the nurse?
   A. diphenhydramine (Benadryl)
   B. atropine
   C. epinephrine (Adrenalin)
   D. fluoxetine (Prozac)

10. Which of the following physical manifestations is related to side effects of anti-cholinergic medications?
    A. diarrhea
    B. vomiting
    C. dry mouth
    D. polyuria

11. The nurse is caring for a patient who is ordered, "haloperidol 4 mg orally now." An oral suspension of "haloperidol 2 mg/mL" is received from pharmacy. How much oral suspension should the nurse administer to the patient?
    A. 0.5 mL
    B. 1 mL
    C. 2 mL
    D. 4 mL

12. The nurse knows that sedation is a side effect of antipsychotics. Therefore, which of the following medications should the nurse question if ordered for a patient taking antipsychotics?
    A. diphenoxylate hydrochloride (Lomotil)
    B. acetaminophen (Tylenol)
    C. verapamil (Calan)
    D. diphenhydramine (Benadryl)

13. The nurse is providing teaching about medications to a patient. The patient states that one pill in particular that must be taken every day causes severe drowsiness. Which of the following options would be most reasonable for the nurse to suggest for management of side effects?
    A. Take the medication with at least 6 ounces of milk.
    B. Take ½ pill in the morning and ½ pill at lunch.
    C. Take the pill at any time, but take 7 pills per week.
    D. Take the pill at bedtime to decrease daytime drowsiness.

14. **The nurse is caring for a patient who experiences postural hypotension related to taking chlorpromazine (Thorazine). The nurse should suggest which of the following interventions for managing the side effect?**
   A. Stay in bed for an hour after taking the medication.
   B. Stand quickly, then wait a moment before walking.
   C. Rise slowly when getting out of bed.
   D. Rise from your left side when getting out of bed.

15. **The nurse is providing education for a patient who experiences constipation related to taking tricyclic antidepressants. Which of the following suggestions could the nurse offer to help resolve the constipation?**
   A. Consume a high-carbohydrate diet.
   B. Increase fluid intake to 3 L per day.
   C. Take furosemide (Lasix) 40 mg per day.
   D. Consume a diet high in iron and B_{12}.

16. **Monoamine oxidase inhibitors (MAOI) can cause numbness, prickling, or tingling feelings, which are referred to as:**
   A. orthostatic hypotension.
   B. paresthesias.
   C. edema.
   D. melancholia.

17. **The nurse is caring for a patient who has been prescribed lithium therapy and now has persistent edema. Which of the following medications could be used to manage the edema?**
   A. docusate sodium (Colace)
   B. digoxin (Lanoxin)
   C. furosemide (Lasix)
   D. albuterol (Proventil)

18. **Which of the following drugs represents a class of medications that is considered to be first-line treatment for depression?**
   A. midazolam (Versed)
   B. nortriptyline (Pamelor)
   C. cyclobenzaprine (Flexeril)
   D. valproic acid (Depakene)

ANSWERS

General

1. **(B)**; The nurse must uphold patient confidentiality. Because there is no way to verify the identity of the caller, the nurse cannot provide any information.

2. **(A)**; Negative symptoms of psychosis involve loss of normal functioning. They include *affective flattening*, alogia (restricted thought and speech), avolution/apathy (lack of behavior initiation), and anhedonia/asociality (inability to experience pleasure or maintain social contacts).

3. **(C)**; Serotonin syndrome is a potentially lethal reaction following the use of serotomimetic agents (SSRIs, TCSs) alone or in combination with MAOIs. Treatment is immediate discontinuation of all serotonergic drugs. Anticonvulsants and drugs to counteract specific symptoms (myoclonus) are given as necessary. Symptoms of serotonin syndrome are confusion, mania, agitation, myoclonus, hyperreflexia, diaphoresis, shivering, ataxia, coma, and low-grade fever.

4. **(B)**; Persons with histrionic personality disorder exhibit excessive emotions and behave in a manner that is attention-seeking. Persons with this type of personality disorder view relationships as closer than they actually are; will do something to be in the center of attention; are often sexually provocative in dress and behavior; seek out compliments; dress in expensive clothing; and crave novelty, stimulation, and excitement.

5. **(A, B, D, E)**; Persons with obsessive-compulsive personality disorder are *rigid, perfectionistic*, indecisive, preoccupied with details, lacking in spontaneity, inflexible, and *reluctant to delegate tasks*. They *crave order*. They do not have a need for admiration and are not manipulative.

6. **(A, B, C)**; An assessment of memory should be done before and after treatment. Short-term memory loss is usually transient. Informed consent is required for treatment of voluntary patients. For involuntary patients, permission can be obtained from the next of kin. The patient must be NPO after midnight prior to the procedure. General anesthesia and paralytic agents have dramatically improved patient comfort and safety during the procedure. Restraints are not applied.

7. **(A, B, C, D)**; ECT is indicated for treatment of major depression, bipolar depressive disorder, lithium-resistant mania, and schizophrenia and schizoaffective disorders. ECT is not indicated for treating personality disorders.

8. **(B)**; The 70-year-old (>65) widower (*male*) with metastatic cancer (*terminal illness*) who talks about saving his pain pills (*plan*) is the patient at highest risk for suicide of those presented. The 21-year-old female who lives with her parents and broke up with a boyfriend has one stress but no significant risks for suicide. The 45-year-old married female with a stressful job also has no significant risk for suicide. Although the 35-year-old married man has a potentially terminal illness, he has social support and significant others, which results in reduced risk for suicide.

9. **(A)**; Appropriate nursing interventions for the patient exhibiting psychomotor agitation include: allowing the patient to have space; decreasing environmental stimuli; *providing calming music or sounds*; and setting limits for the patient. If the patient exceeds the limits, the nurse should administer lorazepam (Ativan) as ordered.

10. **(C)**; The alcohol-dependent patient is likely to develop cirrhosis of the liver.

11. **(B)**; Depression is a comorbidity associated with eating disorders.

12. **(A)**; The nurse realizes that safety is a priority for care of the patient diagnosed with major depression because the patient is likely to be at risk for suicide.

13. **(A)**; Depressed mood and anhedonia (loss of interest or pleasure in activities) are the primary symptoms of major depression.

14. **(A)**; The nurse recognizes that the patient is showing improvement because of both the increased appetite and increasing socialization.

15. **(D)**; Thought broadcasting and thought withdrawal are disturbed thought processes.

16. **(C)**; This patient displays symptoms of obsessive-compulsive personality. Patients with this disorder crave control, value perfection, have excessive devotion to work, experience difficulty relaxing, demonstrate rule-conscious behavior, and have an inability to discard anything.

17. **(C)**; Daily routines and large clocks facilitate patients' functional status.

18. **(D)**; Privacy and autonomy are sacrificed by the patient for the sake of safety.

19. **(A)**; Stalking behaviors should be reported to police promptly for safety purposes.

20. **(B)**; Usual stressors involve work and relationships.

21. **(A, B, C)**; Lasting friendships are a support mechanism and do not increase risk for suicide.

22. **(A)**; Occupational therapy focuses on tasks particular to work and jobs. Electroconvulsive therapy is therapy for mental illness, family therapy deals with family issues, and group therapy focuses on the dynamics within groups.

23. **(B)**; Under the "Tarasoff ruling," the treatment team has a duty to warn the ex-wife of the threat.

24. **(C)**; When a patient has had control of seizures for two years and then begins having seizures again, the nurse should question the patient's compliance with the medication regime.

25. **(C)**; It can take up to 4 weeks for therapeutic effects to occur.

26. **(C)**; Nardil is a monoamine oxidase inhibitor (MAOI). Patients who eat restricted foods may develop a life-threatening hypertensive crisis.

27. **(C)**; The MMSE is used to assess orientation, attention span, recall, and ability to execute simple instructions. Delirium, dementia, and thinking are assessed by the Confusion Assessment Method (CAM), which also assesses acute and fluctuating courses of the condition and altered level of consciousness.

Physical Assessment

1. **(A, B, E, F)**; Extrapyramidal side effects of the central nervous system are involved in the production and control of involuntary and gross motor movements producing *acute dystonia, akathisia, dyskinesia,* and *Parkinsonism.* Amenorrhea, breast secretion, and sexual dysfunction are endocrine-related side effects of the drug.

2. **(A, B, C, D)**; The nurse who is assessing a patient with schizophrenia should perform a detailed assessment of the patient's hallucinations. Questions that the nurse should ask include: *How many different voices speak to you? What do they say? Do you recognize the voices?* When did you first hear the voices? How do you respond to the voices? *What gives you relief?*

3. **(A)**; Safety is a priority, so the nurse must physically search the patient for weapons and harmful materials because the patient made a suicide attempt just prior to arrival. The nurse would not notify the patient's employer because of confidentiality. Lorazepam is not indicated for this patient.

Interpretation of Lab Values

1. **(D)**; A serum lithium level of 2.0 mEq/L is within the toxic range. Lithium has a low therapeutic index, which means that toxicity can occur when levels rise only slightly above normal. For initial therapy of a manic episode, lithium levels may range from 0.8–1.4 mEq/L.

   However, when the therapeutic effect has been achieved, dosage should be decreased to ensure maintenance serum levels of 0.4–1.0 mEq/L.

2. **(C)**; The patient who is intubated and on a ventilator needs to have ABGs drawn periodically to assess for adequacy of ventilation and ability to wean.

Drugs and Treatments

1. **(D)**; The patient indicates that sunscreen is required when going outside on sunny days. This should help the patient to avoid pigmentation changes.

2. **(Neuroleptic malignant syndrome)**; Neuroleptic malignant syndrome occurs in about 0.2 to 1% of patients who take antipsychotic medications. The syndrome is fatal in about 10% of cases. Neuroleptic malignant syndrome is characterized by decreased level of consciousness, muscle rigidity, hyperpyrexia, labile hypertension, tachycardia, tachypnea, diaphoresis, and drooling. Treatment involves early detection and discontinuation of the drug as well as stabilizing the patient medically.

3. **(A)**; Disulfiram works by conditioning the patient not to drink alcohol or the patient will suffer very unpleasant effects from the alcohol–disulfiram reaction. These effects include flushing of the face, sweating, throbbing headache, neck pain, tachycardia, respiratory distress, nausea and vomiting, and a potentially serious drop in blood pressure.

4. **(C)**; Phenelzine (Nardil) is an MAOI drug. Consumption of dietary tyramine by patients taking MAOIs can produce hypertensive crisis. Foods containing high amounts of dietary tyramine include: *avocados*, figs, bananas, *smoked or aged meats*, liver, dried or cured fish, almost all *cheese*, yeast extract, some imported beers, soups, and soy sauce.

5. **(A)**; Persistent *polyuria* and thirst occur in 30 to 50% of patients. Many patients may also develop a persistent *fine hand tremor* that may interfere with writing. Patients who are prescribed lithium therapy should be aware that several adverse effects related to the GI system (nausea, diarrhea, abdominal bloating, anorexia) occur early in treatment but normally disappear with time. About 1 in 3 patients experiences *transient* fatigue, muscle weakness, headache, confusion, and memory impairment.

6. **(C)**; TCAs are lethal in overdose, and SSRIs are fairly safe. Both categories of drugs are equally effective in relieving depressive symptoms. TCAs have more sedative and cardiovascular effects than do SSRIs.

7. **(100 mg in the morning = 4 tablets)**

8. $\left(\dfrac{7.5\,\dfrac{mg}{dose}}{2.5\,\dfrac{mg}{tablet}} = 3 \text{ tablets for the dose} \right)$

9. **(B)**; Atropine has a vagolytic effect and selectively blocks the CNS.

10. **(C)**; Common side effects of anticholinergics include *dry mouth*, blurred vision, urinary retention, and constipation.

11. **(C)**; $\dfrac{4\text{ mg}}{2\frac{\text{mg}}{\text{mL}}} = 2\text{ mL}$

12. **(D)**; Diphenhydramine (Benadryl) is an antihistamine that is likely to enhance the sedative effects of antipsychotic medications. Alcohol and other sleeping aids should also be avoided by the patient taking antipsychotic medications.

13. **(D)**; Taking the pill at night will diminish daytime drowsiness.

14. **(C)**; Sudden position changes lead to dizziness associated with postural hypotension.

15. **(B)**; Increased fluids will help to add bulk to the stool.

16. **(B)**; MAOI-induced paresthesias are a result of vitamin B_6 (pyridoxine) deficiency.

17. **(C)**; Furosemide (Lasix) is a diuretic that could be used to manage edema.

18. **(B)**; Nortriptyline (Pamelor) is a tricyclic antidepressant.

Keep Track

- Percent correct. (Divide the number of questions you answered correctly by the total number of questions you answered.) _____

- Number of questions you missed due to a reading error: _____

- Number of questions you missed due to errors in analysis: _____

- Number of assessment questions you missed: _____

- Number of lab value questions you missed: _____

- Number of drug/treatment questions you missed: _____

Nugget List

Chapter number _____ Topic _____

Practice Test: Nursing Management of Patients with Renal and Urinary Tract Disorders

Karen S. March

PRACTICE TEST

General

ALTERNATE FORMAT

1. The nurse understands that the kidneys are responsible for which of the following bodily functions? SELECT ALL THAT APPLY.
   A. production of erythropoietin
   B. regulation of calcium and phosphate
   C. secretion of mineralocorticoids
   D. elimination of metabolic wastes

2. The nurse is providing care for a patient diagnosed with acute glomerulonephritis. The patient asks the nurse, "What causes this disorder?" The best response by the nurse is which of the following?
   A. "It is caused by inflammation of the walls of the glomerulus."
   B. "It often occurs after a respiratory infection with *streptococcus.*"
   C. "It can result from extremely high intake of dietary protein."
   D. "There are no clearly established risk factors for the disease."

3. The nurse is providing care for a patient who was diagnosed with acute tubular necrosis. It is most important for the nurse to:
   A. practice good aseptic technique at all times.
   B. closely monitor fluid and electrolyte balance.
   C. allow for periods of rest between activity.
   D. encourage foods containing sodium and potassium.

4. The nurse is providing care for a patient who was recently diagnosed with renal carcinoma. In planning care for the patient, the nurse understands which of the following about the prognosis?
   A. Prognosis is very good with surgical resection.
   B. Prognosis is good with surgical removal of the nephron.
   C. Prognosis is uncertain with radiation alone.
   D. Prognosis is poor because disease is advanced.

5. The nurse is providing care for a young female patient with polycystic kidney disease who plans to marry soon. The patient asks the nurse, "Can the polycystic disease be passed on to my children?" The best response by the nurse is which of the following?
   A. "It would be a good idea for you to consider seeking genetic counseling."
   B. "Each of your children will have a 1 in 4 chance of inheriting the disease."
   C. "Your children will not be at risk for the disease unless your spouse has it."
   D. "Polycystic kidney disease is inherited as an autosomal recessive trait."

6. The nurse is providing care for a patient who has a nephrostomy tube. Care of this patient should include which of the following?
   A. flushing the nephrostomy tube every four hours with sterile saline
   B. intermittently clamping the nephrostomy tube to establish continence
   C. assessing skin at the nephrostomy site for irritation due to urine leakage
   D. priming the nephrostomy tubing every 2 hours to maintain flow

7. The nurse is assigned to care for a patient with the diagnosis of pyelonephritis. The nurse provides teaching about prevention of future episodes of pyelonephritis based on the knowledge that:
   A. the disorder occurs more normally in men.
   B. normal GI bacteria cause the disorder.
   C. large amounts of fluid intake can prevent it.
   D. each episode causes prerenal azotemia.

8. The nurse caring for the patient with pyelonephritis must provide education about the disorder. It would be most appropriate for the nurse to focus on which of the following teaching points?
   A. the importance of douching after having sex
   B. wiping front to back after each elimination
   C. taking long-term intravenous antibiotics
   D. collecting a 24-hour urine specimen

ALTERNATE FORMAT

9. The nurse is providing care for a patient who is scheduled for a nephrectomy. The nurse understands that preoperative teaching must include which of the following points? SELECT ALL THAT APPLY.
   A. postoperative coughing and deep breathing
   B. proper use of the incentive spirometer
   C. postoperative pain control
   D. postoperative fluid restrictions

10. The nurse is assigned to care for a patient who has recently returned from the operating room after having had a right nephrectomy. Which of the following indicates a successful outcome for the patient?
    A. The patient is writhing with pain in bed upon arrival from surgery.
    B. The chest X-ray reveals consolidation in the right lower lobe.
    C. Urinary output is 45 to 60 mL per hour on a consistent basis.
    D. The abdomen is slightly distended and silent in all 4 quadrants.

11. The nurse understands that the patient who has undergone a nephrectomy is most at risk for which of the following problems postoperatively?
    A. heart failure
    B. atelectasis
    C. infection
    D. venous thrombosis

12. The nurse is caring for a patient in renal failure who has developed anasarca. Based on this information, the nurse understands that a priority nursing diagnosis for the patient is which of the following?
    A. risk for infection
    B. risk for impaired skin integrity
    C. altered comfort
    D. pain

ALTERNATE FORMAT

13. The nurse is providing care for an elderly patient who was admitted for short-term hospitalization following elective surgery. Upon reviewing the patient's medication record, the nurse becomes concerned about administering which of the following medications to this patient? SELECT ALL THAT APPLY.
    A. furosemide (Lasix)
    B. ketorolac (Toradol)
    C. vancomycin
    D. acetaminophen (Tylenol)

14. The nurse understands that heart failure, hemorrhage, and shock are examples of possible etiologic factors in the development of which type of renal failure?
    A. prerenal
    B. intrinsic
    C. postrenal
    D. prerenal and postrenal

15. The oliguric/anuric stage of acute renal failure begins when the urine output falls below _____ mL/24 hours.
    A. 50
    B. 100
    C. 200
    D. 400

16. The nurse understands that vasospasm of the renal arteries has which of the following effects on blood flow?
    A. results in renal ischemia
    B. results in vasodilation
    C. causes renal artery thrombosis
    D. produces decreased vascular resistance

17. The nurse explains to the patient with prerenal azotemia that the condition:
    A. began at a time prior to the onset of symptoms.
    B. is caused by interference with renal perfusion.
    C. exists between the time of insult and onset of ischemia.
    D. is failure caused by obstruction within the kidneys.

ALTERNATE FORMAT

18. The nurse is providing education to the patient about collection of a 24-hour urine specimen for creatinine clearance. Please place in correct order the steps of the process.
    A. Collect all urine in a bottle on ice at bedside.
    B. Have the patient void to empty the bladder and discard the urine.
    C. Post signs with start and end of collection times.
    D. Instruct the patient not to dump or flush urine during the collection.
    E. Have the patient void to empty the bladder and save the urine.

19. When caring for a patient in renal failure, the nurse would expect elevated levels of which of the following electrolytes?
    A. potassium, phosphate, magnesium
    B. calcium, potassium, phosphate
    C. bicarbonate, calcium, magnesium
    D. chloride, sodium, phosphate

20. The nurse knows that the most common cause of intrinsic renal failure is which of the following?
    A. pyelonephritis
    B. renal calculi
    C. glomerulonephritis
    D. acute tubular necrosis

21. The nurse is caring for a patient who has developed prerenal azotemia. The nurse understands that the primary focus of treatment will be to:
    A. restore renal circulation.
    B. control serum potassium levels.
    C. remove the enlarged prostate.
    D. inspect the urine for gravel and hematuria.

22. The nurse is providing care for a patient who has entered the diuretic phase of acute renal failure. The nurse understands that an important aspect of care during this phase will involve:
    A. relieving symptoms of uremia.
    B. measuring serum potassium levels.
    C. monitoring oxygen saturation.
    D. maintaining fluid and electrolyte balance.

23. The nurse is caring for a patient in acute renal failure. The patient has begun to manifest some muscle twitching and tingling. The EKG reveals some dysrhythmias. The patient is most likely experiencing:
    A. hyperkalemia.
    B. hyperphosphatemia.
    C. hypomagnesemia.
    D. hypocalcemia.

24. The nurse is caring for a patient who has just been diagnosed with acute postrenal failure. The nurse understands that which of the following is a most likely cause?
    A. hemorrhage
    B. prostatic hypertrophy
    C. sepsis
    D. acute pyelonephritis

25. The nurse, who is caring for a patient in acute renal failure, documents in the patient's chart a urine output of 300 mL over the past 24 hours. The nurse understands that the patient is experiencing what phase of acute renal failure?
    A. initiation
    B. oliguric/anuric
    C. diuretic
    D. recovery

26. The nurse understands that a common cause of nephrotoxic intrinsic renal failure is which of the following?
    A. gentamicin
    B. potassium chloride
    C. sepsis
    D. renal calculi

27. The nurse is assigned to a patient who is having a 24-hour urine collected for analysis of creatinine clearance. In the midst of a busy shift and 23 hours into the collection, a voided specimen is inadvertently discarded. The nurse realizes that which of the following measures is required to rectify the situation?
    A. Discard all urine and start the collection again.
    B. Reduce the collection period to 23 hours.
    C. Continue the collection, noting the loss.
    D. Document the exact time and send all urine to the lab.

28. The patient is scheduled for a cystoscopy with biopsy. Prior to the test, the patient asks the nurse for more information about the test. The best response by the nurse is which of the following?
    A. "Cystoscopy allows the physician to look closely at the kidneys and tubules."
    B. "Cystoscopy allows the physician to look closely at the bladder."
    C. "I'll call the radiologist to come and tell you more about the test."
    D. "You will receive more information in the department when you arrive for the test."

29. The nurse is caring for a patient who has been diagnosed with stage III cancer of the bladder. The patient is scheduled for a cystectomy with ureterostomy. Which of the following statements about the patient's follow-up care is correct?
    A. The patient will need to self-catheterize at regular intervals.
    B. The patient will have an abdominal stoma for urinary drainage.
    C. The patient will have a nephrostomy tube placed to drain urine.
    D. The patient will have a number of options available for long-term treatment.

30. The nurse understands that most renal calculi are composed of which of the following materials?
   A. calcium
   B. uric acid
   C. sulfuric acid
   D. sodium chloride

31. The nurse is assigned to care for a patient who is admitted to the hospital with a diagnosis of renal calculi. The nurse anticipates that the patient will exhibit which of the following symptoms?
   A. nausea, headache, fasciculations
   B. anxiety, excruciating pain, ketonuria
   C. dull, diffuse pain, nausea, vomiting
   D. dull, diffuse pain, proteinuria, hematuria

32. The nurse is caring for a patient who has just returned to the floor following extracorporeal shock wave lithotripsy. Which of the following interventions is not appropriate for this patient?
   A. Strain all urine and send gravel to the lab for analysis.
   B. Encourage fluid intake of 2–4 liters per day.
   C. Immediately report hematuria to the physician.
   D. Encourage ambulation to aid passage of calculi fragments.

33. The nurse knows that the most common symptom in patients with cancer of the bladder is which of the following?
   A. diuresis
   B. oliguria
   C. pain
   D. hematuria

34. The nurse understands that the incidence of glomerulonephritis could be decreased if there was more public education about:
   A. proper treatment of pneumonia.
   B. proper treatment of strep throat.
   C. flu vaccine to prevent influenza.
   D. proper hygiene to prevent cystitis.

35. The nurse is providing education to the patient who has had renal calculi composed of uric acid. The nurse knows that the patient should include which of the following foods in the diet?
   A. organ meats, eggs, cheese
   B. dairy products, grains, prunes
   C. peaches, green beans, legumes
   D. peanuts, blueberries, milk

36. During a routine health history a young male patient informs the nurse that he has recently noticed that his urine is a deep yellow color and is very foamy. The nurse immediately recognizes that this may be a sign of which of the following?
   A. hematuria
   B. hyperbilirubinuria
   C. proteinuria
   D. glycosuria

37. The nurse has an order to straight cath a patient for residual urine following each void. The nurse understands which of the following facts about postvoid residual urine volumes?
    A. Volumes less than or = 200 mL indicate normal bladder function.
    B. Volumes greater than 200 mL are anticipated in elderly, incontinent patients.
    C. Volumes less than or = 50 mL indicate near-normal bladder function.
    D. Volumes less than or = 50 mL indicate predisposition to UTI's.

38. The nurse who is caring for a child with nephrotic syndrome should include which of the following as a priority intervention in the plan of care?
    A. Restrict oral fluids to half maintenance.
    B. Prevent palpation of the tumor.
    C. Provide a low-protein, no-salt diet.
    D. Perform urine dipstick test every shift.

39. The nurse realizes that the parents of a child with nephrotic syndrome need further reinforcement of discharge instructions when they state which of the following?
    A. "We will be happy about any weight gain because that is normal."
    B. "We need to provide our toddler with a low salt diet when there's edema."
    C. "We need to test our child's urine for protein frequently at home."
    D. "We should give our child the prednisone with meals or milk."

40. The parent of a child hospitalized with acute glomerulonephritis asks the nurse why blood pressure readings are checked so frequently. The nurse's reply should be based on which of the following points of knowledge about the disease?
    A. Blood pressure fluctuations are a common side effect of antibiotic therapy.
    B. Blood pressure fluctuations indicate when the condition has become chronic.
    C. Acute hypertension is likely and should be treated early and aggressively.
    D. Hypotension leading to sudden shock can develop at any time.

41. The nurse should identify which of the following expected outcomes for the hospitalized toddler with nephrotic syndrome?
    A. The child will have decreased albuminemia.
    B. The child will have decreased proteinuria.
    C. The child will have increased urine specific gravity.
    D. The child will have increased blood urea nitrogen.

Physical Assessment

1. The nurse is caring for a patient who is diagnosed with acute glomerulonephritis. Upon review of laboratory results and assessment of the patient, the nurse would expect to find which of the following?
   A. anuria and +4 pitting edema of the lower extremities
   B. proteinuria, hematuria, and azotemia
   C. BP 190/110; serum creatinine 1.0; U/O 1620 mL/day
   D. urine cultures positive with *pseudomonas* or *streptococcus*

2. In caring for a patient with acute tubular necrosis, the nurse must frequently assess for which of the following complications?
A. diuresis
B. severe dehydration
C. fever
D. hemorrhage

3. The nurse is assigned to care for a patient with newly diagnosed polycystic kidney disease. Upon assessment of the patient, the nurse may expect which of the following signs and symptoms?
A. lumbar pain, tender abdomen, and abdominal pain
B. oliguria, fever > 101.5°F, WBCs in the urinalysis
C. anuria, low-grade fever, presence of ketones in the urine
D. sharp flank pain, hard palpable bladder, hematuria

4. The nurse is assigned to care for a patient diagnosed with pyelonephritis. Based on the diagnosis, the nurse anticipates that the patient will manifest which of the following signs and symptoms?
A. T 102.8°F, chills, flank pain
B. T 100.2°F, abdominal discomfort
C. retroperitoneal discomfort, hematuria
D. bladder tenderness and fullness

5. The nurse assesses the patient for symptoms of hypocalcemia by:
A. tapping the acromion process.
B. tapping the facial nerve.
C. applying a blood pressure cuff to the lower leg.
D. monitoring the patient's blood pressure very closely.

6. The nurse assesses a patient who has experienced weight gain within 24 hours and has edema, jugular venous distention, increased blood pressure, and oliguria. The nurse understands that these findings suggest which type of renal failure?
A. prerenal
B. intrinsic
C. postrenal
D. toxic

7. The nurse is assessing a patient 4 hours after surgery. The patient had an ileal conduit created, and the nurse notes that the stoma is bright red and swollen. Which of the following actions by the nurse is most appropriate?
A. Remove the drainage pouch to increase blood supply to the area.
B. Continue to assess the stoma every hour for the remainder of the shift.
C. Remove the pouch every 2 hours to expose it to air.
D. Notify the surgeon of this abnormal finding immediately.

8. The nurse must assess the patency of a patient's arteriovenous fistula. Which of the following techniques should be used by the nurse for assessment?
A. Auscultate for a bruit, palpate for a thrill.
B. Palpate for a bruit, auscultate for a thrill.
C. Irrigate the access site with normal saline.
D. Assess for the presence of distal pulses.

Interpretation of Lab Values

1. The nurse is caring for a patient with acute glomerulonephritis. Upon reviewing laboratory results, the nurse would expect to find which of the following results on the urinalysis?
   A. clear yellow with occasional bacteria
   B. cloudy yellow with many bacteria
   C. positive RBCs and positive albumin
   D. positive RBCs without albumin

2. The nurse expects which of the following laboratory results from a patient with renal failure?
   A. K$^+$ 5.8 mEq/L; Mg^{++} 3.2 mg/dL; Ca^{++} 7.9 mg/dL
   B. K$^+$ 5.8 mEq/L; Mg^{++} 2.0 mg/dL; Ca^{++} 9.0 mg/dL
   C. K$^+$ 4.2 mEq/L; Mg^{++} 2.2 mg/dL; Ca^{++} 9.2 mg/dL
   D. K$^+$ 4.6 mEq/L; Mg^{++} 2.0 mg/dL; Ca^{++} 11 mg/dL

3. The nurse understands that which of the following lab values provides the most accurate reflection of renal damage?
   A. BUN
   B. serum creatinine
   C. urine osmolality
   D. urinary creatinine clearance

4. The nurse receives urine culture and sensitivity results from a clean catch specimen provided by a female patient. The report indicates that there were 10,000 organisms per mL. The nurse understands that these results:
   A. are diagnostic for urinary tract infection.
   B. suggest contamination of the specimen.
   C. are inconclusive for diagnosis.
   D. should be reported to the physician.

5. The nurse is assigned to care for a 3-year-old child admitted with the tentative diagnosis of nephrotic syndrome. According to the child's mother, the child has not been feeling well for several weeks. The child has been irritable and withdrawn and has not eaten well for the past week. Which of the following clinical profiles would substantiate the tentative diagnosis?
   A. hyperlipidemia, hypertension, hyperthermia
   B. hematuria, hypertension, glycosuria
   C. hyperlipidemia, proteinuria, hypoalbuminemia
   D. proteinuria, polyuria, hyperalbuminemia

Drugs and Treatments

1. The nurse understands that initial treatment of the patient with acute tubular necrosis may include which of the following?
   A. hemodialysis and large doses of diuretics
   B. large volumes of fluid followed by diuretics
   C. fluid restrictions and daily hydrotherapy
   D. fluid challenges and intravenous antibiotics

2. The nurse providing care for a patient diagnosed with pyelonephritis recognizes which of the following medications as common therapy for the disease?
   A. furosemide (Lasix)
   B. levofloxacin (Levaquin)
   C. methylprednisolone (SoluMedrol)
   D. piperacillin and tazobactam (Zosyn)

3. The nurse is assigned to care for a patient with renal carcinoma. The nurse provides teaching with the understanding that treatment will involve which of the following?
   A. surgical removal of the kidney
   B. targeted radiation therapy
   C. continuous chemotherapy regimen
   D. surgery, radiation, and chemotherapy

4. The nurse is assigned to a patient who is diagnosed with acute renal failure. The nurse understands the most effective means of fluid removal in a patient with hemodynamic instability is which of the following?
   A. daily hemodialysis
   B. continuous renal replacement therapy
   C. continuous electrolyte replacement therapy
   D. fluid restriction and diuretics

5. The nurse is providing care for a patient in acute renal failure with a serum potassium level of 6.5 mEq/L. The nurse understands that optimal care for this patient calls for which of the following measures to achieve a normal serum potassium?
   A. administration of IV potassium
   B. administration of IV phosphorus
   C. administration of $D_{50}W$ and IV insulin
   D. administration of IV furosemide (Lasix)

6. The nurse is providing education to the patient with renal failure prior to discharge. The nurse instructs the patient to follow which of the following dietary guidelines to prevent further progression of the disease?
   A. high calorie, low protein, low sodium, low potassium
   B. moderate calorie, low protein, high sodium, low potassium
   C. moderate calorie, moderate protein, high sodium, low potassium
   D. low calorie, high protein, low sodium, high potassium

7. The nurse knows that drugs from all of the following categories are considered to be highly nephrotoxic *except*:
   A. cephalosporins.
   B. aminoglycosides.
   C. cardiac glycosides.
   D. acetaminophen.

8. The nurse is assigned to provide care for a patient who is scheduled for an intravenous pyelogram (IVP) in the morning. In report, the nurse is told that the patient has been NPO in preparation for the test. The nurse understands that, in addition, the prep for the IVP will include which of the following?
    A. ingestion of contrast medium throughout the night prior to the test
    B. administration of enemas to improve visualization of renal structures
    C. a low sodium diet for 24 hours prior to the test to increase hyperosmolarity
    D. insertion of an intravenous line for maintenance of fluid and electrolyte balance

9. When providing discharge teaching for the patient with pyelonephritis, the nurse would include all of the following instructions *except*:
    A. Increase fluid intake to 3–4 L of fluid per day.
    B. Return for re-culture of the urine within one month.
    C. Drink prune juice daily to ensure an acidic urine.
    D. Finish your entire course of antibiotic therapy.

10. The nurse knows that medical management of pyelonephritis consists of administering treatment for infection. The nurse understands that which of the following drugs is not useful for treatment of pyelonephritis?
    A. nitrofurantoin (Macrodantin)
    B. ampicillin and sulbactam (Unasyn)
    C. trimethoprim sulfamethoxazole (Bactrim DS)
    D. ciprofloxacin (Cipro)

ANSWERS

General

ALTERNATE FORMAT

1. **(A, B, D)**; The kidneys help to regulate acid-base balance, *produce erythropoietin*, secrete renin, activate vitamin D, *regulate calcium and phosphate*, regulate extracellular fluid osmolality, and *eliminate metabolic wastes*.

2. **(B)**; Acute glomerulonephritis most commonly occurs within 1 to 3 weeks after an untreated *streptococcus* respiratory infection.

3. **(A)**; The nurse who is caring for the patient with acute tubular necrosis must practice good aseptic technique at all times because infection is life-threatening for patients with acute tubular necrosis.

4. **(D)**; Prognosis is poor for patients with renal carcinoma. About one-fourth of patients have metastases or significantly advanced cancer by the time they develop symptoms and are diagnosed. The cancer is resistant to radiation, and chemotherapy has not been effective.

5. **(A)**; Polycystic kidney disease occurs once in every 500 or so individuals as an autosomal dominant trait. Young adults with polycystic disease should be encouraged to seek genetic counseling because about half of all children born to them will also have the disease.

6. **(C)**; Nursing care for the patient with a nephrostomy tube should include assessment for complications (bleeding, hematuria, fistula formation, and infection), skin integrity (for inflammation, infection, bleeding, urine leakage, and irritation), and tube patency; use of aseptic technique for dressing changes; and encouraging oral intake. A nephrostomy tube should never be clamped and should not be irrigated unless there is a specific order to do so.

7. **(B)**; Because it is normal GI bacteria that typically cause the disorder, women are at greater risk for development than men because of their shorter urethra and the close proximity of the urethra to the rectum.

8. **(B)**; The nurse should reinforce teaching about the importance of wiping from front to back following elimination as a means by which a female patient might decrease the incidence of occurrence of pyelonephritis.

9. **(A, B, C)**; The nurse should discuss with the patient prior to surgery the importance of postoperative coughing and deep breathing, proper use of the incentive spirometer, and a plan for postoperative pain control. The nurse should instruct the patient to request pain medication before the pain becomes severe.

10. **(C)**; Postoperatively, the patient who had a nephrectomy should be able to cough and deep breathe, splint the incision, and use the incentive spirometer as directed. Pain control should be manifested by pain being rated as low (and manageable) on the 0–10 scale. Urine output should be a minimum of 30 mL/hour. The patient should be up and ambulating in the room and hallway as soon as it is tolerable postop. The patient should have clear breath sounds and good oxygenation as demonstrated by SpO_2 > 90%. The patient should have normal, active bowel sounds in all four quadrants.

11. **(B)**; The postoperative nephrectomy patient is most at risk for atelectasis, not only related to general anesthesia, but also as a result of having a flank incision that limits postoperative deep breathing.

12. **(B)**; The nurse understands that a patient with anasarca has total body edema, which implies that skin integrity becomes a priority issue for continued care of the patient.

13. **(B, C, D)**; Individually, ketorolac (Toradol), vancomycin, and acetaminophen (Tylenol) are known nephrotoxic agents. Taken by a postoperative elderly patient, the risk of nephrotoxicity is compounded. Although the risk does not necessarily deem it necessary to discontinue the drugs, it *does* mandate close monitoring of renal function throughout therapy.

14. **(A)**; Heart failure, hemorrhage, and shock all result in decreased perfusion to the kidney and, therefore, are etiologic factors for prerenal failure.

15. **(D)**; Oliguria is defined as urine output of less than 400 mL/24 hr.

16. **(A)**; Vasospasm acts to decrease blood flow to the kidneys and results in ischemia.

17. **(B)**; By definition, prerenal azotemia is caused by situations that result in interference with renal perfusion, such as low cardiac output states.

18. **(D, B, C, A, E)**; The nurse should instruct the patient about the importance of collecting all urine during the test. The nurse should emphasize that any urine lost during

collection means that the test must be started again. The nurse should ask the patient to void to empty the bladder and discard the urine. This will represent the start of the 24-hour collection, which should be noted clearly on signs posted in the room and bathroom. All urine must be collected over the 24-hour period and placed in the bottle on ice at the bedside. The test will end 24 hours from the start time when the nurse again asks the patient to void to empty the bladder. Urine voided at that time is collected to be sent with the full sample to the lab for analysis.

19. **(A)**; The patient in renal failure has hyperkalemia, hyperphosphatemia, and hypermagnesemia.

20. **(D)**; The most common cause of intrinsic renal failure is acute tubular necrosis.

21. **(A)**; Prerenal azotemia develops because there is decreased perfusion to the kidneys. The primary focus for treatment, then, is to restore renal circulation. This may be accomplished by treating hypovolemia, increasing cardiac output, etc.

22. **(D)**; During the diuretic phase, the patient begins to experience increased urine output. When this happens, it is important for the nurse to monitor I&O as well as electrolyte balance.

23. **(D)**; Symptoms of hypocalcemia may include convulsions, carpopedal spasm (positive Trousseau's sign), *dysrhythmias*, EKG changes (prolonged ST segment and QT interval), facial spasm (positive Chvostek's sign), muscle cramps, numbness, tetany, *tingling*, and *muscle twitching*.

24. **(B)**; Of the choices listed, prostatic hypertrophy is the cause of postrenal failure. By definition, conditions that cause postrenal failure cause obstruction to urine flow after the kidney.

25. **(B)**; The patient is in the oliguric/anuric phase of acute renal failure when the total 24-hour urine output is 400 mL or less.

26. **(A)**; Gentamicin is an aminoglycoside, one of the most nephrotoxic classes of drugs. Potassium is not nephrotoxic. Sepsis may cause prerenal failure related to decreased perfusion to the kidneys. Renal calculi may cause postrenal failure related to obstruction of urine flow.

27. **(A)**; When any urine specimen is inadvertently discarded during a 24-hour specimen collection, the entire collection must be discarded and the sample must be started again.

28. **(B)**; The nurse would begin by telling the patient some basic information about the test, such as what information it provides.

29. **(B)**; Stage III means that cancer cells have spread into the outer layer of tissue surrounding the bladder and may have spread to surrounding structures, but it has not spread to lymph nodes or metastasized. Tumors that have infiltrated surrounding tissues require a radical cystectomy—removal of the bladder—and other adjacent structures. A urinary diversion must be created. One frequently used method involves using a segment of ileum to construct a pouch that opens at the skin surface on the abdomen. This is called an ileal conduit.

30. **(A)**; Eighty percent of calculi are composed of calcium.

31. **(C)**; The pain associated with renal calculi can be severe and colicky—traveling from the costovertebral angle to the flank and then to the suprapubic area and genitalia. If the calculi remain in the renal pelvis, however, the pain will be more dull and diffuse in nature. Patients frequently become nauseous and vomit because of the severity of the pain.

32. **(C)**; Slight hematuria is common and expected following lithotripsy. There is no need to notify the physician about hematuria unless bleeding is persistent.

33. **(D)**; The first sign of cancer of the bladder is frequently painless, intermittent hematuria.

34. **(B)**; Glomerulonephritis most commonly follows an infection (usually respiratory) with *streptococcus*. Therefore, if the public were more aware of the importance of appropriate treatment for severe sore throat (probable strep), the incidence of this insult to the kidneys might be reduced.

35. **(C)**; The patient should be encouraged to follow an alkaline–ash diet, which includes *legumes*, milk and milk products, *green vegetables*, rhubarb, and *fruits* (except for cranberries, plums, grapes, and prunes).

36. **(C)**; The nurse recognizes that the foamy description of the urine may mean that the patient is experiencing proteinuria. Under normal conditions, there are no signs or symptoms in the early stages except that it may appear foamy as a patient voids into the toilet.

37. **(C)**; Postvoid residual volumes of more than 50 mL indicate urinary retention.

38. **(D)**; The nurse should check the urine for protein content via dipstick every shift to monitor progress during treatment.

39. **(A)**; It is vital that the parents know the importance of reporting weight gain promptly so that further treatment can be instituted early if necessary.

40. **(C)**; It should be expected that children with acute glomerulonephritis will develop hypertension, and it is important that it is identified early so that definitive treatment can begin.

41. **(B)**; The nurse should expect that, with treatment, the child will have decreased proteinuria—loss of protein in the urine.

Physical Assessment

1. **(B)**; The patient with acute glomerulonephritis will have symptoms that may include oliguria, *proteinuria, hematuria, azotemia,* and mild edema.

2. **(C)**; Patients with acute tubular necrosis are at risk of death from infection. The nurse must frequently assess for fever, and any signs of infection must be treated promptly with appropriate antibiotics.

3. **(A)**; Polycystic kidney disease is challenging to diagnose because early symptoms are nonspecific. Over time, however, the patient will develop signs and symptoms related to kidney enlargement, including lumbar pain, tender abdomen, and abdominal pain that is relieved by lying down.

4. **(A)**; The patient appears acutely ill and usually experiences a high fever, chills, flank pain, and fatigue with pyelonephritis.

5. **(B)**; The nurse can assess the patient for symptoms of hypocalcemia by tapping on the facial nerve to try to elicit a positive Chvostek's sign. The nurse could also apply a blood pressure cuff to the lower forearm, inflate it, and leave it inflated for a brief time to try to elicit a positive Trousseau's sign. The nurse should, of course, also monitor lab results.

6. **(B)**; The patient is manifesting symptoms of intrinsic renal failure.

7. **(B)**; The nurse should continue to assess the stoma hourly for the remainder of the shift. The stoma appearance is normal at this time.

8. **(A)**; The nurse should auscultate (listen) for a bruit and palpate (feel) for a thrill.

Interpretation of Lab Values

1. **(C)**; Glomeruli and nephrons degenerate in acute glomerulonephritis. Remaining glomeruli become permeable and allow RBCs and albumin to appear in the urine. There is no pus formation or any bacteria.

2. **(A)**; The patient in renal failure exhibits the following electrolyte imbalances: ↑ K^+ (> 5.0 mEq/L); ↑ Mg^{++} (> 3.0 mg/dL); and ↓ Ca^{++} (< 8.5 mg/dL).

3. **(D)**; Urinary creatinine clearance provides the most accurate information about the glomerular filtration rate (GFR), which provides insight into the progress and severity of renal failure. When the GFR is impaired, serum creatinine rises and creatinine clearance falls. In the absence of urine output, we look at serum creatinine levels.

4. **(B)**; For female patients, evidence of urinary tract infection is determined based on cultures that yield at least 100,000 bacteria per milliliter. Fewer organisms suggests contamination of the specimen during collection rather than UTI.

5. **(C)**; Classic signs of nephrotic syndrome include hyperlipidemia, massive proteinuria, edema, and hypoalbuminemia.

Drugs and Treatments

1. **(B)**; Initial treatment of acute tubular necrosis may involve administration of large volumes of fluid followed by a diuretic to flush the debris from the renal tubules.

2. **(B)**; Antibiotics commonly used for treatment of pyelonephritis include sulfa drugs (Bactrim), cephalosporins (Maxipime, Ceclor), amoxicillin, *levofloxacin*, and ciprofloxacin.

3. **(A)**; The primary treatment for renal cancer is surgical removal of the kidney. Radiation is not particularly effective in treatment and is used only if the cancer has metastasized to regional lymph nodes. Likewise, chemotherapy has not been effective. There seems to be some promise in biotherapy using lymphokine-activated killer cells with recombinant interleukin-2, but patients suffer severe adverse reactions.

4. **(B)**; Continuous renal replacement therapy is the most desirable method of fluid removal in the hemodynamically unstable patient with acute renal failure. The

method is far more tolerable than hemodialysis because fluid removal is more gradual and controlled.

5. **(C)**; A serum potassium level of 6.5 mEq/L constitutes hyperkalemia, a potentially life-threatening electrolyte imbalance. The nurse understands that measures must be taken to reduce the serum potassium level immediately. The desired result can be achieved by administering $D_{50}W$ and IV insulin, IV calcium, oral or rectal kayexalate (a potassium exchange resin), or by hemodialysis.

6. **(A)**; The nurse should encourage the patient with renal failure to adhere to a high-calorie, low-protein (up to 0.5 g/kg body wt), low-sodium (2–3 g/day) and low-potassium (25–40 mEq/day) diet. The teaching by the nurse should be reinforced with sample menus for the patient and significant other to follow when beginning the dietary regimen.

7. **(C)**; Cephalosporins, aminoglycosides, and acetaminophen are all nephrotoxic drugs. Cardiac glycosides do not exhibit nephrotoxic properties.

8. **(B)**; The patient who is scheduled for an IVP should have a bowel prep of cathartics for 24 hours and an evacuation enema 8 hours prior to the test to cleanse the bowel, thereby providing better visualization of renal structures during the test.

9. **(C)**; The nurse should include instructions to increase fluid intake to help flush out bacteria, to return for re-culture, and to finish the entire course of antibiotics. Prune juice is not prescribed for anything related to pyelonephritis.

10. **(B)**; Unasyn is not indicated for treatment of urinary tract infections. Nitrofurantoin, trimethoprim sulfamethoxazole, and ciprofloxacin are indicated for treatment of urinary tract infections.

Keep Track

- Percent correct. (Divide the number of questions you answered correctly by the total number of questions you answered.) _____

- Number of questions you missed due to a reading error: _____

- Number of questions you missed due to errors in analysis: _____

- Number of assessment questions you missed: _____

- Number of lab value questions you missed: _____

- Number of drug/treatment questions you missed: _____

Nugget List

Chapter number _____ Topic _____

Practice Test: Nursing Management of Patients with Hematologic Disorders

Karen S. March

PRACTICE TEST

General

1. The nurse understands that which of the following factors provides a stimulus for the production of red blood cells (RBCs)?
    A. low Hgb and Hct
    B. normal kidney function
    C. decline of B_{12} levels
    D. tissue hypoxia

2. The nurse knows that red blood cell maturation is dependent upon which of the following vitamins or minerals?
    A. cyanocobalamin
    B. aquaMEPHYTON
    C. thiamine
    D. pyridoxine

3. Which of the following types of blood cells are known for phagocytic activity?
    A. erythrocytes
    B. granulocytes
    C. thrombocytes
    D. lymphocytes

4. The patient asks the nurse why platelets are so important. The best reply by the nurse is which of the following?
    A. "Platelets help the body to fight infection."
    B. "Platelets help to break down clots in the body."
    C. "Platelets plug disruptions in blood vessels."
    D. "Platelets maintain the body's immune status."

5. The nurse is caring for a patient with deep vein thrombosis. The patient asks, "What will happen to the clot?" The best response by the nurse is which of the following?
    A. "The body's fibrinolytic system will work to dissolve the clot eventually."
    B. "The body's hemostatic mechanism will stabilize the clot at its present location."
    C. "The clot will eventually break off in tiny fragments and float into the circulation."
    D. "Treatment with heparin will dissolve the clot and prevent future recurrence."

6. The nurse is caring for a patient who has been diagnosed with liver failure. The nurse anticipates that one of the consequences of the patient's condition is that:
   A. PT is decreased.
   B. PT is increased.
   C. aPTT is decreased.
   D. aPTT is increased.

7. The nurse is providing teaching to a patient about lepirudin (Refludan). Which of the following statements by the patient indicates the need for further instruction?
   A. "I will use a safety razor to shave each day."
   B. "I need to avoid contact sports like football."
   C. "I will wear slippers around the house."
   D. "I will keep my follow-up appointments."

8. The nurse is caring for a patient who will have a bone marrow biopsy obtained from the iliac spine. To which of the following positions should the nurse assist the patient for the test?
   A. ventral decubitus position with legs flexed and arms above the head
   B. lateral decubitus position with top leg flexed and lower leg straight
   C. dorsal recumbent position with both knees flexed and arms at sides
   D. lateral recumbent position with top leg straight and lower leg flexed

9. The nurse is providing education to the patient about bone marrow biopsy. Which of the following teaching points should the nurse be certain to include?
   A. "You won't have discomfort because of heavy sedation for the procedure."
   B. "You will have conscious sedation and minimal discomfort."
   C. "You will experience a sharp, burning pain when the marrow is aspirated."
   D. "You will feel dull, diffuse pain throughout the procedure but it is bearable."

10. The nurse is preparing to administer a unit of packed red blood cells to a patient. Upon carrying the blood into the patient's room, the nurse discovers that the patient's intravenous access is no longer patent. A call is placed to the IV team and the nurse is informed that it will be approximately 30 minutes until someone can come to insert a new line. The most appropriate action by the nurse would be to:
    A. return the unit of packed red blood cells to the laboratory.
    B. place the unit of packed red blood cells in the medication room.
    C. place the unit of packed red blood cells in the refrigerator.
    D. leave the unit of packed red blood cells at the patient's bedside.

ALTERNATE FORMAT

11. The nurse is preparing to administer a unit of packed red blood cells to a patient. Please indicate which of the following must be verified with another nurse:
    SELECT ALL THAT APPLY.
    A. the patient's ID number
    B. the patient's room number
    C. the patient's name
    D. the patient's blood type
    E. the Rh match

12. The nurse is caring for a patient with iron deficiency anemia. During teaching, the nurse should encourage the patient to increase consumption of which of the following foods?
    A. spinach, pinto beans, liver
    B. oranges, cranberries, avocado
    C. whole grain bread, fish, tomatoes
    D. whole milk, cheese, grapes

13. The nurse is caring for a patient who is newly diagnosed with pernicious anemia. The nurse recognizes this as a deficiency of:
    A. thiamine.
    B. riboflavin.
    C. pyridoxine.
    D. cyanocobalamin.

14. The patient with pernicious anemia should be encouraged to include which of the following foods in the diet?
    A. milk, eggs, meat
    B. celery, sweet potato, spinach
    C. green beans, squash, salmon
    D. fish, cheese, citrus fruits

15. The nurse is providing discharge education for the patient with aplastic anemia. Which of the following statements by the patient indicates comprehension of the material?
    A. "I need to maintain a good level of activity to prevent deep vein thrombosis."
    B. "If I have a bad headache, I can take aspirin or ibuprofen to get rid of it."
    C. "I can avoid infection by eliminating uncooked foods from my diet for now."
    D. "If it becomes harder to breathe than usual, I should lie down and rest."

16. The nurse is assigned to care for a patient with sickle cell crisis. The nurse knows that the priority nursing diagnosis for this patient is which of the following?
    A. risk for infection
    B. pain
    C. fluid volume overload
    D. impaired mobility

17. The nurse is providing discharge education for the patient with sickle cell crisis. Which of the following statements by the patient indicates the need for further teaching?
    A. "I should try to drink at least 4 to 6 liters of fluid per day."
    B. "I need to learn stress-reduction strategies and use them effectively."
    C. "Physical activity is good for me but I need to avoid overexertion."
    D. "It is okay for me to work at a sawmill during the winter time."

18. The nurse knows that therapeutic management of sickle cell crisis can include all of the following *except*:
    A. pain management.
    B. therapeutic hypothermia.
    C. oxygen administration.
    D. oral hydration.

19. The nurse understands that the abnormality responsible for secondary polycythemia vera lies in:
    A. overproduction of erythrocytes.
    B. excessive production of erythropoietin.
    C. abnormal myelosuppression.
    D. overproduction of leukocytes.

20. The nurse caring for a patient with polycythemia vera knows that nursing measures to prevent complications for this patient should include which of the following?
    A. maintaining adequate hydration
    B. administer packed cells as ordered
    C. administer fresh frozen plasma as ordered
    D. monitor strict intake and output

21. The nurse is providing discharge instructions to the patient with thrombocytopenia. Which of the following statements by the patient indicates understanding of the instructions?
    A. "I won't worry if I get a nosebleed now that I have been treated."
    B. "I will call the doctor if I notice that I get nauseated at mealtimes."
    C. "I will call the doctor if I notice any bruising on my chest or abdomen."
    D. "I have nothing more to worry about because I had my spleen removed."

22. The nurse is providing care for a patient with hemophilia A. The nurse realizes that the patient's deficiency is related to which of the following clotting factors?
    A. VII
    B. VIII
    C. IX
    D. X

23. The nurse is caring for a patient with hemophilia A who is admitted with hemiarthrosis. The nurse anticipates that which of the following will be a priority in therapeutic management of this patient?
    A. monitor for signs of abnormal clotting
    B. administration of aspirin as an analgesic
    C. application of warm soaks for pain control
    D. application of ice to reduce pain

24. The nurse is providing care for a patient with disseminated intravascular coagulation (DIC). The nurse understands that this disorder:
    A. involves abnormal clotting in the periphery.
    B. is precipitated by widespread tissue damage.
    C. occurs only in patients with clotting factor deficiency.
    D. is effectively controlled by infusions of packed cells.

25. The nurse is caring for a patient with neutropenia. A priority nursing diagnosis for this patient would be:
    A. risk for infection.
    B. impaired tissue perfusion.
    C. impaired gas exchange.
    D. decreased cardiac output.

26. The nurse is caring for a patient with neutropenia. Care for the patient will include all of the following *except*:
    A. monitor for temperature elevations.
    B. enforce strict handwashing.
    C. use a private room with HEPA filtration.
    D. add fresh flowers to brighten the room.

Physical Assessment

1. The nurse is caring for a patient following bone marrow aspiration. Upon follow-up assessment, the nurse finds the pressure dressing over the site soaked with blood. Which of the following should the nurse do first?
   A. Remove the original dressing and apply a new pressure dressing.
   B. Notify the physician of excessive bleeding at the site of aspiration.
   C. Assist the patient to a prone position to increase pressure on the dressing.
   D. Assist the patient to a lateral recumbent position to expose the site.

2. The nurse is caring for a patient who is receiving a blood transfusion. About 5 minutes into the transfusion, the patient develops difficulty breathing, pruritis, and urticaria. Vital signs are stable. What should the nurse do first?
   A. Immediately discontinue the entire intravenous site.
   B. Immediately notify the physician and the blood bank.
   C. Immediately stop the infusion and change the IV tubing.
   D. Immediately discard the remaining blood in the unit.

3. The nurse is assessing the patient with pernicious anemia. During assessment the nurse must be especially attentive to deficits within which of the following body systems?
   A. neurologic
   B. gastrointestinal
   C. hepatic
   D. cardiovascular

4. The nurse must assess a patient with folic acid deficiency. Based on the diagnosis, the nurse anticipates which of the following signs or symptoms during assessment?
   A. paresthesias, visual deficits, gait disturbance
   B. progressive weakness, pallor, shortness of breath
   C. constipation, anxiety, forgetfulness
   D. nausea, vomiting, diarrhea

5. The nurse is assigned to care for a patient diagnosed with aplastic anemia. Based on the diagnosis, the nurse would anticipate which of the following signs or symptoms upon assessing this patient?
   A. atypical chest pain
   B. purpura
   C. development of deep vein thrombosis
   D. severe pounding headache

6. **The nurse is assigned to care for a patient with polycythemia vera. Which of the following clinical manifestations does the nurse anticipate?**
   A. distended superficial veins
   B. skin is pink, warm, and dry
   C. dry mucous membranes
   D. pale yellow cast to skin

7. **The nurse caring for a patient with thrombocytopenia anticipates which of the following findings upon performing physical assessment?**
   A. peripheral edema
   B. petechiae
   C. dyspnea
   D. angina

8. **The nurse is caring for a patient with leukemia. Which of the following clinical manifestations would the nurse expect to find upon physical assessment?**
   A. angina, dyspnea, fatigue
   B. petechiae, muscle aching, splenomegaly
   C. insomnia, shortness of breath, hematuria
   D. night sweats, gingival bleeding, ecchymoses

9. **The nurse is providing care for a patient with Hodgkin's lymphoma. The nurse expects to identify which of the following clinical manifestations of the disease upon performing a physical assessment?**
   A. painless enlarged lymph nodes in the groin
   B. painless enlarged lymph nodes in the abdomen
   C. painless enlarged lymph node under the arm
   D. painless enlarged lymph node on the neck

Interpretation of Lab Values

1. **The nurse is caring for a patient who has had blood drawn for a prothrombin time. The nurse realizes that prothrombin time:**
   A. is often used rather than INR to evaluate clotting.
   B. evaluates the intrinsic coagulation pathway.
   C. evaluates the extrinsic coagulation pathway.
   D. should range between 60–70 seconds normally.

2. **The nurse is caring for a patient who has had blood drawn for an activated partial thromboplastin time. The nurse understands that activated partial thromboplastin time:**
   A. is decreased during anticoagulation therapy.
   B. is closely correlated with prothrombin time.
   C. evaluates the extrinsic coagulation pathway.
   D. has a normal range of 30 to 45 seconds.

3. The nurse is reviewing the following lab work on a patient:

Red blood cells (RBC)	2.8 million/µL
White blood cells (WBC)	3800/µL
Platelets	68,000/µL
Hemoglobin	8.8 g/dL
Hematocrit	25.4%

   The nurse realizes that the laboratory findings are consistent with which of the following?
   - A. thrombocytosis
   - B. leukocytosis
   - C. pernicious anemia
   - D. pancytopenia

4. The nurse is reviewing lab work for a patient with polycythemia vera. The nurse expects which of the following results?
   - A. decreased platelets and WBCs
   - B. decreased platelets and increased WBCs
   - C. increased Hgb and erythrocytes
   - D. increased Hgb and decreased erythrocytes

5. The nurse caring for a patient with thrombocytopenia understands that the patient is at grave risk for cerebral and pulmonary hemorrhage if platelet counts fall below:
   - A. $10,000/mm^3$
   - B. $40,000/mm^3$
   - C. $75,000/mm^3$
   - D. $98,000/mm^3$

6. The nurse is caring for a patient with disseminated intravascular coagulation (DIC). The nurse would expect which of the following laboratory findings?
   - A. low D-dimer
   - B. prolonged partial thromboplastin time
   - C. decreased prothrombin time
   - D. increased platelet count

7. The nurse understands that a patient would be diagnosed with neutropenia if the neutrophil count is which of the following?
   - A. $< 2000/mm^3$
   - B. $4500–10,000/mm^3$
   - C. $12,000–14,000/mm^3$
   - D. $> 20,000/mm^3$

8. The nurse is caring for a patient with Hodgkin's lymphoma. The nurse understands that the disease is diagnosed based upon the presence of which of the following types of cells?
   - A. undifferentiated neutrophils
   - B. Reed-Sternberg
   - C. Greenburg-Stein
   - D. highly differentiated lymphocytes

Drugs and Treatments

1. The nurse is caring for a patient who developed heparin-induced thrombocytopenia. Which of the following medications will be required for anticoagulation?
   A. heparin
   B. warfarin (Coumadin)
   C. vitamin K (AquaMEPHYTON)
   D. lepirudin (Refludan)

2. The nurse is teaching the patient with iron deficiency anemia about taking supplemental iron at home. Which of the following instructions should the nurse be sure to include?
   A. Crush the pills and mix in applesauce to improve the taste.
   B. Take the supplemental iron 1 hour before meals.
   C. Take the medication immediately following meals.
   D. Supplemental iron may cause severe diarrhea.

3. The nurse is providing education to the patient with pernicious anemia. Which of the following statements by the patient indicates comprehension of the information?
   A. "I will need to take vitamin B_{12} replacement for the rest of my life."
   B. "Once I get over this episode, I will not have to take the medicine regularly."
   C. "If I add vitamin B_{12} foods to my diet consistently, I don't need medication."
   D. "I have a higher chance of developing Alzheimer's because of B_{12} deficiency."

4. The nurse is providing care for a patient with hemophilia A who has been admitted with signs of bleeding. The nurse understands that treatment for the patient will involve which of the following?
   A. sandostatin
   B. albumin infusions
   C. immune globulin
   D. cryoprecipitate

ALTERNATE FORMAT

5. The nurse who is caring for a patient with disseminated intravascular coagulation (DIC) would anticipate the need for which of the following factors and/or blood products? SELECT ALL THAT APPLY.
   A. cryoprecipitate to replace fibrinogen
   B. platelets for thrombocytopenia
   C. factor VIII
   D. factor X
   E. fresh frozen plasma

6. The nurse is caring for a patient with neutropenia. The nurse understands that which of the following medications will be administered to stimulate production of neutrophils?
   A. epoetin alfa (Epogen)
   B. filgrastim (Neupogen)
   C. enoxaparin (Lovenox)
   D. neutrophil stimulating factor

ANSWERS

General

1. **(D)**; In response to tissue hypoxia, erythropoietin is released by the kidneys. Erythropoietin stimulates the production of erythrocytes (red cells) in the bone marrow.

2. **(A)**; Cyanocobalamin (vitamin B_{12}) is referred to as a maturation factor for red blood cells. When individuals lack this vitamin, their erythrocytes become larger and irregularly shaped. The cells also have a shorter life span. AquaMEPHYTON is vitamin K, thiamine is vitamin B_1, and pyridoxine is vitamin B_6.

3. **(B)**; Granulocytes are phagocytic cells. Erythrocytes are red blood cells, which are largely responsible for carrying oxygen to tissues. Thrombocytes are also known as platelets, and they are important in the processes of hemostasis and coagulation. Lymphocytes are a type of leukocyte that are important to immunity.

4. **(C)**; Platelets help to maintain hemostasis and coagulation by plugging disruptions in the integrity of blood vessels. When an injury occurs to a blood vessel, platelets collect at the edge of the break and, by adhering to one another, plug the injured area and limit blood loss. If the platelet number is inadequate, the response will be sub-therapeutic and the patient may lose a lot of blood.

5. **(A)**; In the body, fibrinolysis is a process by which a clot is broken down over time. This process is effective at breaking down clots that are not immediately life-threatening.

6. **(D)**; The nurse understands that patients with liver failure have an inadequate supply of clotting factors and therefore anticipates that the aPTT is increased.

7. **(A)**; The most common side effect of this medication is bleeding. Therefore, the patient must be cautioned to use an electric razor for shaving, not a safety razor. Also, the patient must not participate in contact sports and should be sure to wear slippers at home. It is also important for the nurse to emphasize the need for follow-up assessments.

8. **(B)**; The patient should be assisted to a lateral decubitus position with the top leg flexed and the lower leg straight, a position that provides optimal exposure of the iliac crest. This position also provides stabilization with the lower leg.

9. **(C)**; The patient should be warned in advance to expect a sharp, burning pain when the marrow is aspirated. The patient will not be heavily sedated for the procedure. Typically, the skin and periosteum are anesthetized with lidocaine to decrease pain, but the patient will feel discomfort.

10. **(A)**; Because the nurse knows that the delay will be more than 20 minutes, the unit of packed red blood cells should be immediately returned to the laboratory where it will be properly maintained until it can be transfused. It is not a good idea to keep the blood on the unit in the hopes that the IV team will arrive earlier than expected because blood should be administered immediately upon arrival from the laboratory.

11. **(A, C, D, E)**; Two nurses must verify the patient's name, ID number, blood type, and Rh match prior to administering blood products. Both nurses must sign the form from the blood bank to verify that the checks were completed.

12. **(A)**; The nurse should encourage the patient to increase consumption of iron-rich foods, including *organ meats*, *green leafy vegetables*, *beans*, molasses, raisins, and other meats.

13. **(D)**; The patient with pernicious anemia has a deficiency of vitamin B_{12}, cyanocobal-amin. Thiamine is vitamin B_1; riboflavin is vitamin B_2; and pyridoxine is vitamin B_6.

14. **(A)**; The patient with pernicious anemia should be encouraged to include vitamin B_{12}-rich foods in the diet, including dairy products, animal proteins, and eggs.

15. **(C)**; The patient can help to avoid infections by not eating uncooked foods—no fresh fruits or vegetables. Patients with aplastic anemia should not take aspirin or ibuprofen because both drugs can increase bleeding tendency. Patients with aplastic anemia are not at risk for deep vein thrombosis because of inadequacy of platelets. The patient should notify the physician if/or when activity becomes increasingly intolerable.

16. **(B)**; The patient who is in sickle cell crisis is in severe pain, which typically requires large doses of narcotic (opioid) analgesics for control.

17. **(D)**; Among strategies to prevent sickle cell crisis, the patient should be encouraged to drink 4 to 6 liters of fluid per day, to avoid overexertion, to use stress-reduction techniques, and to avoid exposure to the cold. Having a job at a sawmill in the winter may not be desirable because of constant exposure to a cold environment.

18. **(B)**; Patients in sickle cell crisis should have pain management, administration of oxygen, oral hydration, monitoring for complications, and management of infection. Therapeutic hypothermia is not desirable for the patient with sickle cell crisis. In fact, exposure to cold is a stressor that can provoke sickle cell crisis.

19. **(B)**; Secondary polycythemia vera occurs because of overproduction of erythropoietin in response to hypoxia. Hypoxia stimulates the kidneys to release erythropoietin.

20. **(A)**; Nursing measures for the patient with polycythemia vera include maintaining adequate hydration to decrease blood viscosity, encouraging early ambulation, educating the patient about performing passive leg exercises when on bed rest, and avoiding crossing of the legs.

21. **(C)**; The patient should notify the healthcare provider if *any* signs of bleeding are noticed at home. Although splenectomy is one part of therapeutic management for idiopathic thrombocytopenia purpura, the patient must be alert to signs of bleeding post-splenectomy.

22. **(B)**; Patients with hemophilia A, the most common form of the disorder, are deficient in Factor VIII.

23. **(D)**; The nurse anticipates assisting with management of pain associated with the hemiarthrosis. These measures include joint immobilization, application of ice, and administration of analgesics (no aspirin because of its effects on coagulation).

24. **(B)**; The nurse understands that DIC (a disorder of abnormal clotting and hemorrhage) is precipitated by conditions resulting in widespread tissue damage like trauma, sepsis, hypoxia, extensive burns, and obstetric complications.

25. **(A)**; The patient with neutropenia is at significant risk for infection because normal phagocytic activity is lacking.

26. **(D)**; Fresh flowers, fruits, and standing water should not be permitted in the patient's room because they carry microorganisms, and the patient does not have normal immune mechanisms.

Physical Assessment

1. **(A)**; The nurse should first remove the original dressing and apply a new pressure dressing. Next, the nurse should assist the patient to a supine position to enhance pressure over the aspiration site and then notify the physician of excessive bleeding.

2. **(C)**; The nurse's initial immediate action should be to stop the infusion and change the IV tubing. The site should be preserved and kept open with a normal saline infusion because it may be needed for administration of emergency medications. As soon as possible, the nurse should notify the physician and the blood bank of the signs and symptoms exhibited by the patient. The remaining blood should not be discarded. It must be returned to the lab for further analysis of the event.

3. **(A)**; The nurse should be especially attentive when assessing the patient's neurologic function because deficiency of vitamin B_{12} can disrupt function of the brain, spinal cord, and nerves.

4. **(B)**; The patient with folic acid deficiency is likely to have some of the following manifestations: pallor, progressive weakness, fatigue, shortness of breath, cardiac palpitations, severe diarrhea. Patients do not have neurological symptoms.

5. **(B)**; The nurse would want to carefully assess for purpura and signs of bleeding from the gums, nose, vagina, or rectum. Additionally, the nurse should assess for pallor, fatigue, palpitations, exertional dyspnea, infections of the skin and mucous membranes, and retinal hemorrhage.

6. **(A)**; Patients with polycythemia vera may have the following clinical manifestations: plethora (ruddy color to hands, face, feet, ears, etc.), headaches, vertigo, blurred vision, *distended superficial veins*, itching unrelieved by antihistamines, angina, dyspnea, erythromelalgia, and splenomegaly.

7. **(B)**; Upon performing a physical assessment on the patient with thrombocytopenia, the nurse anticipates finding petechiae and purpura on the thorax, arms, neck, and ankles. Other possible findings might include epistaxis and gingival bleeding.

8. **(D)**; Upon physical assessment of the patient with leukemia, the nurse would anticipate finding that the patient suffers from *night sweats, gingival bleeding, ecchymoses,* weakness, fatigue, anorexia, shortness of breath, decreased activity tolerance, epistaxis, pallor, and splenomegaly or hepatomegaly.

9. **(D)**; Characteristically, the patient with Hodgkin's disease will present with a painless enlarged lymph node on one side of the neck.

Interpretation of Lab Values

1. **(C)**; Prothrombin time (PT) reflects how fast the blood clots. Normal values range from 11 to 16 seconds. PT evaluates the extrinsic pathway of the coagulation cascade.

2. **(D)**; Activated partial thromboplastin time (aPTT) is used to monitor heparin therapy. Normal results range from 30 to 45 seconds. Results are increased during anticoagulation therapy. aPTT is used to evaluate the intrinsic coagulation pathway.

3. **(D)**; The lab results reveal decreased RBCs, WBCs, and platelets. This condition is referred to as pancytopenia, which is consistent with aplastic anemia.

4. **(C)**; The nurse anticipates that lab work for the patient with polycythemia vera would reveal *increased hemoglobin and erythrocyte* count, increased platelets, and increased WBCs.

5. **(A)**; The nurse understands that the patient with thrombocytopenia is at grave risk for cerebral and pulmonary hemorrhage if the platelet counts fall below $10,000/mm^3$.

6. **(B)**; The nurse who is caring for a patient with DIC would expect to find that partial thromboplastin time is prolonged, prothrombin time is prolonged, platelet count is decreased, and D-dimer is elevated.

7. **(A)**; The nurse understands that a patient with a neutrophil count of less than $2000/mm^3$ is considered to be neutropenic.

8. **(B)**; Hodgkin's disease is diagnosed based on identification of an invasive tumor (Reed-Sternberg cell) found in bone biopsy.

Drugs and Treatments

1. **(D)**; Lepirudin is an anticoagulant used to treat patients with heparin-induced thrombocytopenia. Heparin is contraindicated and vitamin K improves clotting ability, which is not desirable.

2. **(B)**; The nurse should instruct the patient to take the medication 1 hour before meals because there is decreased absorption of iron when taken with food. Also, patients who will take oral liquid iron should be aware that the liquid can stain the teeth. Therefore, patients should always use a straw and brush the teeth thoroughly after the medicine.

3. **(A)**; The patient's acknowledgment of the need to take replacement B_{12} for an entire lifetime indicates comprehension of material taught.

4. **(D)**; The nurse knows that the patient with hemophilia who has clinical manifestations of bleeding will be treated with cryoprecipitate containing factor VIII every 12 hours until bleeding stops.

5. **(A, B, E)**; The nurse who is caring for a patient with DIC should anticipate the need to administer cryoprecipitate to replace fibrinogen, platelets for thrombocytopenia, and fresh frozen plasma to replace all clotting factors except platelets.

6. **(B)**; Filgrastim (Neupogen) is administered to the neutropenic patient to stimulate production of neutrophils.

Keep Track

- Percent correct. (Divide the number of questions you answered correctly by the total number of questions you answered.) _____

- Number of questions you missed due to a reading error: _____

- Number of questions you missed due to errors in analysis: _____

- Number of assessment questions you missed: _____

- Number of lab value questions you missed: _____

- Number of drug/treatment questions you missed: _____

Nugget List

Chapter number _____   Topic _____

Practice Test: Nursing Management of Patients with Musculoskeletal Disorders

Karen S. March

PRACTICE TEST

General

1. Which of the following is the most common radiological test used to assess musculoskeletal problems?
   A. EMG
   B. MRI
   C. CT
   D. X-ray

2. The patient is scheduled for an EMG. Which of the following statements by the patient indicates understanding of the purpose of the test?
   A. "This test will help my doctor know if my nerves are working correctly."
   B. "The doctor will be able to fix the problem with my arm during this test."
   C. "I cannot eat or drink for at least 10 hours before I have this test."
   D. "I will have to remain flat on my back throughout the test."

3. The patient is scheduled for an arthroscopy in 24 hours. Which of the following statements by the patient indicates an understanding of the purpose of the procedure?
   A. "The doctor will insert a tiny camera through small incisions around my knee."
   B. "The doctor will be able to see if I have signs of rheumatoid arthritis."
   C. "I cannot eat or drink for at least 10 hours before the procedure."
   D. "I will not have much pain afterward because the scope is so small."

4. The nurse is providing post-procedural teaching to the client who has had an arthroscopy. Which of the following statements by the patient indicates a need for further teaching?
   A. "I can do any activity that I want and take analgesics for pain control."
   B. "I will need to monitor for the development of any hematomas."
   C. "I will do a neurovascular assessment on my leg several times per day."
   D. "If I develop a fever or warmth at the site, I will call my doctor."

5. The nurse is providing pre-procedural teaching to a client who will have an arthrogram. Which of the following statements by the patient indicates understanding of the education?
   A. "I will notice a decrease in my urine output for a while after the procedure."
   B. "When the dye is injected, I will feel a sensation of icy cold and a salty taste."
   C. "I will have to move my joint a number of times for X-rays."
   D. "I can expect that my leg will be very cool and pale after the procedure."

6. The nurse is caring for a patient who is scheduled for an MRI of the lumbar spine. Which of the following information should the nurse provide to the patient before the procedure?
   A. "You can have a mild sedative before the procedure to help keep you calm."
   B. "This test will be done in the X-ray department of the hospital."
   C. "You will not be a candidate for this test if you have had cataract surgery."
   D. "You will be able to watch television while the test is done."

7. The nurse is working in a same day procedure unit with patients scheduled for different types of procedures. Which of the following patients would be a candidate for an MRI?
   A. a patient with a history of hip replacement
   B. a patient who has a mechanical aortic valve
   C. a patient who has abdominal pain
   D. a patient who has an automated internal defibrillator

ALTERNATE FORMAT

8. The nurse is caring for a patient who will undergo a bone scan. Which of the following statements by the patient indicates understanding of this procedure? SELECT ALL THAT APPLY.
   A. "I will have to drink the contrast material before the test begins."
   B. "A special camera will scan my entire body."
   C. "There will be better absorption of the contrast in healthy bone."
   D. "Increased absorption of contrast indicates abnormal areas."

ALTERNATE FORMAT

9. The nurse is caring for a patient admitted with Buck's traction in place. Which of the following facts should the nurse teach the patient about skin traction? SELECT ALL THAT APPLY.
   A. Buck's is a type of skin traction.
   B. The traction should be in place for a short time.
   C. The traction will help decrease muscle spasms and pain.
   D. The traction may cause an uncomfortable pulling sensation.

10. The nurse is providing teaching to a patient who has had a cast applied to the left arm. Which of the following statements by the patient indicate understanding of the teaching?
    A. "I should call the doctor if my fingers become cold and I cannot move them."
    B. "If I have itching under the cast, I can carefully use a butter knife to scratch."
    C. "If my fingers swell, I should just put an ice bag on and stay in bed."
    D. "If I have tingling under my cast, I need to move my fingers more."

11. The nurse is caring for a patient post-laminectomy. The nurse will include which of the following in the patient's plan of care?
    A. Encourage early ambulation to decrease risk for DVT.
    B. Provide ample fluids for oral intake to promote dye excretion.
    C. Logroll the patient with the assistance of at least two others.
    D. Report any tingling of extremities to the physician.

12. **The nurse is providing discharge teaching for the patient who has had a laminectomy. Which of the following statements by the patient indicates a need for further teaching?**
    A. "I will notify the doctor if I feel any tingling in my legs."
    B. "It is important that I maintain proper spine alignment."
    C. "I can use pillows under my thighs when I lie on my back."
    D. "I should use pillows between my legs when I am on my side."

13. **The nurse is providing discharge teaching for a patient who has undergone total hip replacement. Which of the following statements by the patient indicate a need for more teaching?**
    A. "I will notify my doctor if I notice any foul smelling drainage from my incision."
    B. "I will have to go to an outpatient laboratory for weekly testing of my PT."
    C. "When I can walk without a walker, I can stop attending physical therapy."
    D. "I will need to use a reacher to get things I drop on the floor."

14. **The nurse is providing teaching to a patient who has had an amputation of the left lower leg. Which of the following statements by the patient indicates understanding of proper care for the incision and left upper leg?**
    A. "I can use powder inside my limb sock to keep it cool."
    B. "I need to lie on my abdomen for 30 minutes several times per day."
    C. "I will have some foul-smelling drainage because I had gangrene."
    D. "I can elevate my stump on 2 or 3 pillows to help decrease edema."

ALTERNATE FORMAT

15. **The nurse is providing care for a patient diagnosed with osteoporosis. The nurse recognizes which of the following as being risk factors for development of osteoporosis? SELECT ALL THAT APPLY.**
    A. thin, small body frame
    B. large body frame
    C. Asian-American ethnicity
    D. African-American ethnicity
    E. smoking
    F. female
    G. male

16. **A patient asks the nurse, "What can I do to decrease my risk of developing osteoporosis?" The best response by the nurse is which of the following?**
    A. "Do weight-bearing exercises on a regular basis."
    B. "You should take in 250 mg of Ca^{++} per day."
    C. "Increase your intake of red and yellow vegetables."
    D. "Drink a glass of red wine daily."

17. **The nurse is caring for a patient who has had a total hip replacement. The patient asks the nurse, "Why is it important to notify all care providers about my hip surgery?" The best response by the nurse is which of the following?**
    A. "It is important that all of your care providers know your full medical history."
    B. "You will need to take prophylactic antibiotics before any invasive procedures."
    C. "It is important that they all understand why you are using a walker."
    D. "You will want them to be able to continue to give you good medical advice."

18. The patient asks the nurse what type of organism causes osteomyelitis. The best response by the nurse is:
    A. *klebsiella.*
    B. *candida.*
    C. *staphylococcus.*
    D. *streptococcus.*

19. Which type of fracture results when the bone is broken into multiple pieces?
    A. avulsion
    B. comminuted
    C. compressed
    D. spiral

20. Which type of fracture is common in children?
    A. impacted
    B. depressed
    C. spiral
    D. greenstick

21. The nurse is caring for a patient admitted with a right hip fracture. Based on the diagnosis, the nurse realizes that the priority nursing diagnosis for this patient is:
    A. risk for peripheral neurovascular dysfunction.
    B. risk for fluid volume deficit.
    C. decreased cardiac output.
    D. anxiety.

22. The nurse is providing information about activity limitations upon discharge to a patient following repair of a hip fracture. Which of the following statements by the patient indicates the need for further teaching?
    A. "I can go up the stairs as soon as I feel ready."
    B. "I should not sit on very low chairs."
    C. "I will need to use a raised toilet seat."
    D. "I will not be able to bend more than 90 degrees."

23. The nurse is caring for a patient admitted with an initial diagnosis of gout. Which of the following is a priority nursing diagnosis for this patient?
    A. anxiety
    B. pain
    C. depression
    D. risk for altered nutrition

24. The nurse is caring for a patient diagnosed with gout. When providing teaching about managing exacerbations, the nurse should include which of the following statements?
    A. Allopurinol (Zyloprim) helps to decrease inflammation.
    B. Use a bed cradle during an episode.
    C. Drink a glass of red wine each evening.
    D. Maintain active range of motion.

25. The patient has a cast in place following a fracture to the ulna. The patient informs the nurse that he cannot feel his fingers. The best initial response by the nurse is to:
    A. notify the physician immediately.
    B. remove excess cast padding to decrease pressure.
    C. assure the patient that this feeling is normal.
    D. check for capillary refill in the fingers.

26. A patient's left knee appears to be swollen. To further evaluate the situation, the nurse should first:
    A. compare it to the right knee.
    B. perform range of motion on the knee.
    C. test muscle strength in the extremity.
    D. palpate for crepitus.

27. The nurse is providing care for a patient who sustained a crush injury to the left leg with significant tissue edema. Within 36 hours of the injury, the patient begins complaining of tingling in the leg. Which of the following complications should the nurse suspect?
    A. comminuted fracture
    B. fat embolism
    C. compartment syndrome
    D. impacted fracture

Physical Assessment

1. The nurse is caring for a patient who had a cast applied within the past 24 hours. Which of the following assessment findings should the nurse report immediately?
   A. temperature of 100.4°F
   B. burning under the cast
   C. mild edema
   D. itching under the cast

2. The nurse is caring for a patient at risk of developing osteomyelitis. Which of the following symptoms would indicate presence of the condition?
   A. increased urine output
   B. elevated serum Ca^{++}
   C. pain unrelieved by analgesics
   D. temperature of 100.4°F

3. The nurse is caring for a patient with a suspected ankle fracture following a motor vehicle accident. Which of the following assessment findings would support the initial diagnosis?
   A. ability to walk briskly
   B. loss of sensation
   C. crepitation
   D. tingling in the foot

4. The nurse is caring for a patient who has experienced a soft tissue injury. Which of the following signs or symptoms would alert the nurse to the possible development of compartment syndrome?
   A. 2+ peripheral pulses
   B. capillary refill < 3 seconds
   C. loss of sensation
   D. pain relieved by acetaminophen

5. The nurse is caring for a patient who has a history of a fractured tibia and fibula. Which of the following symptoms would suggest the possibility that a fat embolism is present?
   A. chest pain and dyspnea
   B. calf tenderness and swelling
   C. leg pain and tenderness
   D. bradycardia and hypertension

6. The nurse suspects that a patient may have osteoarthritis based on physical assessment along with a history of pain that is:
   A. sharp and stabbing.
   B. worse at the end of the day.
   C. worse in the morning.
   D. not affected by the weather.

7. The patient is admitted to a nursing unit with acute osteomyelitis. Which of the following symptoms would the nurse expect to find upon physical examination?
   A. nausea and vomiting
   B. erythema and fever
   C. paresthesia of the extremity
   D. generalized bone pain

8. The nurse is caring for a patient who sustained multiple fractures in an automobile accident. Two days after admission the patient develops confusion, dyspnea, and a fever of 102.6°F. Based on the presentation, the nurse should strongly suspect:
   A. sepsis.
   B. fat embolism.
   C. pulmonary embolism.
   D. compartment syndrome.

9. A patient is admitted through the emergency department with classic signs of hip fracture. The nurse should anticipate which of the following findings upon assessment of the patient?
   A. The injured leg is externally rotated and shorter.
   B. The injured leg is internally rotated and shorter.
   C. Pedal pulses are absent and the skin is ruddy.
   D. Pedal pulses are intact and the skin is pale.

10. A patient is admitted with gout. The nursing assessment will reveal which of the following?
    A. abdominal pain
    B. swollen great toe
    C. flank pain
    D. shoulder pain

Interpretation of Lab Values

1. **Which of the following laboratory studies can be used to suggest the presence of antibodies against one's own tissues?**
   A. ESR
   B. ANA
   C. RF
   D. WBC

2. **The nurse is caring for a patient who has had lab work done during a hospital admission. The patient's erythrocyte sedimentation rate (ESR) is 45 mm/hr. Which of the following interpretations by the nurse is correct?**
   A. The value is within the normal range.
   B. The value indicates the presence of inflammation.
   C. The test result is inconclusive.
   D. The result indicates a red blood cell problem.

Drugs and Treatments

1. **The patient is scheduled for myelography. Which of the following questions should the nurse be certain to ask the patient before the procedure?**
   A. "Do you need to use the restroom before the test begins?"
   B. "Did you take any medications this morning?"
   C. "Are you allergic to iodine or shellfish?"
   D. "Did you eat a good breakfast this morning?"

2. **The nurse is providing patient teaching related to use of estrogen replacement therapy to a female patient. Which of the following statements by the patient indicates the need for further teaching about this treatment option?**
   A. "The medication will help to prevent osteoporosis after menopause."
   B. "This medication can decrease my risk for endometrial cancer."
   C. "I will have to take a pill or apply a skin patch to use this medication."
   D. "When I use this medication, I will be at risk for deep vein thrombosis."

3. **The patient has been prescribed calcitonin (Miacalcin). Which of the following statements by the patient indicates an understanding of side effects of this medication?**
   A. "Calcitonin can increase the risk of spinal and hip fractures."
   B. "The medication can cause flushing of the face and hands."
   C. "The medication can cause impaired thyroid function."
   D. "Calcitonin can increase the level of pain in weight-bearing joints."

4. **The nurse is providing care for a patient with osteomyelitis. In preparing to teach the patient about medications, the nurse should plan to focus on which medication categories?**
   A. diuretics and calcium channel blockers
   B. antibiotics and analgesics
   C. anesthetics and glucocorticoids
   D. antihelmintics and stool softeners

5. Treatment for compartment syndrome includes which of the following?
    A. elevation of the extremity
    B. acetaminophen
    C. non-steroidal anti-inflammatory medications
    D. fasciotomy

ALTERNATE FORMAT

6. The nurse knows that which of the following interventions will facilitate management of pain associated with osteoarthritis? SELECT ALL THAT APPLY.
    A. teaching the patient about relaxation techniques
    B. encouraging the patient to participate in water aerobics
    C. encouraging alternating periods of rest with activity
    D. using a dry heating pad to soothe discomfort

7. A patient with rheumatoid arthritis is likely to be on all of the following medications for control of the condition except:
    A. aspirin.
    B. ibuprofen (Motrin).
    C. prednisone.
    D. furosemide (Lasix).

8. The nurse is providing education about medications to a patient with gout. The nurse explains that allopurinol (Zyloprim) acts by:
    A. inhibiting uric acid production.
    B. increasing excretion of uric acid.
    C. decreasing excretion of purines.
    D. raising the serum level of purines.

ANSWERS

General

1. **(D)**; X-ray is commonly used for assessment in patients with musculoskeletal problems.

2. **(A)**; The electromyogram (EMG) reveals electrical activity within the muscles during contraction. It is useful in discriminating between muscular dysfunction and nerve dysfunction.

3. **(B)**; Arthroscopy can be used to diagnose disorders such as rheumatoid arthritis, osteoarthritis, and internal joint injuries. Although options A and D are accurate responses, they do not answer the question about the *purpose* of the procedure.

4. **(A)**; Following arthroscopy, the patient should be instructed to *limit* activity and take analgesics for comfort.

5. **(C)**; An arthrogram is a diagnostic test in which contrast media (dye) or air is injected into a joint to visualize structures. The patient is required to move the joint several times throughout the test for X-rays. After the procedure, the patient should be advised to increase fluid intake to help eliminate contrast from the body. The patient should

also be advised to expect a feeling of warmth, nausea, headache, salty taste in the mouth, itching, hives, or rash as the dye is injected.

6. **(A)**; Many patients become anxious and feel claustrophobic when having this test. Therefore, a mild sedative should be offered to the patient before the test.

7. **(C)**; The only patient who would be a candidate for an MRI is the one with abdominal pain. Each of the other patients has contraindications. Patients with artificial joints, mechanical heart valves, or automated internal defibrillators are not candidates because metal distorts the MRI image and can affect the magnetic field.

8. **(B, D)**; A bone scan requires injection of a small amount of radioactive material. Then a specialized camera is used to scan the entire body to identify any areas of increased uptake of the radioactive material. Increased absorption of contrast indicates abnormality. This test is useful in helping to diagnose osteomyelitis, osteoporosis, fractures, Paget's disease, and cancer of the bone.

9. **(A, B, C)**; Buck's traction is a type of skin traction that is used short-term, often following hip fracture. The traction will usually use 5 to 10 pounds of weight to help decrease muscle spasms and pain. Pain is more severe without the traction.

10. **(A)**; Patients with casts must be taught to do neurovascular assessments and to notify the physician if there is any abnormality. Patients should not insert any foreign objects under the cast for any reason. Ice application is most helpful at reducing edema during the first 24 hours. After that time, increased edema could be a sign of a significant complication and therefore should be reported to the physician. If the patient develops any other signs or symptoms of compartment syndrome (increasing pain, excessive swelling, burning or tingling under the cast, sores or foul odor under the cast), the doctor must be notified immediately.

11. **(C)**; The nurse should logroll the patient with the assistance of at least two others because it is critical to maintain proper alignment of the spine at all times postoperatively.

12. **(A)**; The patient should be told not to expect immediate relief from numbness and tingling of the extremities. It may take time for these symptoms to go away.

13. **(C)**; The patient should be informed that the goal of physical therapy is to facilitate return to normal function. Typically patients use a walker first and then use a cane before final transition to ambulation without an assistive device.

14. **(B)**; The patient should lie prone three or four times daily for 30 minutes or so. This position will help to decrease the chances of developing contractures. It is not advisable to use lotions or powder on the stump. Foul-smelling drainage should be reported to the physician. The patient should be advised not to elevate the stump on pillows because it will lead to contractures.

15. **(A, C, E, F)**; Risk factors for osteoporosis include female gender, Caucasian or Asian-American ethnicity, thin or small body frame, smoking, anorexia, steroid medications, and more.

16. **(A)**; Weight-bearing exercises can force Ca^{++} back into the bone, which decreases risk for osteoporosis.

17. **(B)**; Patients who have had joint replacements are at risk for development of osteo-myelitis. Therefore, it is important for them to take prophylactic antibiotics prior to any invasive procedures, including dental work, for the rest of their lives.

18. **(C)**; Osteomyelitis is an infection of the bone that is usually caused by *staphylococcus aureus*.

19. **(B)**; A comminuted fracture is one in which the bone breaks into multiple pieces.

20. **(D)**; Greenstick fractures involve an incomplete break in the bone. One side of the bone usually splinters, and the other may remain intact. This type of fracture is more common in children.

21. **(A)**; The patient with a right hip fracture is at risk for peripheral neurovascular dys-function related to bone and tissue trauma.

22. **(A)**; The patient with repair of a hip fracture will not be ready to go up the stairs for a period of time post-operatively. The initial focus will be on returning to normal walk-ing and building strength and endurance.

23. **(B)**; Pain is a priority diagnosis for the patient with gout because it is quite painful.

24. **(B)**; The nurse should teach the patient to use a bed cradle or footboard to control pain during exacerbations. Corticosteroids and NSAIDs are used to help decrease inflammation. Patients should refrain from alcohol intake while on medications for treatment of gout. Patients should also remain on bed rest with extremity immobiliza-tion during exacerbations.

25. **(D)**; The patient may be developing compartment syndrome. It is essential that the nurse perform a neurovascular assessment before notifying the physician.

26. **(A)**; As a baseline, it is best to compare both knees. Only after doing this can the nurse make an informed decision about whether the left knee looks different.

27. **(C)**; Onset of tingling in an extremity with a history of crush injury with significant tissue edema should prompt the nurse to suspect compartment syndrome.

Physical Assessment

1. **(B)**; The nurse must notify the physician if the patient complains of burning under the cast because this is a sign of compartment syndrome, a serious complication.

2. **(C)**; Symptoms of osteomyelitis include fever with chills, restlessness, severe pain unre-lieved by rest or analgesics, swelling, redness, and warmth at the site of infection.

3. **(C)**; Crepitation is a sound created by the movement of broken bone on bone. It can sound like grating or popping.

4. **(C)**; Compartment syndrome occurs when there has been extreme swelling within a tissue compartment resulting in increased pressure and impaired circulation. Manifes-tations include pallor, decreased or absent pulses, tingling or decreased sensation, loss of sensation, and coolness of the extremity.

5. **(A)**; A fat embolism may occur following fracture of the long bones. Signs and symptoms include chest pain, dyspnea, tachycardia, apprehension, petechiae over the trunk and axilla, altered level of consciousness, and decreased O_2 saturation.

6. **(B)**; The pain of osteoarthritis is associated with movement and weight-bearing and is therefore worse at the end of the day.

7. **(B)**; Erythema and fever are symptoms associated with acute osteomyelitis.

8. **(B)**; The nurse should strongly suspect that the patient has developed a fat embolism based on the occurrence of altered level of consciousness, dyspnea, and fever—all of which are classic, textbook symptoms.

9. **(A)**; In a patient with a classic presentation of hip fracture, the injured leg is externally rotated and shorter than the other.

10. **(B)**; During an exacerbation of gout, a common assessment finding is a swollen great toe.

Interpretation of Lab Values

1. **(B)**; Antinuclear antibodies (ANA) provide a sensitive screening tool for detection of autoimmune disease. Antinuclear antibodies are present in patients with autoimmune diseases such as rheumatoid arthritis, scleroderma, and lupus.

2. **(B)**; ESR is a test that indicates the rate at which red blood cells settle out of unclotted blood. Elevated levels indicate that an inflammatory process is present.

Drugs and Treatments

1. **(C)**; The nurse should ask about allergies to iodine or shellfish because an affirmative response would indicate the need to modify the usual protocol.

2. **(B)**; Estrogen replacement therapy is used for prevention of osteoporosis after menopause. Its use can increase the risk for both breast and endometrial cancer.

3. **(B)**; Calcitonin (Miacalcin) is a hormone secreted by the thyroid. It can cause the following side effects: flushing of the face and hands, urinary frequency, nausea. Rhinorrhea can result from use of the nasal spray, and skin rash may result from the injectable form.

4. **(B)**; A patient with osteomyelitis will need information on antibiotics and analgesics. Antibiotics are used to treat the infection. Analgesics are used to help to control pain.

5. **(D)**; Fasciotomy involves a deep incision into the fascia to relieve pressure within the compartment. Timing of this treatment is crucial. Done too early, the patient will lose a lot of blood. Done too late, tissue death will occur.

6. **(A, B, C)**; Management of pain for the patient with osteoarthritis may be accomplished through a variety of mechanisms. The nurse should teach the patient about relaxation therapy, encourage participation in water aerobics, and encourage alternating periods

of rest with activity. Additionally, maintenance of ideal body weight prevents excess stress on the joints.

7. **(D)**; The patient with rheumatoid arthritis is likely to be treated with aspirin, ibuprofen, and prednisone. Furosemide (Lasix) is not part of the treatment regimen for rheumatoid arthritis.

8. **(A)**; Allopurinol (Zyloprim) acts by inhibiting uric acid production.

Keep Track

- Percent correct. (Divide the number of questions you answered correctly by the total number of questions you answered.) _____

- Number of questions you missed due to a reading error: _____

- Number of questions you missed due to errors in analysis: _____

- Number of assessment questions you missed: _____

- Number of lab value questions you missed: _____

- Number of drug/treatment questions you missed: _____

Nugget List

Chapter number _____ Topic _____

Practice Test: Nursing Management of Patients with GI and Biliary Tract Disorders

Karen S. March

PRACTICE TEST

General

1. The nurse is caring for a patient who was recently diagnosed with oral cancer. The nurse explains to the patient the purpose of having radiation treatments pre-operatively. Which of the following statements by the patient indicates under-standing of the teaching?
   A. "I will have radiation to cure the cancer before surgery."
   B. "Radiation will help to shrink the tumor before surgery."
   C. "Radiation will reduce the pain associated with the tumor."
   D. "I may not have to have surgery if the radiation works well."

2. From a health promotion perspective, the nurse is aware that which of the follow-ing is the single most important factor in reducing risk of oral cancer?
   A. eliminating tobacco use
   B. controlling alcohol use
   C. eliminating analgesics
   D. smoking cessation

3. The nurse is caring for a patient with acute diverticulitis. Prior to discharge the nurse should instruct the patient to increase which of the following foods in the diet?
   A. cucumbers, popcorn, cantaloupe
   B. asparagus, carrots, shredded wheat
   C. peas, strawberries, corn
   D. tomatoes, peas, corn

4. The nurse is caring for a patient with acute diverticulitis. Prior to discharge the nurse should instruct the patient to avoid which of the following foods in the diet?
   A. squash, potatoes, brown rice
   B. chicken, hamburger, peanut butter
   C. poppy seeds, strawberries, cucumbers
   D. salmon, grilled vegetables, pears

5. The physician has ordered insertion of a nasogastric tube. Which of the following actions by the nurse would make insertion more difficult?
   A. lubricating the tube with a water-soluble lubricant
   B. asking the patient to swallow while the tube is passed
   C. placing the coiled tube in ice chips prior to insertion
   D. asking the patient to turn the head during insertion

6. The nurse is caring for a patient with an NG tube attached to suction. Which of the following actions should the nurse take if the patient complains of nausea?
   A. Irrigate the tube with normal saline to ensure patency.
   B. Provide oral care with a toothbrush and mouthwash.
   C. Immediately administer a prescribed antiemetic medication.
   D. Increase the amount of suction on the nasogastric tube.

7. The nurse is caring for a patient with peptic ulcer disease. During patient teaching, the patient admits to having considerable stress at work. The nurse instructs the patient that, if the stress is unavoidable, the patient must:
   A. consider changing jobs to something less stressful.
   B. identify the stressors at work and then try to reduce them.
   C. plan for periods away from work throughout the day.
   D. improve the ability to cope with identified stressors.

8. The patient has had a gastric resection for adenocarcinoma of the stomach. During surgery, a nasogastric tube was placed. The nurse understands that the purpose for tube placement is to:
   A. prevent excessive pressure on suture lines.
   B. monitor for the occurrence of bloody drainage.
   C. allow for early postoperative feeding of the patient.
   D. allow for antacid administration to promote healing of the suture line.

9. The nurse is providing care for a patient who had gastric surgery. Which of the following signs and symptoms would alert the nurse to leakage at the site of anastomosis?
   A. pain, fever, and dyspnea following oral fluids
   B. diarrhea with the presence of fat in the stool
   C. palpitations, pallor, and diaphoresis after eating
   D. feeling of fullness and nausea after eating

10. The nurse working in a primary care office sees a patient who came in for evaluation of gastroesophageal reflux disease (GERD). When documenting the patient's history, the nurse expects the patient to report that symptoms are worse when:
    A. exercising.
    B. bending over.
    C. sitting.
    D. walking.

11. The nurse is providing teaching about dietary modifications to a patient with gastroesophageal reflux disease (GERD). The nurse should suggest elimination of which of the following foods or substances for this patient?
    A. chocolate, oranges, tomatoes
    B. lettuce, carrots, whole wheat
    C. potatoes, grapes, squash
    D. juices, ice cream, asparagus

12. The nurse understands that the most common symptom of gastroesophageal reflux disease (GERD) is which of the following?
    A. sour taste in the morning
    B. dysphagia
    C. belching
    D. heartburn

13. The nurse is assigned to care for a patient with achalasia. The nurse understands that the patient is likely to have which of the following clinical manifestations related to this diagnosis?
    A. frequent nausea and diarrhea
    B. dysphagia and chest pain
    C. slow peristalsis and constipation
    D. silent abdomen and lower quad pain

14. The nurse is providing care for a patient who is receiving total parenteral nutrition (TPN). Which of the following interventions is most appropriate to prevent infection?
    A. Change the total parenteral nutrition tubing every 2 days.
    B. Culture the insertion site of the infusion device every 48 hours.
    C. Administer other intravenous medications in a separate line.
    D. Maintain a closed system and do not change the TPN tubing.

15. The nurse is providing preoperative teaching to a patient who will undergo surgery to create a temporary colostomy. The patient asks the nurse about the difference between colostomies and ileostomies. The best response by the nurse is:
    A. "A colostomy occurs in the GI tract, and an ileostomy occurs in the urinary tract."
    B. "A colostomy is temporary, and an ileostomy is always permanent."
    C. "A colostomy is in the large intestine, and an ileostomy is in the small intestine."
    D. "Dietary restrictions are required for the patient with an ileostomy but not a colostomy."

16. The nurse working in the emergency department realizes that which of the following patients with acute abdominal pain is most likely to have acute appendicitis?
    A. an 8-month-old female
    B. a 14-year-old male
    C. an 85-year-old woman
    D. a 70-year-old male

17. The nurse is caring for a patient who has ulcerative colitis with orders for bed rest with bathroom privileges. The nurse understands the rationale for the activity restriction is:
    A. to conserve energy.
    B. to reduce intestinal peristalsis.
    C. to promote rest and comfort.
    D. to prevent injury.

18. The nurse is teaching a patient with an ileostomy about methods used to reduce flatus and odor. Which of the following methods would be least effective in achieving the desired results?
    A. Advise the patient to avoid eating broccoli and cabbage.
    B. Utilize deodorizing drops in the bottom of the appliance.
    C. Put a tiny pinhole in the appliance to allow flatus to escape.
    D. Empty feces and gas from the appliance as often as necessary.

19. The nurse is caring for a patient with an acute exacerbation of Crohn's disease. Which of the following nursing interventions is least appropriate for this patient?
    A. Encourage bed rest with bathroom privileges.
    B. Encourage strict NPO status.
    C. Administer prescribed stool softeners.
    D. Place a deodorizer in the patient's room.

20. The nurse is assigned to care for a patient with a GI bleed. The physician suspects that there is a bleeding lesion in the colon. The nurse realizes that the most likely initial approach to treatment will involve which of the following procedures?
    A. exploratory laparotomy
    B. esophagogastrocolonoscopy
    C. esophagogastroduodenoscopy
    D. colonoscopy

21. Assessment of the patient's gag response is a priority nursing intervention following which of the following procedures?
    A. colon biopsy
    B. small bowel biopsy
    C. barium enema
    D. colonoscopy

22. The nurse is performing a health history on a patient who is hospitalized with esophageal reflux. Which of the following factors reported is least likely to predispose the patient to esophageal reflux?
    A. "I have an occasional drink socially."
    B. "I use NoDoz every day to keep me going at work."
    C. "I drink about 6 to 10 cups of coffee per day."
    D. "I've smoked two packs per day for 20 years."

23. Following administration of a bolus tube feeding to a patient, the nurse must:
    A. encourage the patient to lie flat for at least 45 minutes.
    B. elevate the head of the bed 30 degrees for at least an hour.
    C. encourage the patient to lie on the right side for 45 minutes.
    D. have the patient sit upright in bed for at least 5 minutes.

24. The nurse is reviewing dietary teaching with a patient diagnosed with chronic gastritis. The nurse realizes that teaching has been effective when the patient makes which of the following statements?
    A. "I can take ibuprofen for my arthritis pain."
    B. "I can still eat my favorite Cajun foods."
    C. "I can have jello and toast for snacks."
    D. "I can have beer and pizza for dinner."

25. The nurse is managing the care of a patient who will undergo diagnostic tests of the GI tract including EGD, barium swallow, and barium enema. The nurse schedules the tests in which order, taking into consideration the nursing implications for each procedure?
    A. barium swallow, barium enema, EGD
    B. barium swallow, EGD, barium enema
    C. EGD, barium enema, barium swallow
    D. barium enema, barium swallow, EGD

26. Early signs of cancer of the colon include which of the following?
    A. abdominal pain
    B. abdominal distention
    C. alternating constipation with diarrhea
    D. nausea and vomiting

27. The nurse is preparing to administer medications to a patient via a nasogastric feeding tube. Which of the following actions by the nurse is not indicated during administration of medications via a feeding tube?
    A. Elevate the HOB at least 20 degrees during medication administration.
    B. Check feeding tube placement with air auscultation before administration.
    C. Irrigate the tube with water before, during, and after medication administration.
    D. Elevate the HOB 45 degrees during and for 30 to 60 minutes after administration.

28. The nurse understands that which of the following nursing diagnoses is highest priority for the patient who has had an upper or lower GI study? Risk for:
    A. activity intolerance r/t fatigue.
    B. constipation r/t presence of barium in the GI tract.
    C. altered comfort r/t abdominal cramps and diarrhea.
    D. anxiety r/t insufficient knowledge or post-test care.

29. The nurse intends to participate in a health screening clinic and is preparing teaching materials about colorectal cancer. The nurse should plan to include which of the following in a list of risk factors for colorectal cancer?
    A. age older than 30 years
    B. high fiber, low fat diet
    C. distant relative with colorectal cancer
    D. personal history of GI polyps

30. The nurse is caring for a patient following a gastric resection and is monitoring the patient closely for signs of dumping syndrome. Which of the following symptoms is indicative of dumping syndrome?
    A. abdominal cramping and right lower quadrant pain
    B. bradycardia and indigestion
    C. double vision and chest pain
    D. orthostatic hypotension and diaphoresis

31. The nurse is caring for an 8-month-old admitted to the hospital with dehydration. The nurse knows that which of the following factors predisposes the infant to fluid imbalance?
    A. decreased body surface area in comparison with an adult
    B. lower metabolic rate than an adult
    C. inability of the kidneys to dilute or concentrate urine
    D. decreased daily exchange of extracellular fluid

32. The nurse understands that which of the following is a viral pathogen that frequently causes acute diarrhea in young children?
    A. giardia
    B. shigella
    C. rotavirus
    D. salmonella

33. The nurse knows that acute diarrhea in children is often caused by which of the following?
    A. celiac disease
    B. antibiotic therapy
    C. vitamin deficiency
    D. protein malnutrition

34. Which of the following is a high fiber food that the nurse could recommend for a child who has chronic constipation?
    A. popcorn
    B. pancakes
    C. muffins
    D. ripe bananas

35. The nurse is caring for a 4-month-old infant with gastroesophageal reflux (GER). After feeding and burping the infant, the nurse should place the infant in which of the following positions?
    A. secured upright in an infant carrier
    B. supine with a pillow under the head
    C. on the right side with a blanket roll
    D. prone with head elevated 30 degrees

36. The nurse is caring for a 4-year-old child with celiac disease. The nurse expects to find which of the following manifestations of the disease while assessing the child and obtaining the health history from the patient's mother?
    A. anorexia, abdominal distention, steatorrhea
    B. vomiting, diarrhea, abdominal pain, jaundice
    C. constipation, abdominal cramping, flatulence
    D. nausea, vomiting, diarrhea

37. When caring for a child with probable appendicitis, the nurse must be alert to recognize which of the following signs of perforation?
    A. nausea and vomiting
    B. anorexia
    C. sudden relief from pain
    D. decreased abdominal distention

38. The nurse is caring for a patient with pancreatic enzyme insufficiency. The nurse understands that the patient will have which of the following symptoms without treatment?
    A. steatorrhea and weight loss
    B. nausea and vomiting
    C. peripheral edema and weight gain
    D. muscle wasting and anorexia

39. The nurse is caring for a patient with hepatitis A. The nurse understands that this patient most likely acquired the disease from which of the following sources?
    A. donating blood within the past three months
    B. having hemodialysis treatments for renal failure
    C. eating food contaminated by an infected individual
    D. sharing needles for intravenous drug use

40. The nurse is caring for a patient with hepatitis B. The nurse understands that high risk groups for acquiring this virus include which of the following?
    A. food workers
    B. college students
    C. elderly patients
    D. hemodialysis nurses

41. **The nurse is providing dietary teaching for a patient with hepatitis. The nurse realizes that the material has been understood when the patient makes which of the following statements?**
    A. "I will eat more whole grains, egg whites, and fat-free yogurt."
    B. "I will increase my intake of sausage, butter, and whole milk."
    C. "I will still be able to have a few beers each day."
    D. "I will try to reduce my alcohol intake to 2 liters per day."

42. **The nurse is providing care for a patient with acute pancreatitis. Which of the following nursing interventions would be most appropriate to achieve patient comfort?**
    A. assisting the patient to turn side to side every hour
    B. administration of hydromorphone via PCA
    C. administration of morphine by infusion device
    D. administration of meperidine (Demerol) via PCA

43. **The nurse is caring for a patient who will undergo paracentesis. Which of the following instructions should the nurse be sure to provide prior to the procedure?**
    A. "You must not eat or drink for 12 hours before the procedure."
    B. "You will need to empty your bladder before the procedure."
    C. "You will be on strict bed rest for 6 hours after the procedure."
    D. "You will need to empty your bowel before the procedure."

44. **The nurse is caring for a patient with end-stage cirrhosis who is admitted to the hospital with vomiting. The nurse must be alert to the possibility of which of the following complications for this patient?**
    A. intrahepatic bile stasis
    B. bleeding esophageal varices
    C. decreased bilirubin excretion
    D. plasma accumulation in the peritoneum

45. **The nurse understands that which of the following patients would be most at risk for development of liver cancer?**
    A. 58-year-old patient with history of diabetes mellitus
    B. 28-year-old patient with history of blunt liver trauma
    C. 65-year-old patient with history of cirrhosis
    D. 80-year-old patient with history of malnutrition

46. **The nurse is caring for a patient who has undergone a laparoscopic cholecystectomy and now complains of gas pains. The best action by the nurse would be to:**
    A. assist with ambulation.
    B. assist to cough and deep breathe.
    C. encourage bed rest with legs elevated.
    D. insert a rectal tube to facilitate flatus passage.

Physical Assessment

1. **The nurse is caring for a patient with an ileostomy. The nurse anticipates that a normal stoma should appear:**
   A. pale pink.
   B. reddish pink.
   C. red with white edges.
   D. purple.

2. The nurse is caring for a patient with peptic ulcer disease. Which of the following clinical manifestations would be most likely if the ulcer perforates?
   A. projectile vomiting
   B. frequent belching
   C. diarrhea
   D. board-like abdomen

3. The nurse is caring for a patient who will undergo an endoscopic procedure (EGD) of the upper GI tract so the physician can visualize the location and severity of an ulcer. Upon return of the patient to the unit, priority assessment by the nurse would include checking vital signs and:
   A. the gag reflex.
   B. breath sounds.
   C. bowel sounds.
   D. intake and output.

4. The nurse is caring for a patient who had a gastric resection 24 hours ago. The nurse expects to assess normal drainage from the nasogastric tube. Which of the following would be considered normal at this point postoperatively?
   A. brown
   B. bright red
   C. black
   D. cloudy white

5. The nurse is providing care for a patient who is admitted in the prodromal phase of hepatitis. Upon assessment, the nurse expects to find which of the following symptoms?
   A. fever, petechiae, easy bruising
   B. flu-like symptoms, malaise, fatigue
   C. ascites, jaundice, hemangiomas
   D. splenomegaly, hypoalbuminemia, GI bleeding

6. The nurse is providing care for a patient who is in the icteric phase of acute hepatitis. The nurse expects which of the following findings upon assessment and care of the patient?
   A. anorexia and vomiting
   B. fever and elevated WBC
   C. jaundice and dark-colored urine
   D. ascites and dark-colored stools

7. The nurse is caring for a patient with suspected cholecystitis. Which of the following assessment findings would be most significant for this patient?
   A. right upper quadrant pain
   B. skin color is pale
   C. bowel function is normal
   D. rebound abdominal tenderness

8. The nurse is caring for a patient with acute pancreatitis and is aware that, upon performing an abdominal assessment, it is particularly important to:
   A. inspect the abdomen for presence of peristalsis.
   B. auscultate for high-pitched, rushing bowel sounds.
   C. assess for severe epigastric pain that radiates to the back.
   D. palpate the epigastric region for pancreatic enlargement.

9. The nurse is assisting a physician to perform a paracentesis. Following the procedure, it is important for the nurse to monitor the patient for signs of which of the following?
   A. intake and output
   B. hypovolemia
   C. systemic vasoconstriction
   D. rebound hypertension

Interpretation of Lab Values

1. The nurse knows that a patient who is receiving total parenteral nutrition (TPN) has the potential for systemic imbalances related to administration of electrolytes and nutritional components. Which of the following must be monitored closely during the initiation of therapy?
   A. serum glucose
   B. serum potassium
   C. serum sodium
   D. blood gases

2. The nurse is reviewing lab work for a patient who is receiving total parenteral nutrition. Which of the following lab results might be interpreted as a complication of therapy?
   A. serum Na^+ 137 mEq/L
   B. fasting glucose: 101 mg/dL
   C. serum K^+ 5.0 mEq/L
   D. white blood count: 16,000

3. The nurse is reviewing the results of an arterial blood gas specimen from a 3-month-old child who has a 3-day history of diarrhea. The results are as follows: pH 7.30; pCO_2 35 mm Hg; and HCO_3 17 mEq/L. The nurse recognizes that the infant is in:
   A. metabolic acidosis.
   B. metabolic alkalosis.
   C. respiratory acidosis.
   D. respiratory alkalosis.

4. The nurse is caring for a patient with liver dysfunction and an elevated ammonia level. Nursing interventions should be based on the understanding that an elevated ammonia level:
   A. is due to chronic ingestion of large amounts of alcohol.
   B. results from disrupted protein metabolism.
   C. is related to impaired glycogenolysis.
   D. results in impaired synthesis of clotting factors.

5. The nurse is providing treatment for a patient with hepatic encephalopathy. Which of the following clinical manifestations indicates that the patient's condition is deteriorating?
   A. frequent liquid diarrhea
   B. decreased serum ammonia levels
   C. increased serum potassium levels
   D. asterixis

Drugs and Treatments

1. The nurse is caring for a patient with gastroesophageal reflux disease (GERD). In preparation for discharge, the nurse must teach the patient about omeprazole (Prilosec). Which of the following statements by the patient indicates understanding of the material?
   A. "Prilosec coats the lining of my esophagus to reduce tissue irritation."
   B. "Prilosec neutralizes stomach acid and reduces the amount of reflux."
   C. "Prilosec decreases the acidity in the esophagus to normal levels."
   D. "Prilosec reduces production of almost all gastric acid within 2 hours."

2. A young patient with a history of severe ulcerative colitis is admitted to the hospital for surgery. Preoperatively the physician orders a clear liquid diet, neomycin, and GoLYTELY. The nurse understands that the purpose of the bowel prep is to:
   A. decrease the risk of postoperative sepsis.
   B. decrease ileal drainage following surgery.
   C. prevent excess bleeding during surgery.
   D. prevent dehydration following surgery.

3. The nurse must instruct the patient about how to self-administer GoLYTELY. Which of the following directions provided by the nurse would be appropriate?
   A. "You will need to drink a full cup every 10 minutes for a few hours."
   B. "You will be able to take one pill every hour for the next four hours."
   C. "Drink this liquid over the next 30 minutes for results by morning."
   D. "Drink 1 cup of this liquid every hour until your stools are clear."

4. The nurse is caring for a patient with heart failure who needs antacid therapy. The nurse knows that which of the following antacids would be the best choice for this patient?
   A. Amphojel
   B. AlternaGEL
   C. Maalox
   D. Riopan

5. The physician prescribes sucralfate (Carafate) 1 gram four times per day for 8 weeks for the patient with a duodenal ulcer. The nurse instructs the patient to take the medication:
   A. with meals and at bedtime.
   B. 1 hour before meals and at bedtime.
   C. with an antacid four times per day.
   D. after meals and at bedtime.

ALTERNATE FORMAT

6. The nurse understands that the patient with gastroesophageal reflux disease (GERD) may treat the condition with which of the following over-the-counter drugs? SELECT ALL THAT APPLY.
   A. famotidine (Pepcid)
   B. calcium carbonate (Tums)
   C. propranolol (Inderal)
   D. verapamil (Calan)
   E. ranitidine (Zantac)

7. The nurse is providing care for a patient who will have a barium enema. The nurse anticipates that the patient will receive which medication following the barium enema?
   A. bisacodyl (Dulcolax)
   B. serum of ipecac
   C. aluminum hydroxide (AlternaGEL)
   D. acetylcysteine (Mucomyst)

8. The nurse understands that a medicine used to neutralize gastric acid is:
   A. metoclopramide (Reglan).
   B. ranitidine (Zantac).
   C. misoprostol (Cytotec).
   D. aluminum and magnesium hydroxide (Maalox TC).

9. The nurse knows that histamine (H_2) receptor antagonists work by:
   A. forming a protective barrier in the gut.
   B. decreasing motility within the gut.
   C. reducing acid production in the gut.
   D. increasing acid neutralization in the gut.

10. The nurse knows that ondansetron (Zofran) is used:
    A. to suppress chemotherapy-induced emesis.
    B. as an antimicrobial agent to treat bacterial pneumonia.
    C. may cause significant hemodynamic effects in patients.
    D. to treat patients with Zollinger-Ellison syndrome.

11. The nurse is caring for a patient with severe Crohn's disease who has an order for infliximab (Remicade). The nurse knows that this drug works by reducing:
    A. the number of stools per day.
    B. pain associated with Crohn's.
    C. symptoms and inducing remission.
    D. the likelihood for surgery.

12. The nurse in a community health clinic is preparing public health information about exposure to hepatitis. The nurse knows that which of the following groups should be vaccinated against both hepatitis A and hepatitis B virus?
    A. residents of elderly housing
    B. day care workers
    C. library workers
    D. computer programmers

13. The nurse who received an accidental needlestick injury while drawing blood from a patient with hepatitis B should receive what type of postexposure care?
    A. two doses of immune globulin—within 1 week of exposure and at 1 month
    B. two doses of immune globulin—within 2 weeks of exposure and at 3 months
    C. hepatitis B vaccine booster shot with a dose of immune globulin
    D. hepatitis B vaccine booster shot with two doses of immune globulin

14. The nurse is providing care for a patient with blood-clotting problems related to hepatic dysfunction. Based on this knowledge, the nurse anticipates the need for which of the following interventions?
    A. administration of salt-poor albumin
    B. administration of protamine sulfate
    C. administration of total parenteral nutrition
    D. administration of parenteral vitamin K

15. The nurse is providing care for a patient who has hepatic encephalopathy with orders for lactulose to be administered via a nasogastric tube. Within 24 hours of the start of therapy, the patient develops diarrhea. The best response by the nurse is to:
    A. withhold further doses of lactulose and notify the physician.
    B. discontinue the lactulose because diarrhea is a severe side effect.
    C. continue to administer lactulose as ordered for this desired effect.
    D. hold the current dose and obtain further orders from the physician.

ANSWERS

General

1. **(B)**; Although excision of the tumor is usually the treatment of choice, radiation may be used to help to reduce the size and vascularity of the tumor before surgery.

2. **(A)**; The nurse should be aware that risk factors for oral cancer include tobacco use (chewing and smoking), heavy alcohol consumption, and marijuana use. Tobacco contains known carcinogens. This is especially hazardous because the carcinogens are absorbed directly through the oral mucosa into the bloodstream. Elimination of all forms of tobacco use is the single most significant factor in reducing risk for oral cancer.

3. **(B)**; The patient should be instructed to increase foods that are high fiber when the acute inflammation has subsided. These high-fiber foods include such things as wheat bran, oat bran, *shredded wheat*, oatmeal, whole-wheat bread, multigrain bread, cooked *asparagus*, broccoli, squash, spinach, lettuce, *carrots*, peaches, apples, and oranges.

4. **(C)**; The patient with acute diverticulitis should be instructed to avoid foods with small seeds, nuts, and foods with skins—like raisins, grapes, corn, *strawberries*, raspberries, blueberries, and figs; rye bread with caraway seeds; popcorn; sesame seeds; *poppy seeds*; sunflower seeds; nuts; *cucumbers*; and okra. Avoidance of these foods will help to decrease exacerbations of diverticulitis.

5. **(D)**; The nurse will succeed in making the task of inserting the nasogastric tube more difficult by asking the patient to turn the head during insertion. Each of the other options would facilitate tube insertion.

6. **(A)**; When caring for a patient with an NG tube who develops nausea, the nurse should first attempt to irrigate the tube to determine patency.

7. **(D)**; The nurse instructs the patient about stress management techniques to help the patient deal with the stress without internalizing it.

8. **(A)**; A nasogastric tube was placed during surgery and will remain in place post-operatively to prevent excessive pressure on suture lines.

9. **(A)**; If a patient has leakage at the surgical anastomosis following gastric surgery, the patient would experience pain, fever, and dyspnea following oral fluids because the fluids leak into the peritoneum, setting the stage for development of peritonitis.

10. **(B)**; Gastroesophageal reflux symptoms are most pronounced with activities that increase intraabdominal pressure, such as bending, straining, lifting, and lying down.

11. **(A)**; The nurse should encourage the patient to eliminate chocolate, oranges, and tomatoes from the diet because they increase the risk of GERD symptoms. Patients experience symptoms of GERD following oral intake of substances that decrease lower esophageal stricture (LES) pressure. These substances include alcohol, caffeine, nicotine, *chocolate*, fatty foods, *citrus fruits*, onions, *tomatoes*, and peppermint.

12. **(D)**; Heartburn is the most common symptom of GERD. Other symptoms that may occur include dysphagia, belching, coughing, chest pain, and sour taste in the morning.

13. **(B)**; Patients with achalasia develop symptoms related to the failure of the lower esophageal sphincter (LES) to relax properly following swallowing. The patient develops chronic and progressive dysphagia, regurgitation, and chest pain.

14. **(C)**; The nursing intervention that is most important in prevention of infection for patients with TPN is to administer intravenous medications via a separate line. Every time the intravenous line is accessed, there is potential for introduction of bacteria into the highly desirable (high glucose content) environment.

15. **(C)**; The nurse should explain that the name of the ostomy arises from the region that is surgically brought to the surface of the abdominal wall. Hence, when the colon (large intestine) is the site of surgery, the site is referred to as colostomy (colon + ostomy). When the ileum (small intestine) is the site of surgical intervention, the abdominal stoma is referred to as ileostomy (ileum + ostomy).

16. **(B)**; The patient with acute abdominal pain who is most likely to have acute appendicitis is the 13-year-old male.

17. **(B)**; Patients with ulcerative colitis tend to have severe diarrhea. Activity restriction may help to reduce intestinal peristalsis and diarrhea.

18. **(C)**; The nurse might suggest to the client to avoid eating broccoli and cabbage; to empty feces and gas from the appliance frequently throughout the day, and to utilize deodorizing drops in the bottom of the appliance. Putting pinholes in the appliance is not an effective means of reducing flatus, and it would most certainly not limit odor.

19. **(C)**; The patient with an exacerbation of Crohn's disease may be having 6–12 or more stools per day. It is absolutely not appropriate to administer stool softeners to this patient.

20. **(D)**; A colonoscopy is a test that requires insertion of a flexible scope into the rectum. The scope is carefully advanced until it enters the colon. It can provide direct visualization of the inside of the colon and helps to identify the exact cause and location of bleeding.

21. **(B)**; A small bowel biopsy may be done during an esophagogastroduodenoscopy. This examination involves insertion of a flexible scope through the esophagus (esophago), into the stomach (gastro), and then into the small bowel (duodenoscopy). The patient's throat is anesthetized prior to insertion of this scope. Therefore, it is important for nurses to assess gag reflex when the patient returns to the nursing unit before administering any fluids by mouth.

22. **(A)**; Although caffeine, nicotine, and alcohol can each predispose a patient to esophageal reflux, the fact that the patient drinks only occasionally would be the factor least likely to predispose to reflux. NoDoz is an over-the-counter stimulant substance that is composed primarily of caffeine, and the patient admits to drinking 6–10 cups of coffee in addition.

23. **(B)**; The patient should have the head of the bed elevated at least 30 degrees for at least an hour after a bolus feeding to reduce the risk of aspiration.

24. **(C)**; The nurse would encourage the patient to avoid spicy foods, alcohol, and other known irritants, such as ibuprofen.

25. **(C)**; It is essential for the EGD to occur prior to the barium swallow because traces of barium left after the swallow would interfere with visualization of the GI tract with the scope. It does not really matter whether the barium swallow or the barium enema occurs next. What matters most is that the patient increases fluid intake and receives laxatives to facilitate elimination of the barium following the two exams.

26. **(C)**; Cancer of the colon is often asymptomatic until it is quite advanced. Early symptoms are most commonly vague or may include changes in bowel habits, such as alternating diarrhea with constipation. The symptom that most frequently results in a trip to see the healthcare provider is blood in the stools.

27. **(A)**; The HOB should be elevated at least 30–45 degrees for at least 30–60 minutes to reduce the risk of aspiration following administration of medications via an NG feeding tube.

28. **(B)**; The patient is at risk for constipation related to the presence of barium in the GI tract.

29. **(D)**; The patient with a personal history of GI polyps is at risk for colon cancer. Additional risk factors include diets high in animal protein, fat, and calories; daily alcohol consumption; and elevated levels of C-reactive protein.

30. **(D)**; Dumping syndrome is a common problem following gastric resections. It occurs because the food bolus enters the duodenum or jejunum very quickly. Water is pulled into the lumen of the gut to dilute the food bolus. This fluid shift causes a rapid decrease in blood volume and a reflex response by the sympathetic nervous system that results in tachycardia, orthostatic hypotension, dizziness, flushing, and diaphoresis. Patients may also have nausea, epigastric pain, cramping, and loud, hyperactive bowel sounds within 5 to 30 minutes after a meal. Diarrhea occurs soon afterward.

31. **(C)**; Kidneys of infants are immature and do not have the ability to dilute or concentrate urine or to regulate electrolyte loss. This makes infants prone to developing dehydration.

32. **(C)**; Rotavirus frequently causes acute diarrhea in young children.

33. **(B)**; Diarrhea is a very common side effect of antibiotic therapy in children.

34. **(A)**; Popcorn is high in fiber, and children will eat it as a snack, which may help to relieve constipation.

35. **(D)**; The infant should be positioned in a prone position with the head and chest elevated 30 degrees to reduce the likelihood of reflux.

36. **(A)**; Clinical manifestations of celiac disease include *steatorrhea*, foul-smelling stools, malnutrition, muscle wasting, anemia, *anorexia, abdominal distention*, irritability, fretfulness, uncooperativeness, and apathy.

37. **(C)**; If the appendix perforates, the child will develop peritonitis. Initial signs of peritonitis include fever, sudden relief from pain after perforation with later increase in diffuse pain, abdominal distention, tachycardia, rapid shallow breathing, pallor, chills, and irritability.

38. **(A)**; The patient with pancreatic enzyme insufficiency will be unable to digest fats, and therefore fats will be excreted in the stool. Over time the inability to digest fats will result in weight loss.

39. **(C)**; Hepatitis A is usually transmitted by the fecal–oral route. Patients commonly acquire this type of hepatitis by drinking contaminated water, eating uncooked food washed in sewage-contaminated water, or eating food contaminated by an infected person who did not wash his or her hands after using the toilet. Hepatitis A may be transmitted by oral sex and can be transmitted through infusion of infected blood.

40. **(D)**; Hepatitis B virus is found in blood, semen, cervical secretions, saliva, and wound drainage. Transmission is through direct contact with the blood or body fluids. Specific modes of transmission include working with blood and blood products, sexual contact, and contact with contaminated inanimate objects (the virus can survive up to a week on environmental surfaces). High-risk populations include healthcare workers—especially those who work in the blood bank or hemodialysis—IV drug abusers, homosexual men, and people with multiple sexual partners.

41. **(A)**; The nurse recommends a low-fat, high-calorie diet for the patient with hepatitis. Based on the statement, the patient understands that good low-fat sources of protein should include *egg whites*, tofu, beans, and *fat-free dairy* products. *Whole wheat*, fruits, and vegetables are good complex carbohydrate choices.

42. **(D)**; Meperidine (Demerol) is the drug of choice for pain control in acute pancreatitis. There is speculation that it produces less spasm of the sphincter of Oddi than morphine.

43. **(B)**; The patient must empty the bladder before the paracentesis to decrease the risk of inadvertant trauma to the bladder during needle insertion.

44. **(B)**; Esophageal varices develop as a consequence of portal hypertension and are prone to bleeding with coughing, sneezing, *vomiting*, or ingestion of foods high in fiber.

45. **(C)**; Most primary liver cancer in the United States is related to alcoholic cirrhosis.

46. **(A)**; Patients who undergo laparoscopic cholecystectomy suffer gas pain postoperatively related to insufflation of the abdomen with CO_2 during surgery. The patient should be encouraged and assisted (if necessary) to ambulate to facilitate dissipation of the gas.

Physical Assessment

1. **(B)**; A normal stoma should be reddish pink in appearance.

2. **(D)**; When a patient with peptic ulcer disease experiences perforation of an ulcer, the nurse will assess for signs and symptoms. Classic manifestations include a board-like abdomen and absence of bowel sounds, which occur almost immediately following perforation. Diagnosis is more challenging in the older adult, who may exhibit more nonspecific symptoms.

3. **(A)**; The nurse must be certain to check for a gag reflex before allowing the patient any fluids by mouth. The throat was anesthetized prior to the procedure to improve patient tolerance, and the patient may or may not have a gag reflex present upon return. Introducing fluids prior to the return of the gag reflex would put the patient at risk for aspiration.

4. **(A)**; By 24 hours postoperatively, nasogastric drainage should contain only small amounts of old blood, which results in brownish drainage.

5. **(B)**; The prodromal phase of acute hepatitis occurs between time of exposure and onset of jaundice. Symptoms are often vague but may include flu-like symptoms with anorexia, nausea, vomiting, malaise, myalgia, arthralgia, and easy fatigue.

6. **(C)**; The icteric phase of acute hepatitis begins with the onset of jaundice. Because of high levels of conjugated bilirubin, the nurse expects that the urine may be very dark colored during this phase.

7. **(A)**; Clinical manifestations of cholecystitis include sudden onset of severe and steady right upper quadrant pain that radiates to the scapula or shoulder, nausea, vomiting, heartburn, flatulence, fever, and chills.

8. **(C)**; Clinical manifestations of acute pancreatitis include the onset of steady and severe epigastric pain that radiates to the back following ingestion of alcohol or a fatty meal.

9. **(B)**; Following removal of a significant amount of ascitic fluid, the nurse must monitor the patient closely for signs of hypovolemia.

Interpretation of Lab Values

1. **(A)**; Serum glucose or point-of-care glucose testing should be done at least every 4 hours for 48 hours at the onset of TPN therapy to track whether or not the patient will require supplemental insulin to maintain normal glucose levels.

2. **(D)**; The white blood count of 16,000 is indicative of infection, which could be related to administration of TPN.

3. **(A)**; The pH is acidotic at 7.30, and HCO_3 is very low at 17 mEq/L. The combination of these features with a low normal pCO_2 implies metabolic acidosis.

4. **(B)**; In the patient with a liver disorder, an elevated ammonia level represents disrupted protein metabolism.

5. **(D)**; The occurrence of asterixis (flapping tremor of the fingers and wrists) in a patient with hepatic encephalopathy indicates worsening of the patient's condition.

Drugs and Treatments

1. **(D)**; Omeprazole (Prilosec) is a very powerful drug used to suppress production of gastric acid. The drug reduces baseline acid levels and blocks production of nearly all stimulated acid production within 2 hours of an oral dose of medication.

2. **(A)**; Administration of the bowel prep includes neomycin (an aminoglycoside) to suppress bowel flora prior to surgery and GoLYTELY (a polyethylene glycol electrolyte solution) as a laxative. Together the drugs help to decrease the risk of postoperative sepsis in the patient undergoing bowel surgery.

3. **(A)**; The nurse should explain to the patient that there will be a large volume of fluid to drink (about 4 L) and that it is best to drink about 1 cup every 10 minutes or so for a few hours.

4. **(D)**; Riopan is the best choice of antacid for the patient with heart failure because it has very low sodium content in contrast to the others, which are aluminum-containing antacids.

5. **(B)**; Sucralfate (Carafate) is a mucosal protective agent that should be taken on an empty stomach. Doses should be taken 1 hour before meals and at bedtime.

6. **(A, B, E)**; Patients often self-treat GERD. Over-the-counter medications that are used by patients to treat symptoms of GERD include cimetidine (Tagamet), *ranitidine (Zantac)*, *famotidine (Pepcid)*, nizatidine (Axid), omeprazole (Prilosec), and a variety of *antacids*.

7. **(A)**; Following a barium enema, the patient will receive a laxative, such as Dulcolax, to aid in evacuating the barium from the bowel.

8. **(D)**; Antacids neutralize gastric acid. None of the other medications listed work by the same mechanism.

9. **(C)**; Histamine (H$_2$) receptor antagonists work by blocking H$_2$ receptor sites and reducing acid production.

10. **(A)**; Ondansetron (Zofran) was the first medication approved to suppress chemotherapy-related emesis. It can be administered either orally or intravenously.

11. **(C)**; Infliximab (Remicade) is a monoclonal antibody that binds with and inactivates *tumor necrosis factor-alpha*. In studies it reduced symptoms and induced remission for patients with Crohn's.

12. **(B)**; The nurse knows that people in high-risk groups should be vaccinated against hepatitis A and B. Therefore, the nurse should recommend vaccination to healthcare workers, day care workers, correctional facility employees, IV drug users, male homosexuals, patients on hemodialysis, and household and sexual contacts of individuals with hepatitis B virus.

13. **(A)**; Upon exposure to hepatitis B, the nurse should receive postexposure prophylaxis with two doses of immune globulin. One dose must be administered within 1 week of initial exposure, and the second is administered 1 month after exposure. The nurse may also receive hepatitis B vaccine with the immune globulin following exposure.

14. **(D)**; Patients with hepatic dysfunction are deficient of vitamin K. The liver normally produces bile, which is necessary for formation of fat-soluble vitamins, including vitamin K. When liver function is impaired, deficiency of fat-soluble vitamins is likely.

15. **(C)**; The nurse should continue to administer the lactulose to the patient. Lactulose is a hyperosmolar laxative that blocks absorption of ammonia in the large intestine and produces diarrhea. Diarrhea helps to limit production of ammonia by limiting the amount of time that the feces is in the presence of bacteria in the intestine.

Keep Track

- Percent correct. (Divide the number of questions you answered correctly by the total number of questions you answered.)   _____

- Number of questions you missed due to a reading error: _____

- Number of questions you missed due to errors in analysis: _____

- Number of assessment questions you missed: _____

- Number of lab value questions you missed: _____

- Number of drug/treatment questions you missed: _____

Nugget List

Chapter number _____ Topic _____

Practice Test: Nursing Management of Patients with Endocrine Disorders

Karen S. March

PRACTICE TEST

General

1. The nurse is providing teaching to a pregnant female with gestational diabetes. Which statement by the patient indicates understanding of the long-term prognosis?
   A. "Soon after I deliver, I won't have these high blood glucose levels."
   B. "I will continue to check my blood glucose levels twice per day."
   C. "This means that my baby will have Type I diabetes at birth."
   D. "This means that I will have Type II diabetes for the rest of my life."

2. The nurse has been providing teaching to a pregnant woman with Type I diabetes. Which of the following statements by the patient indicates an understanding of the impact of pregnancy on insulin needs?
   A. "Because pregnancy increases my metabolism, I'll need less insulin."
   B. "Hormone production during my pregnancy increases my insulin needs."
   C. "Because my blood glucose levels are stable, I'll check them only once per day."
   D. "My placenta continually produces insulin, which decreases my blood glucose."

3. The nurse is providing teaching to a pregnant female with diabetes. Which of the following statements by the patient indicates an understanding of plans for delivery?
   A. "I will have a cesarean delivery before my due date."
   B. "I will have a cesarean delivery scheduled on my due date."
   C. "I plan to use natural childbirth strategies without drugs."
   D. "I will receive drug injections to help my baby's lungs to mature."

4. The nurse is caring for a patient with Type II diabetes. Which of the following statements by the patient indicates understanding of predisposing factors for the disease?
   A. "Both of my parents and one grandparent had diabetes."
   B. "My youngest child was diagnosed with Type I diabetes."
   C. "I got diabetes because I've eaten too many sweets over the years."
   D. "My pancreas stopped making insulin, which caused my disease."

5. The nurse is caring for a hospitalized non-diabetic patient with a fasting blood glucose level of 145 mg/dL. The patient asks, "How can that be? I don't have diabetes." The best response by the nurse is:
   A. "The doctor will be in later to discuss these test results with you."
   B. "It is not unusual to have elevated blood glucose during acute illness."
   C. "We will need to check your blood glucose again in a week."
   D. "Your glucose can best be managed by dietary modification."

6. The nurse is providing teaching to a patient who has been diagnosed with Type I diabetes. Which statement by the patient indicates an understanding of key characteristics of the disease?
   A. "I may be able to decide if I take insulin or oral medications."
   B. "I probably developed this disease because I am overweight."
   C. "Newly diagnosed patients get very ill very quickly with Type I."
   D. "Part of the problem is that my body has developed insulin resistance."

7. The nurse is assigned to care for a preoperative patient with Type II diabetes. Which of the following statements by the patient confirms expected characteristics with this type of diabetes?
   A. "I was up five times through the night to urinate."
   B. "I've been feeling good and have had no recent problems."
   C. "My blood sugar seems to be all over the place."
   D. "I have always been thin throughout my life."

8. The nurse is providing information about insulin resistance to a patient with Type II diabetes. Which of the following statements by the patient indicates that teaching has been effective?
   A. "I have normal or high levels of insulin in my bloodstream."
   B. "My body is not producing any insulin, so I have to take shots."
   C. "My blood glucose is high because my pancreas isn't working."
   D. "My muscles and subcutaneous fat readily absorb insulin."

9. The nurse is caring for a patient who is newly diagnosed with Type II diabetes. The patient is visibly upset about the diagnosis and states, "Now I'll never be able to keep my job as a teacher. I've heard that diabetes causes blindness." The best response by the nurse is:
   A. "You may need to have an appointment with a career counselor."
   B. "Blindness is a risk only for patients with Type I diabetes."
   C. "Controlling glucose and blood pressure reduces risk for blindness."
   D. "Blindness does not occur frequently in patients with diabetes."

10. The nurse is caring for a patient who was recently diagnosed with Type I diabetes. The patient asks the nurse if it would be possible to convert from insulin to treatment with oral hypoglycemics because, "I really hate shots." The best response by the nurse is:
    A. "Try to think about being somewhere you enjoy before giving your shot."
    B. "Oral medications will not work for you because your body makes no insulin."
    C. "We can talk to the doctor about using both oral medications and insulin."
    D. "Somewhere down the road it might be an option for us to consider."

11. A patient with Type I diabetes asks the nurse if it is okay to eat foods that contain sugar. The best reply by the nurse is:
    A. "You can eat some sugary foods as long as you reduce other carbs for the day."
    B. "Unfortunately, you will need to eat things with a sugar substitute only."
    C. "You can eat as much sugar as you want as long as you cover it with insulin."
    D. "It is important to use sugar substitutes as your primary sweetening agent."

12. A patient with Type I diabetes reveals to the nurse that his blood glucose levels "have been all over the place lately." The patient then says, "I'm just not sure what to do. I know I have to exercise every day to stay healthy." The best response by the nurse is:
    A. "Let's look at your food diary to review what you have been eating lately."
    B. "Yes, you should exercise. That is an essential part of your treatment plan."
    C. "Until we get your blood glucose regulated, you should not exercise."
    D. "If you are going to exercise, you will need to consume more calories."

13. The nurse is caring for a patient in the emergency department who was admitted with a serum glucose level of 857 mg/dL. The patient is nauseated, vomiting, lethargic, and polyuric. Vital signs are BP 78/50; P 125; R 28. A priority nursing diagnosis for this patient would be:
    A. altered nutrition—more than body requirements.
    B. altered mental status.
    C. fluid volume deficit.
    D. impaired gas exchange.

ALTERNATE FORMAT

14. The nurse is providing teaching about hypoglycemia to a patient with diabetes. Which of the following statements by the patient indicates an appropriate understanding of this information? SELECT ALL THAT APPLY.
    A. "My symptoms will depend upon how fast my glucose level falls."
    B. "I should always carry some sugar-free Life Savers and candy."
    C. "I may feel jittery or nervous if my glucose level falls fast."
    D. "It may be hard for me to tell when my blood sugar is low."

15. Laboratory results for patients with hyperosmolar hyperglycemic state (HHS) are similar to those for patients with diabetic ketoacidosis (DKA), with a few major exceptions. The nurse expects to see which of the following results for the patient with HHS in comparison to results for the patient with DKA?
    A. higher serum glucose, higher bicarbonate, greater ketosis
    B. higher serum glucose, milder ketosis, higher pH
    C. lower serum glucose, lower pH, greater ketosis
    D. lower serum glucose, higher pH, milder ketosis

16. A patient presents to the emergency department with symptoms of diabetic ketoacidosis. The nurse would identify which of the following nursing diagnoses as a priority for this patient?
    A. disrupted sleep pattern
    B. impaired health maintenance
    C. imbalanced nutrition: less than body requirements
    D. deficient fluid volume

17. The nurse is providing care for a patient who was recently diagnosed with hypothyroidism. When the patient asks the nurse how long he will have to take the medication, the best response by the nurse is:
    A. "That will depend on your serum blood levels."
    B. "You will have to take medication for the rest of your life."
    C. "You will need the medication until after surgery."
    D. "We will make that decision in a few months."

ALTERNATE FORMAT

18. The nurse is caring for an infant with the diagnosis of hypothyroidism. When the mother asks about the prognosis for the child, the best response by the nurse is: SELECT ALL THAT APPLY.
    A. "Hypothyroidism in infants cannot be treated, so we will wait to treat."
    B. "Outcomes are best when the child is treated within a few days of birth."
    C. "Unfortunately, your child will probably not survive to one year of age."
    D. "Your child will have some degree of mental retardation."

19. The nurse is caring for a patient with hyperthyroidism. Which of the following statements by the patient indicates inadequate control of the disease?
    A. "I just feel so nervous and sweaty all of the time that I don't know what to do."
    B. "I feel pretty good, but I just don't have much of an appetite lately."
    C. "I keep gaining weight no matter what I try, and I cannot seem to lose."
    D. "I am so tired that I just want to sleep all the time."

20. The nurse is caring for a patient with Graves' disease. When the patient asks the nurse how the disease is normally treated, the best response by the nurse is:
    A. "You will receive artificial thyroid stimulating hormone to normalize your levels."
    B. "You will receive oral catecholamines to help to normalize your metabolism."
    C. "You may require surgical removal of some or all of your thyroid gland."
    D. "You may require treatment with intravenous potassium."

21. The nurse is assigned to care for an acutely ill patient with thyrotoxicosis. Which of the following assessment findings by the nurse would indicate worsening of the patient's condition?
    A. The heart rate is 100 beats per minute.
    B. The patient is displaying symptoms of angina.
    C. The temperature is 98.6°F.
    D. The patient is sleeping soundly.

22. The nurse is caring for a patient with Graves' disease who asks why both surgery and medication are required for treatment of the disease. The best response by the nurse is:
    A. "The medication decreases the vascularity of the thyroid before surgery."
    B. "Your situation is especially dangerous, so both methods are necessary."
    C. "It is important to increase your thyroid hormone levels before surgery."
    D. "A multifaceted approach is most effective to treat your disease."

23. The nurse is assigned to care for a patient who has been admitted with new onset of diabetes insipidus. Based on the diagnosis, the nurse would expect which of the following to be the priority nursing diagnosis?
    A. fluid volume deficit
    B. anxiety
    C. alteration in comfort
    D. impaired gas exchange

24. The nurse is providing discharge instructions for the patient who is being treated for diabetes insipidus. Which of the following instructions must the nurse include for this patient?
    A. "You will need to take this medication for at least 14 days."
    B. "It is important for you to measure and record your urine output."
    C. "You should try to drink at least 3000 mL of fluid every day."
    D. "It is likely that your urine output will increase with treatment."

25. The nurse is assigned to care for a patient with a diagnosis of adrenal crisis. Which of the following situations is likely responsible for this diagnosis?
    A. abrupt withdrawal from chronic glucocorticoid therapy
    B. inadequate supply of antidiuretic hormone
    C. impaired release of corticotropin releasing factor
    D. elevated levels of adrenocorticotropic hormone

26. Goiter is associated with which of the following states?
    A. symptomatic hyperthyroidism
    B. compensated hyperthyroidism
    C. symptomatic hypothyroidism
    D. compensated hypothyroidism

27. The nurse must schedule administration of hormones on the medication administration record. The nurse plans to administer a large dose of hormone in the morning and a smaller dose in the evening every day because:
    A. patients must maintain constant hormone levels throughout the day.
    B. patients are more likely to remember to take medications twice per day.
    C. the physiologic effect will mimic the body's normal hormone levels.
    D. the patient requires a periodic boost to its inherent hormone levels.

28. The nurse is teaching a patient about hormonal regulation and includes information that which of the following provides the mechanism for hormonal level maintenance?
    A. cell wall integrity
    B. enzymatic activity
    C. negative feedback
    D. the renin–angiotensin–aldosterone system

29. The nurse is caring for a patient with a disorder of calcium metabolism. The nurse recognizes that which of the following glands is most likely responsible for this problem?
    A. adrenal cortex
    B. thyroid gland
    C. parathyroid gland
    D. posterior pituitary

30. The nurse is caring for a patient who has iatrogenic endocrine disease. Which factor in the patient's history is least likely to have contributed to the development of her disease?
    A. hormonal replacement therapy
    B. irradiation of a gland
    C. high blood pressure
    D. surgical removal of a gland

31. The nurse is providing preoperative teaching for a patient who will undergo a partial thyroidectomy. Which of the following information should the nurse be sure to include in the teaching plan?
    A. The patient will definitely require lifetime hormone replacement therapy.
    B. Until surgery, the client should avoid iodine-containing substances.
    C. Adequate preparation for surgery may take two to three months.
    D. There is a need for weight reduction prior to scheduling surgery.

32. The nurse is caring for a patient following thyroidectomy. Which of the following symptoms, as reported by the patient, should alert the nurse to the development of postoperative complications?
    A. abdominal discomfort
    B. an odd sensation around the mouth
    C. loss of appetite
    D. increased thirst

33. The nurse is planning for discharge teaching with a patient with Addison's disease. On which of the following should the nurse place the highest priority for teaching purposes?
    A. strategies for coping with a chronic disease
    B. strategies for maintaining compliance with therapy
    C. strategies for preventing hypertension
    D. strategies for achieving long-term weight loss

34. The nurse is caring for a patient diagnosed with pheochromocytoma. Based on this information, the nurse realizes that which of the following assessments is critical to providing appropriate care for this patient?
    A. blood pressure
    B. daily weight
    C. abdominal girth
    D. pulse regularity

35. The nurse is caring for a patient who will have a transsphenoidal hypophysectomy. Which aspect of normal postoperative care will the nurse modify for this patient?
    A. oxygen administration
    B. leg exercises
    C. nutrition
    D. oral care

36. The nurse is preparing to care for a patient who is diagnosed with syndrome of inappropriate ADH (SIADH). The nurse must carefully assess this patient for signs and symptoms of:
    A. hypercalcemia.
    B. hypernatremia.
    C. magnesium overload.
    D. water intoxication.

Physical Assessment

ALTERNATE FORMAT

1. The nurse is assigned to care for a patient with diabetic gastroparesis. The nurse anticipates that this patient will have which of the following manifestations of this syndrome? SELECT ALL THAT APPLY.
   A. nausea
   B. vomiting
   C. diarrhea
   D. abdominal bloating

2. An emergency department nurse receives a patient who is comatose. The patient is wearing a MedicAlert bracelet that reveals that the patient is diabetic. A priority for care of this patient must involve:
   A. assessment of serum glucose level.
   B. placing an oral airway.
   C. putting the patient on a monitor.
   D. administering IV glucose.

3. A patient presents to the emergency department with the following symptoms: polydipsia, polyuria, abdominal pain, nausea, and fruity breath. The emergency department nurse immediately recognizes these symptoms as typical for patients with:
   A. Addison's disease.
   B. diabetic ketoacidosis.
   C. hyperosmolar hyperglycemic state.
   D. myxedema coma.

4. The nurse is assigned to care for a patient who has been admitted with hypothyroidism. Based on this information, which of the following findings would the nurse anticipate?
   A. flat affect
   B. fever
   C. pink, warm, dry skin
   D. hyperalertness

5. The nurse is assigned to care for a patient with Addison's disease. Based on the diagnosis, the nurse would expect which of the following characteristic symptoms when assessing this patient?
   A. weakness and hyperglycemia
   B. hypoglycemia and hyperkalemia
   C. hypertension and bradycardia
   D. emaciation and tachycardia

6. The nurse is assigned to care for a patient with Cushing's disease. Based on the diagnosis, the nurse would expect which of the following characteristic findings during assessment of this patient?
   A. hypertension and impaired immunity
   B. hypoglycemia and tachycardia
   C. hyperthermia and thin skin
   D. osteoporosis and polyphagia

7. The nurse must assess the patient for signs of hypoparathyroidism. Which of the following assessments would provide important information?
   A. checking the size of the patient's pupils
   B. instructing the patient to dorsiflex the foot
   C. tapping the side of the patient's face
   D. monitoring the patient's blood pressure

Interpretation of Lab Values

ALTERNATE FORMAT

1. A nurse working in a primary practice office is reviewing laboratory results for a group of patients. The nurse becomes concerned about a patient with a fasting blood glucose of: SELECT ALL THAT APPLY.
   A. 45 mg/dL
   B. 72 mg/dL
   C. 98 mg/dL
   D. 110 mg/dL
   E. 130 mg/dL
   F. 134 mg/dL

2. The nurse is providing teaching for a patient who was diagnosed with Type II diabetes just a few weeks ago. The nurse asks how frequently the patient performs self-monitoring of blood glucose at home. The patient replies that self-monitoring is done daily but that the glucose levels seem to vary considerably throughout each day. When the patient asks if there will be follow-up testing at the laboratory, the nurse responds:
   A. "You will need to have a hemoglobin A1c measured at least once per year."
   B. "You will need to have fructosamine levels drawn every month or so."
   C. "If your blood glucose is under control, hemoglobin A1c is drawn twice per year."
   D. "As long as you continue to do your self-monitoring, you won't need lab work."

3. The nurse is caring for a patient who was admitted through the emergency department with a serum glucose level of 857 mg/dL. The patient is nauseated, vomiting, and polyuric. Vital signs are BP 78/50; P 125; R 28. After an insulin drip infused for one hour, the serum glucose level rose to 975 mg/dL. When a family member of the patient asks how the glucose could rise while the patient is receiving insulin, the best response by the nurse would be:
   A. "I will check to be sure that nothing is wrong with the IV line."
   B. "Sometimes insulin will cling to tubing, which weakens its effect."
   C. "We are investigating other possible reasons for the high glucose."
   D. "I will change the IV and tubing to ensure that everything is primed well."

4. Which of the following sets of laboratory results best reflects those anticipated in a patient with diabetic ketoacidosis?

	pH	HCO$_3$	Blood glucose
A.	7.28	34 mEq/L	260 mg/dL
B.	7.18	13 mEq/L	120 mg/dL
C.	7.26	14 mEq/L	450 mg/dL
D.	7.38	24 mEq/L	620 mg/dL

5. Which of the following statements by the nurse best describes the rationale for administering potassium supplements with insulin therapy?
   A. "Potassium replaces losses incurred with diuresis."
   B. "It is necessary because the patient is malnourished."
   C. "IV potassium renders the infused solution isotonic."
   D. "Insulin drives potassium back into the cells."

ALTERNATE FORMAT

6. The nurse is caring for a patient who is being worked up for thyroid dysfunction and has the following lab results:

Test	Patient value	Normal value
Serum total thyroxine (T4)	14 µg/dL	4.5–12.0 µg/dL
Serum total triiodothyronine (T3)	220 ng/dL	70–190 ng/dL
Serum thyrotropin (TSH)	1.2 µU/mL	0.4–4.8 µU/mL

   Based on the lab results, the nurse realizes which of the following? SELECT ALL THAT APPLY.
   A. The anterior pituitary gland is working excessively.
   B. The anterior pituitary gland is working normally.
   C. The thyroid gland is producing excessively.
   D. The thyroid gland is producing normally.

ALTERNATE FORMAT

7. The nurse is assigned to care for a patient who is being assessed for thyroid dysfunction and has the following lab results:

Test	Patient value	Normal value
Serum total thyroxine (T4)	2.4 µg/dL	4.5–12.0 µg/dL
Serum total triiodothyronine (T3)	62 ng/dL	70–190 ng/dL
Serum thyrotropin (TSH)	8.0 µU/mL	0.4–4.8 µU/mL

   Based on the lab results, the best interpretation by the nurse is which of the following? SELECT ALL THAT APPLY.
   A. The patient has hypothyroidism.
   B. The patient has Graves' disease.
   C. The patient's thyroid gland is producing normally.
   D. The patient's anterior pituitary gland is producing excessively.

8. The following lab work for a patient with thyroid dysfunction is reviewed by the nurse:

Test	Patient value	Normal value
Serum total thyroxine (T4)	14 μg/dL	4.5–12.0 μg/dL
Serum total triiodothyronine (T3)	220 ng/dL	70–190 ng/dL
Serum thyrotropin (TSH)	7.2 μU/mL	0.4–4.8 μU/mL

Based on these results, the nurse realizes:
   A. that the patient has primary hyperthyroidism.
   B. that the patient has secondary hyperthyroidism.
   C. that the dysfunction occurs in the thyroid gland.
   D. that the patient has a pituitary adenoma.

Drugs and Treatments

1. Which of the following statements by a patient with diabetic gastroparesis indicates understanding of expected treatment?
   A. "I will take metoclopramide (Reglan) to reduce my symptoms."
   B. "Strict control of my blood glucose will correct this problem."
   C. "When I have an exacerbation, I will need artificial nutrition."
   D. "I need to increase my exercise daily to improve my condition."

2. The nurse is providing baseline education to a patient who was recently diagnosed with Type II diabetes. The patient is 66 inches tall and weighs 115 pounds and has been started on glipizide (Glucotrol) for control of blood glucose. When asked by the patient why glipizide (Glucotrol) was ordered instead of metformin (Glucophage), the nurse's best reply is:
   A. "The choice really comes down to physician preference."
   B. "Glucotrol promotes insulin release from the pancreas."
   C. "Glucophage is a second-line drug for treatment."
   D. "We can talk to the doctor about changing to Glucophage."

3. The nurse is caring for a patient who is to receive 6 units of lispro (Humalog) insulin with breakfast. The nurse knows that the ideal time of administration for Humalog is:
   A. when the patient's breakfast tray arrives.
   B. 30 to 60 minutes prior to breakfast.
   C. up to two hours after breakfast.
   D. with all of the morning medications.

ALTERNATE FORMAT

4. The nurse is caring for a patient who must receive 5 units of insulin aspart (NovoLog) with breakfast and a morning dose of 20 units of NPH insulin. Which of the following provides sound rationale about how the insulin should be administered? SELECT ALL THAT APPLY.
   A. NovoLog cannot be mixed with any other form of insulin.
   B. NovoLog must be administered immediately before eating.
   C. Both insulins can be mixed in one U-50 syringe.
   D. Both insulins can be administered simultaneously.

5. The nurse reviews a patient's medication administration record to discover the following orders for insulin:

---

1. Sliding scale insulin coverage AC and HS with regular insulin:

If blood glucose is:	Administer:
150–199	2 units S.C.
200–224	3 units S.C.
225–249	4 units S.C.
250–274	5 units S.C.
275–299	6 units S.C.
300–324	7 units S.C.
325–349	8 units S.C.

Call physician for 350 or greater

2. Insulin glargine (Lantus) 24 units at HS

Based on experience, the nurse plans to administer the HS doses of regular insulin and insulin glargine:
   A. combined in the same syringe.
   B. in two separate syringes.
   C. at least one hour apart.
   D. at least 30 minutes apart.

6. If the patient's dose of NPH insulin was administered at 8 a.m., the nurse should be particularly alert to signs of hypoglycemia:
   A. between 11 a.m. and noon.
   B. between 3 p.m. and 5 p.m.
   C. between 11 p.m. and midnight.
   D. between 3 a.m. and 5 a.m.

7. The nurse is assigned to care for a patient admitted with diabetic ketoacidosis. Realizing that the patient will require an insulin drip for treatment, the nurse knows that which insulin will be used?
   A. regular
   B. insulin glargine (Lantus)
   C. insulin detemir (Levemir)
   D. insulin lispro (Humalog)

ALTERNATE FORMAT

8. The nurse must administer 15 units of regular insulin and 35 units of NPH insulin to a patient. Please place in order the steps that the nurse will take in preparing the injection.
   A. Draw up the 15 units of regular insulin.
   B. Draw up the 35 units of NPH insulin.
   C. Wipe the top of the vial with alcohol.
   D. Verify insulin order on medication administration record.
   E. Verify the correct patient by using at least 2 forms of identification.
   F. Administer insulin subcutaneously.

9. The patient with Type II diabetes is ordered the following medications during hospitalization:

Medication administration record
Hydrocortisone sodium succinate (Solu-Cortef) 100 mg IV every day
Metformin (Glucophage) 850 mg PO T.I.D.
Hydrochlorothiazide (HCTZ) 25 mg PO B.I.D.
Enteric coated aspirin 81 mg PO every day

Which of the following statements by the patient indicates understanding of interactions between the ordered medications?

A. "I take a high dose of metformin because I am on Solu-Cortef and HCTZ."
B. "I take HCTZ to help me get rid of excess fluid caused by metformin."
C. "The aspirin helps me to keep healthy immunity while I'm on the others."
D. "The Solu-Cortef increases my blood glucose levels."

10. The nurse is providing discharge teaching for the patient with Type II diabetes who has been ordered the following medications prior to discharge:

Medication administration record
Atenolol (Tenormin) 25 mg PO daily
Metformin (Glucophage) 850 mg PO T.I.D.
Hydrochlorothiazide (HCTZ) 25 mg PO B.I.D.
Enteric coated aspirin 81 mg PO every day
Glipizide SR (Glucotrol XL) 10 mg PO B.I.D.

Which of the following statements by the patient indicates understanding of the implications of drug interactions between these medications?

A. "I need to monitor my glucose levels at home so I know if the meds are working."
B. "I may not always know if I am becoming hypoglycemic because of these meds."
C. "I need the HCTZ because the metformin and aspirin make my ankles swell."
D. "I need the atenolol because the metformin and glipizide cause my heart to race."

11. The patient with diabetes takes glipizide SR 10 mg every morning to control blood glucose levels. Which of the following statements by the patient indicates an understanding of its mechanism of action?
A. "The medicine acts by stimulating my pancreas to release insulin."
B. "The medication causes decreased production of glucose by my liver."
C. "The medication helps my muscles use my body's insulin better."
D. "The medication makes all of the cells in my body respond better."

12. A patient with Type II diabetes informs a nurse that he has not felt well since beginning therapy with metformin (Glucophage). When asked to provide more detail, the patient relates that he has been experiencing nausea and diarrhea consistently. The best reply by the nurse would be:
A. "We will have to discuss some alternatives with the doctor."
B. "Your symptoms might be related to a contagious influenza."
C. "Your symptoms are normal and should decrease with time."
D. "We will have to run some tests to find out what is going on."

13. **A patient with Type II diabetes asks the nurse why he cannot drink alcohol while he takes metformin (Glucophage) for his disease. The best response by the nurse is:**
    A. "Drinking alcohol will raise your blood glucose levels."
    B. "Alcohol will chemically deactivate the metformin."
    C. "Drinking alcohol will increase your chances of hypoglycemia."
    D. "Alcohol increases your risk of developing lactic acidosis."

14. **The patient with diabetes is to receive 8 units of insulin intravenously. Which of the following actions by the nurse represents good judgment?**
    A. The nurse obtains and draws up 8 units of insulin detemir (Levemir).
    B. The nurse obtains and draws up 8 units of Humulin 70/30.
    C. The nurse obtains and draws up 8 units of insulin glargine (Lantus).
    D. The nurse obtains and draws up 8 units of regular insulin.

15. **The nurse is assigned to care for a patient with diabetic ketoacidosis. When asked by a significant other about treatment for this problem, the best response by the nurse is:**
    A. "The patient will have carefully controlled infusion of potassium."
    B. "The patient will receive large doses of oral hypoglycemic agents."
    C. "The patient will receive large bolus doses of intravenous insulin."
    D. "The patient will remain NPO throughout the entire treatment process."

16. **Which therapeutic intervention should be initiated first for the patient in a hyperosmolar hyperglycemic state?**
    A. rapid rehydration
    B. vital sign monitoring
    C. high dose insulin boluses
    D. hourly blood glucose readings

17. **A nurse is providing diabetic education follow-up for a patient with recently diagnosed Type I diabetes. When the patient asks the nurse how long insulin can be used from an open vial, the best response by the nurse is:**
    A. "Date the vial when you open it and then use it for not more than 1 month."
    B. "You may use it for up to six weeks if it is stored at room temperature."
    C. "If you keep it in the refrigerator, you can use it until the expiration date."
    D. "You should not use insulin from a vial that has been opened longer than 60 days."

18. **The nurse is providing teaching for a patient with newly diagnosed hypothyroidism. The patient asks the nurse why therapy involves only administration of T_4 and not T_3. The best response by the nurse is:**
    A. "You don't need T_3 because that is the inactive form of the hormone."
    B. "We will add T_3 after your T_4 levels have become normal."
    C. "T_4 is the more potent hormone and, therefore, the most important."
    D. "Some of the T_4 gets converted to T_3, so you actually get both."

19. **The nurse is providing education about medication to a patient who was newly diagnosed with hypothyroidism. Which of the following statements by the patient indicates understanding about treatment with levothyroxine (Synthroid)?**
    A. "I will not realize the full effect of the drug for several weeks."
    B. "I need to be very certain to take all three doses each day."
    C. "I should always take this medication with food."
    D. "I may gain weight while taking this drug if I do not exercise."

20. The nurse is providing teaching to a patient about radioactive iodine (^{131}I) therapy. Which of the following statements by the patient indicates understanding of the information?
    A. "This treatment is very expensive."
    B. "I will know within one week if it works."
    C. "There are no known disadvantages to this."
    D. "It is possible that I will develop hypothyroidism."

21. The nurse is assigned to care for a patient who has begun treatment with desmopressin for diabetes insipidus. Which of the following assessment findings by the nurse indicates that the treatment has begun to work?
    A. The serum blood glucose level is 106 mg/dL.
    B. The urine output is 1256 mL over 24 hours.
    C. The patient has crackles in both lungs.
    D. The patient drinks 3 liters of fluid in 24 hours.

22. The nurse is providing education about glucocorticoid therapy for a patient with Addison's disease. Which of the following statements by the patient indicates understanding of the instructions?
    A. "I need to have a supply of my drugs at home at all times."
    B. "I will take two-thirds of my daily dose at 9 a.m. and one-third at 5 p.m."
    C. "I will perform self-monitoring of blood glucose at least four times daily."
    D. "I might develop increased muscle mass after I've taken this for a while."

ANSWERS

General

1. **(B)**; Gestational diabetes frequently resolves following delivery of the baby.

2. **(B)**; During pregnancy, production of hormones increases a woman's insulin needs.

3. **(A)**; The patient should be scheduled for a cesarean delivery before her due date because fetal death frequently occurs near term.

4. **(A)**; Family history of Type II diabetes is a strong predictor. Patients do not get the disease as a result of intake of sweets. The pancreas still produces insulin with Type II diabetes.

5. **(B)**; The nurse should explain that part of the body's response to stress includes elevation of blood glucose. Therefore, it is not unusual for non-diabetic patients to have elevated blood glucose during acute illness.

6. **(C)**; Because there is absolutely no insulin production by the pancreas in Type I diabetes, patients with the disease become very ill very quickly. Patients must take insulin to survive.

7. **(B)**; For a normal preoperative patient with Type II diabetes, the nurse would anticipate that the patient is asymptomatic and feeling good. If the blood glucose is not adequately managed, the patient would not likely be a surgical candidate.

8. **(A)**; Patients with Type II diabetes have normal or high levels of circulating insulin. The problem for them is not lack of insulin production; it is that their tissues are resistant to the insulin—the tissues do not use insulin effectively.

9. **(C)**; Although blindness is certainly a risk, the nurse should inform the patient that controlling blood glucose and blood pressure significantly reduces one's risk for blindness. Therefore, with appropriate self-management of the diabetes, the patient should be able to continue working as a teacher long term.

10. **(B)**; Oral medications will not work for patients with Type I diabetes because all oral medications work by influencing aspects of insulin metabolism—there is no insulin production in Type I diabetes.

11. **(A)**; Patients with diabetes can eat some amount of any food of their choice as long as they adjust their carbohydrate intake. Therefore, if a patient eats something with sugar, the amount of carbohydrate in that food must be subtracted from the usual allotment for that particular meal.

12. **(C)**; The patient needs some further teaching about management of blood glucose if the levels have been "all over the place." Also, it is not advisable for patients with diabetes to exercise when blood glucose levels are higher than 250 mg/dL. The patient should not exercise until the blood glucose is regulated.

13. **(C)**; The patient is hyperglycemic, nauseated, vomiting, and polyuric. The priority nursing diagnosis would be *fluid volume deficit*.

14. **(A, C)**; The patient's symptoms of hypoglycemia will depend, at least to some degree, on how fast the glucose level falls. When the glucose falls very rapidly, it is likely that the patient may feel very jittery or nervous. Patients with very tight glucose control may have more difficulty identifying symptoms of hypoglycemia until blood glucose is very low.

15. **(B)**; The patient with hyperosmolar hyperglycemic state (HHS) will tend to have higher serum glucose with milder ketosis and higher pH than a patient with diabetic keto-acidosis (DKA). In comparison to DKA in which the pH is <7.30 and HCO_3 is <15 mEq/L, the pH in HHS is >7.30 with HCO_3 >20 mEq/L.

16. **(D)**; The patient who is experiencing diabetic ketoacidosis is extremely dehydrated—perhaps even in hypovolemic shock. Therefore, the priority nursing diagnosis is *deficient fluid volume*.

17. **(B)**; Patients who are diagnosed with hypothyroidism will have to take medicine throughout their lifetime.

18. **(B, D)**; Infants born with hypothyroidism will have some degree of mental retardation; however, outcomes are best when the condition is diagnosed and the child is treated within a few days of birth.

19. **(A)**; If the patient with hyperthyroidism is feeling nervous, jittery, and sweaty all of the time, this is a sign that therapy is inadequately controlling symptoms.

20. **(C)**; Graves' disease is a form of hyperthyroidism. Treatment is likely to involve removal of some or all of the thyroid tissue to reduce hormone production.

21. **(B)**; Symptoms of angina indicate worsening of symptoms of thyrotoxicosis, which may include severe tachycardia, fever, insomnia, restlessness, delirium, agitation, psychosis, heart failure, and angina.

22. **(A)**; The patient with Graves' disease will receive medication prior to surgical removal of thyroid tissue. The antithyroid medication helps to decrease the size and vascularity of the thyroid gland, which reduces the likelihood of hemorrhage during or after surgery.

23. **(A)**; Patients with diabetes insipidus experience extreme polyuria, which makes the priority diagnosis *fluid volume deficit*.

24. **(B)**; Throughout treatment for diabetes insipidus, it is important for the patient to monitor urine output; therefore, the nurse should encourage measurement of urine output at home so that the patient can have some parameters for notifying the healthcare provider if medication is not adequately controlling the condition.

25. **(A)**; Abrupt withdrawal from chronic glucocorticoid therapy is a frequent cause of adrenal crisis. Therefore, teaching should always include this critical information for patients.

26. **(D)**; Goiter is associated with compensated hypothyroidism.

27. **(C)**; The nurse plans to administer a large dose of hormone in the morning and a smaller dose in the evening every day because the physiologic effect will mimic the body's normal hormone levels.

28. **(C)**; The patient recognizes that negative feedback is the mechanism by which hormonal regulation occurs in the body.

29. **(C)**; The parathyroid gland is most responsible for calcium metabolism.

30. **(C)**; High blood pressure is not a risk factor for endocrine disease; however, hormone replacement therapy, irradiation of a gland, or surgical removal of a gland can certainly affect endocrine function.

31. **(C)**; It is important for the patient to realize that preparation for surgery will require medication therapy to reduce the size and vascularity of the thyroid gland, a process that will require about 2 to 3 months.

32. **(B)**; If the patient reports an odd sensation around the mouth, the nurse must assess for hypocalcemia, which could result from inadvertent removal of parathyroid tissue during the surgery.

33. **(A)**; Addison's disease is a chronic disease, so the nurse should focus on living with a chronic disease and maintaining an optimal state of wellness.

34. **(A)**; Blood pressure must be monitored closely in the patient with pheochromocytoma.

35. **(D)**; Alternative oral care should be practiced for at least 10 days postop to avoid the risk of meningitis.

36. **(D)**; The nurse must carefully assess this patient for signs and symptoms of water intoxication.

Physical Assessment

1. **(A, B, D)**; Patients with diabetic gastroparesis are prone to nausea, vomiting, and abdominal bloating. They do not experience diarrhea.

2. **(A)**; When a patient with known diabetes is comatose, it is critically important to know the serum glucose level to identify appropriate treatment.

3. **(B)**; The symptoms described (polydipsia, polyuria, abdominal pain, nausea, and fruity breath) are classic signs of diabetic ketoacidosis.

4. **(A)**; Manifestations of hypothyroidism include dry, puffy skin; thin hair; hoarseness; large tongue; bradycardia; shallow, slow respirations; chronic constipation; slow mentation; and slow reflexes.

5. **(B)**; Patients with Addison's disease would have hypoglycemia and hyperkalemia.

6. **(A)**; Patients with Cushing's disease experience a vast array of symptoms, including hypertension and impaired immunity.

7. **(A)**; By tapping on the side of the patient's face, the nurse can assess Chvostek's sign, an indicator of hypoparathyroidism.

Interpretation of Lab Values

1. **(A, E, F)**; The nurse should be concerned about fasting glucose levels of <60 and >126 mg/dL.

2. **(C)**; Patients who maintain good control of blood glucose, as demonstrated by hemoglobin A1c <7, should have the test twice per year. If control is less than adequate, A1c should be drawn every three months.

3. **(B)**; During IV infusion, some amount of insulin is likely to adhere to the tubing, which means that less is available to lower blood glucose.

4. **(C)**; The patient with diabetic ketoacidosis is likely to have pH <7.30; HCO_3 <15 mEq/L; and elevated serum glucose.

5. **(D)**; Patients who receive IV insulin require potassium replacement because the insulin drives potassium back into the intracellular space, thus leaving the patient with a dangerously low serum K+ level.

6. **(B, C)**; This patient's anterior pituitary gland is working normally (normal TSH), but the thyroid gland is producing excessive amounts of hormone ($\uparrow$ T_3 and T_4).

7. **(A, D)**; This patient has hypothyroidism ($\downarrow$ T_3 and T_4 despite $\uparrow$ TSH).

8. **(B)**; This patient has hyperthyroidism secondary to overproduction of TSH.

Drugs and Treatments

1. **(A)**; Metoclopramide (Reglan) is typically used to increase gastric motility in patients with diabetic gastroparesis.

2. **(B)**; Glipizide (Glucotrol) is a sulfonylurea. These medications are useful in thin patients with Type II diabetes because they promote insulin release from the pancreas.

3. **(A)**; The nurse knows that, ideally, the patient should receive 6 units of lispro (Humalog) insulin when the breakfast tray arrives. Because the insulin has a very rapid onset, the nurse should be certain that the patient will eat immediately.

4. **(B, C, D)**; These insulins can be mixed in one syringe. Because the total number of units of insulin is 25, they may be mixed in one U-50 syringe. The insulins should be administered immediately before the patient begins to eat because of NovoLog's very rapid onset of action.

5. **(B)**; Lantus insulin should not be mixed with any other type of insulin, so the insulins must be administered in two different syringes.

6. **(B)**; If the patient received NPH insulin at 8 a.m., the nurse should be alert to signs of hypoglycemia in this patient between 3 p.m. and 5 p.m. because the effects of the insulin would peak by that time and it is not yet dinner time.

7. **(A)**; Regular insulin is the only insulin that should *ever* be used in an insulin drip.

8. **(D, C, A, B, E, F)**; First, the nurse must verify the insulin order on the MAR. Next, the top of the vial should be disinfected with alcohol. Then, the nurse should draw up the 15 units of regular insulin, followed by the 35 units of NPH insulin. Prior to administration, the nurse must verify the correct patient by at least two forms of identification, and finally, the nurse can administer the insulin subcutaneously.

9. **(A)**; The patient is ordered the highest possible dose of metformin. It is likely that the patient requires such a high dose because both Solu-Cortef and HCTZ tend to produce elevated glucose levels.

10. **(B)**; This patient may not always be aware of episodes of hypoglycemia because the atenolol (Tenormin) tends to mask the signs.

11. **(A)**; Glipizide acts by stimulating the pancreas to release insulin.

12. **(C)**; Many patients experience GI symptoms at the onset of metformin therapy; however, the symptoms typically subside with time.

13. **(D)**; Lactic acidosis is a very serious potential adverse effect of metformin (Glucophage). Alcohol consumption with metformin increases the patient's risk of developing lactic acidosis.

14. **(D)**; The nurse must choose regular insulin for intravenous administration.

15. **(A)**; Treatment for diabetic ketoacidosis requires intensive treatment with monitoring throughout. Patients will require carefully controlled infusions of potassium in addition to an intravenous insulin drip. Oral hypoglycemics are not useful in treating DKA. When blood glucose levels get down to about 250–300 mg/dL, the patient may take food or fluids by mouth.

16. **(A)**; Patients in a hyperosmolar hyperglycemic state (HHS) are extremely dehydrated and often shocky. Volume resuscitation is a priority.

17. **(C)**; Insulin kept in the refrigerator has a very long shelf life. It can be used until the expiration date noted on the vial.

18. **(D)**; Physiologically, some of the T_4 gets converted to T_3 automatically, so by administering T_4, both deficits may be corrected with one drug.

19. **(A)**; When patients take levothyroxine (Synthroid), it is important for them to understand that they will not realize maximal beneficial effects for several weeks.

20. **(D)**; The patient who receives radioactive iodine (^{131}I) should be aware that treatment may result in hypothyroidism.

21. **(B)**; When the patient's urine output has normalized, the nurse knows that the desmopressin has begun to work.

22. **(B)**; Glucocorticoids should be administered by two-thirds of the total daily dose in the morning and the remaining one-third in the evening.

Keep Track

- Percent correct. (Divide the number of questions you answered correctly by the total number of questions you answered.) _____

- Number of questions you missed due to a reading error: _____

- Number of questions you missed due to errors in analysis: _____

- Number of assessment questions you missed: _____

- Number of lab value questions you missed: _____

- Number of drug/treatment questions you missed: _____

Nugget List

Chapter number _____ Topic _____

Practice Test: Nursing Management of Patients with Reproductive System Disorders

Karen S. March

PRACTICE TEST

General

1. The nurse is caring for a patient following prostate surgery. Upon assessment, the nurse notes that the patient has a urinary catheter that is secured very snugly to the inner thigh. The nurse understands that the catheter:
    A. is positioned to help prevent hemorrhage.
    B. may be repositioned if the patient is uncomfortable.
    C. should be repositioned at least every few hours.
    D. will normally drain urine with large clots.

2. The nurse is caring for a patient following prostate surgery who has an indwelling catheter. The patient informs the nurse that he feels like he needs to void. Which of the following is the best response by the nurse?
    A. Inform the patient that the feeling is normal, but discourage straining to try to void.
    B. Tell the patient that he can try to void if it will make him feel more comfortable.
    C. Encourage the patient to go ahead and try to void because it may help to pass a clot.
    D. Notify the surgeon immediately because this is a sign of impending hemorrhage.

3. The nurse is providing care for a patient with continuous bladder irrigation (CBI) following removal of the prostate. The nurse understands that the CBI should be adjusted as needed to result in catheter outflow of which of the following types?
    A. cloudy yellow
    B. light pink
    C. amber with clots
    D. cherry colored with clots

ALTERNATE FORMAT

4. The nurse must calculate intake and output for the patient with continuous bladder irrigation at the end of the shift. At the beginning of the shift, the patient had 1800 mL of irrigation fluid in the bag. By the end of the shift, 1250 mL remains. The total catheter output throughout the shift was 1000 mL. How much urine output did the patient have throughout the shift?

5. The nurse caring for a patient with continuous bladder irrigation realizes that the irrigation is running too slowly if:
    A. less than 500 mL of irrigation is used per shift.
    B. the patient develops bladder spasms.
    C. the output remains yellow without any clots.
    D. the output remains light pink in color.

6. **The nurse is caring for a patient following a mastectomy. The nurse knows to position the patient in which position upon return from surgery?**
   A. supine or with affected arm elevated
   B. supine or on the affected side
   C. prone with the affected arm elevated
   D. prone or on the affected side

7. **The nurse caring for a patient following a mastectomy understands the importance of encouraging early range of motion exercises to:**
   A. prevent development of deep vein thrombosis.
   B. prevent respiratory compromise from atelectasis.
   C. prevent contractures and lymphedema.
   D. prevent muscle atrophy from disuse.

8. **The nurse is caring for a patient with multiple sclerosis who suffers from priapism. The nurse anticipates that a priority nursing diagnosis for this patient is which of the following?**
   A. altered sexual function
   B. pain
   C. impaired tissue perfusion
   D. knowledge deficit

9. **The nurse is providing care for a patient admitted with testicular cancer. The nurse understands that clinical manifestations of the disease generally include which of the following?**
   A. painless, hard area or lump found during self-examination
   B. painless mass identified during screening ultrasound
   C. painful, lumpy testes identified during self-examination
   D. painful, swollen testes identified during self-examination

10. **The nurse is providing care for a patient with benign prostatic hypertrophy. Clinical manifestations, as described by the patient, include:**
    A. urinary frequency with strong stream.
    B. difficulty starting and stopping the stream.
    C. daytime urinary frequency with incontinence.
    D. fever, chills, nausea, and vomiting.

11. **The nurse who is assigned to care for the patient with pelvic inflammatory disease realizes that the priority nursing diagnosis for this patient is:**
    A. pain.
    B. fluid volume excess.
    C. impaired tissue perfusion.
    D. risk for infection.

12. **The nurse assigned to care for the patient with syphilis is providing education. Which of the following statements by the patient indicates a need for further education?**
    A. "If I have sex with someone who has syphilis, I need to be treated immediately."
    B. "I am not supposed to have sex for at least 1 month after I am treated for syphilis."
    C. "I need to talk to my sexual partners to have them come in for treatment, too."
    D. "I am not at risk for other sexually transmitted diseases because I've been treated."

13. The nurse is providing education to the patient who is diagnosed with genital herpes. Which of the following statements by the patient indicates understanding of factors that tend to trigger recurrent outbreaks?
    A. "After I have been treated for this disease, I will be cured."
    B. "I may have recurrent outbreaks of the disease more often in winter."
    C. "When I am under a lot of stress, I am likely to have another outbreak."
    D. "I will have another outbreak immediately following sexual intercourse."

14. The nurse is providing care to a patient with stage IV ovarian cancer. The nurse understands this means that cancer cells are found:
    A. on the ovaries, and there is metastasis to the liver.
    B. on the ovaries, and the cancer has spread to the lymph nodes.
    C. on the ovaries and into the pelvis.
    D. only on one or both of the ovaries.

Physical Assessment

1. The nurse knows that which of the following findings would be normal during examination of the prostate?
   A. wide and tender gland with multiple nodules
   B. narrow and non-tender gland with a large protrusion
   C. wide and non-tender gland that is smooth and rubbery
   D. narrow and tender gland that is smooth and rubbery

2. The nurse is teaching a patient about breast self-examination. Which of the following statements by the patient indicates comprehension of the information?
   A. "I should palpate both breasts at any time during the month *every* month."
   B. "I should palpate both breasts during my menses while I am in the shower."
   C. "It is a good idea to do breast self-examination at the same time every month."
   D. "Breast self-examination is important but not vital because I get a yearly mammogram."

3. The nurse is teaching a patient about testicular self-examination. Which of the following statements by the patient indicates understanding of assessment technique?
   A. "I should roll my testicle between my thumb and forefinger during a warm shower."
   B. "While lying down on the bed, I should gently touch all surfaces of each testicle."
   C. "While standing in front of a mirror, I should check for symmetrical position."
   D. "I should have my partner perform the testicular examination for me."

4. The nurse is caring for a patient with a diagnosis of phimosis. Based on the diagnosis, the nurse anticipates which of the following findings upon physical assessment?
   A. an infected, circumcised penis
   B. a penis with a large, loose foreskin
   C. a penis with a constricted foreskin
   D. a very small, retracted penis

5. The nurse caring for a patient with orchitis would anticipate finding which of the following clinical manifestations upon physical assessment?
   A. scrotal edema, pain, redness
   B. sudden sharp pain, scrotal nodules
   C. pruritis, mumps, petechiae
   D. penile inflammation and infection

6. The nurse is providing care for a patient with continuous bladder irrigation (CBI) following prostatectomy. Which of the following output characteristics, if found on the first postop day, would be considered abnormal?
   A. clear to pale pink output
   B. pale pink output with occasional clots
   C. bright red output
   D. light red output

7. The nurse who is providing care for a patient with pelvic inflammatory disease would anticipate finding which of the following clinical manifestations upon assessing the patient?
   A. abdominal tenderness and distention
   B. fever and foul-smelling vaginal discharge
   C. urinary tract infection and malaise
   D. pain that abates with movement

8. The nurse is providing care for a patient with uterine prolapse. The nurse antici-pates finding which of the following clinical manifestations during physical assessment of the patient?
   A. swelling in the lower pelvis
   B. a lump protruding from the rectum
   C. a lump protruding from the vagina
   D. sharp pain upon palpation near the vagina

Interpretation of Lab Values

1. The nurse understands that serum human chorionic gonadotropin (hCG) is used for which of the following purposes?
   A. to determine adequacy of hormone production in early pregnancy
   B. to measure hormone levels in females undergoing fertility testing
   C. as an index for likelihood of cervical ripening for fertilization
   D. as an indicator of erectile sustainability in male fertility workups

2. The nurse is reviewing patient lab work and notes results from a PSA test. The nurse understands that the PSA test:
   A. is indicative of infectious prostatitis in young men aged 20 to 50 years.
   B. can be used to evaluate the therapeutic response to treatment for prostate cancer.
   C. can be used as an indicator for benign prostatic hypertrophy in middle-aged men.
   D. is diagnostic for the presence of benign prostatic hypertrophy in men of all ages.

3. Which of the following tests is useful in evaluating male fertility?
   A. prostate-specific antigen (PSA)
   B. serum testosterone levels
   C. semen analysis
   D. ultrasonography

4. Which of the following diagnostics are used as markers to monitor therapeutic response to treatment for testicular cancer?
   A. alpha fetoprotein and hCG
   B. scrotal ultrasound
   C. prostate-specific antigen
   D. serum testosterone

Drugs and Treatments

1. **Which of the following examinations allows visualization of the inside of the uterus and can be useful early in workups for infertility?**
   A. colposcopy
   B. hysteroscopy
   C. laparoscopy
   D. Papanicolaou smear

2. **The nurse is caring for a patient who has a mass in the right breast that was identified by mammography. The nurse is preparing the patient to undergo an aspiration biopsy. Which of the following statements by the patient indicates understanding of what is involved with an aspiration biopsy of the breast?**
   A. "The doctor will use a needle to remove cells from my breast for examination."
   B. "The doctor will remove a piece of tissue from around the mass for examination."
   C. "The doctor will remove the entire mass from my breast during surgery."
   D. "The doctor will use a large needle to enter the mass using fluoroscopy."

3. **The nurse is providing education about medications for a patient with erectile dysfunction. Which of the following statements by the patient indicates understanding of the instructions?**
   A. "I can't use sildenafil (Viagra) because I take ACE inhibitors for my blood pressure."
   B. "Sildenafil (Viagra) could cause severe hypertension in conjunction with nitrates."
   C. "Because I have leukemia, it is possible that sildenafil (Viagra) may cause priapism."
   D. "Sildenafil (Viagra) is a drug that must be self-administered by penile injection."

4. **The nurse is providing education about medication side effects to a patient with erectile dysfunction. The nurse informs the patient that the drug sildenafil (Viagra) should be discontinued and the healthcare provider notified if:**
   A. the patient decides to use a vacuum constriction device.
   B. the patient develops chest pain or shortness of breath.
   C. the patient's problem is related to fear of failure.
   D. the patient no longer chooses to engage in sexual activity.

5. **The nurse, who is caring for a patient with orchitis, knows that drugs from which category are commonly used to treat the condition?**
   A. antibiotics
   B. ACE inhibitors
   C. vasodilators
   D. corticosteroids

6. **The nurse who is assigned to care for a patient with primary syphilis is providing education to the patient about medications. The nurse expects that treatment will involve which of the following medications?**
   A. intravenous penicillin G
   B. rifampin
   C. acyclovir (Zovirax)
   D. piperacillin and tazobactam (Zosyn)

7. The nurse is providing care to a patient with trichomoniasis. The nurse knows that treatment normally involves administration of:
   A. penicillin.
   B. metronidazole (Flagyl).
   C. ampicillin and sulbactam (Unasyn).
   D. acyclovir (Zovirax).

8. The nurse is providing education about treatment for candidiasis. In response, the patient recognizes which of the following as a means by which the normal vaginal flora can be restored?
   A. Eat 8 ounces of yogurt daily.
   B. Take daily doses of antibiotics.
   C. Use vinegar douches daily.
   D. Use miconazole (Monistat) as ordered.

ANSWERS

General

1. **(A)**; The nurse understands that traction is applied to an indwelling catheter to prevent hemorrhage following surgery. When traction is applied, the catheter should not be repositioned because the balloon near the end of the catheter exerts pressure to prevent bleeding.

2. **(A)**; The nurse should let the patient know that the feeling he describes is normal but that he should not strain to try to void because that may cause bleeding. The nurse should assure the patient that the catheter is draining normally and that the output will be monitored continually to ensure proper function.

3. **(B)**; The nurse understands that the goal is to have outflow that is light pink without clots. CBI must be titrated accordingly to achieve the desired outcome.

4. **(450 mL)**; The nurse first must calculate how much irrigation fluid infused by subtracting what remains (1250 mL) from what was available to start the shift (1800 mL). That means that 1800 – 1250 = 550 mL infused. Next, the nurse must subtract the amount of CBI infused from the total output to find the true urine output: 1000 mL total output – 550 mL CBI = 450 mL true urine output.

5. **(B)**; The nurse realizes that continuous bladder irrigation (CBI) is infusing too slowly if the patient develops bladder spasms or output that contains frank blood.

6. **(A)**; The nurse should position the patient who has had a mastectomy supine or on the unaffected side with the affected arm elevated.

7. **(C)**; The nurse caring for a patient following mastectomy understands that early range of motion exercises help to prevent contractures and lymphedema.

8. **(B)**; Priapism is a painful erection that lasts at least 4 hours and is not associated with sexual arousal. Conditions like sickle cell anemia, multiple sclerosis, and metastatic tumors may lead to its occurrence.

9. **(A)**; Clinical manifestations of testicular cancer may include a painless, hard area or lump found during self-examination. There is no screening ultrasound testing.

10. **(B)**; The patient with benign prostatic hypertrophy describes clinical manifestations of the disorder that include urinary frequency, nocturia, weak stream, difficulty starting and stopping the stream, and dribbling.

11. **(A)**; The priority nursing diagnosis for the patient with pelvic inflammatory disease is pain. Treatment can include antibiotic therapy, surgical removal of abscesses if present, and application of heat to the abdomen to relieve pain.

12. **(D)**; When the patient states that there is no risk for other sexually transmitted diseases following treatment for syphilis, the nurse must recognize this statement as an indication of the need for further teaching.

13. **(C)**; The patient verbalizes understanding that stress may cause outbreaks. Other factors that may cause recurrent outbreaks include heat, intercourse, anxiety, emotional upset, menstruation, or ovulation. The disease is controlled by anti-viral drugs. It cannot be cured.

14. **(A)**; A diagnosis of stage IV ovarian cancer means that there is cancer on the ovaries and evidence of distant metastasis.

Physical Assessment

1. **(C)**; The prostate gland is evaluated by inserting a gloved, lubricated index finger into the rectum. Normally, the prostate should be wide, non-tender, smooth, and rubbery.

2. **(C)**; It is best to perform breast self-examination at the same time every month, ideally about 5 days after the menstrual period begins. Assessment at the same time each month ensures that regular changes that may occur throughout the month do not confound the findings.

3. **(A)**; The patient should be encouraged to perform testicular self-examination at least once per month by gently rolling each testicle between the thumb and forefinger of each hand. The examination should be done with soapy hands in a warm bath or shower.

4. **(C)**; The patient with phimosis has a penis with a very tight, constricted foreskin. Patients frequently manifest signs of infection, such as swelling, redness, purulent discharge, and pain related to inability to perform adequate hygiene. The condition can also cause painful urination with decreased urine flow and the need to strain to void.

5. **(A)**; Orchitis is infection or inflammation of one or both of the testicles. Clinical manifestations include fever, chills, and sudden pain in the testes, as well as tenderness, redness and warmth, scrotal edema, and presence of other infections, such as urinary tract infection or epididymitis.

6. **(C)**; On the first postop day, bright red output could indicate arterial bleeding. The nurse should check the CBI flow rate, check vital signs, and notify the surgeon. Clear to pale pink, pale pink with occasional clots, or light red output would be considered within normal limits on the first postop day.

7. **(B)**; Patients with pelvic inflammatory disease have clinical manifestations that include fever, nausea, malaise, severe lower abdominal pain, dysuria, nausea and vomiting, and purulent and foul-smelling vaginal discharge.

8. **(C)**; The patient with a uterine prolapse will have a painless lump protruding from the vagina that has gradually increased in size over time. The lump is usually more pronounced when the patient stands or strains to urinate or defecate.

Interpretation of Lab Values

1. **(A)**; Serum hCG helps to detect early pregnancy and is used to determine adequacy of hormone levels in a high-risk pregnancy.

2. **(B)**; PSA or prostate-specific antigen is used to track the progression of prostate cancer and/or its response to the therapeutic regimen. It is frequently used as a screening tool for prostate cancer in men older than 50 years of age. It should be used in conjunction with digital rectal examination.

3. **(C)**; Semen analysis can be used to evaluate male fertility, to help substantiate the effectiveness of a vasectomy, or to detect semen on the body or clothing of a rape victim. It is collected by the patient.

4. **(A)**; Elevated levels of both alpha fetoprotein (AFP) and hCG provide strong evidence of testicular cancer. These levels are useful in monitoring the patient's response to therapy.

Drugs and Treatments

1. **(B)**; Hysteroscopy is an endoscopic exam that allows visualization of the inside of the uterus via the cervical canal. It can be used as an early diagnostic test for female infertility workups.

2. **(A)**; Aspiration biopsy involves using a fine needle to remove cells or fluid from the mass in the patient's breast for examination.

3. **(C)**; Patients with sickle cell anemia, leukemia, multiple sclerosis, and metastatic tumors may develop priapism following administration of phosphodiesterase type 5 inhibitors like sildenafil (Viagra). Patients should be cautioned about this potential side effect.

4. **(B)**; Phosphodiesterase inhibitors should be discontinued and the healthcare provider notified immediately if the patient develops chest pain or shortness of breath during use of the drug.

5. **(D)**; Orchitis is infection or inflammation of one or both testicles. The nurse realizes that corticosteroids are used to treat inflammation related to orchitis.

6. **(A)**; Intravenous penicillin G is used to treat primary syphilis. Treatment is based on the length of illness and the stage of the disease.

7. **(B)**; Treatment of trichomoniasis typically requires a single dose of metronidazole (Flagyl).

8. **(A)**; The patient can help to restore the normal vaginal flora by consuming 8 ounces of yogurt with live active cultures daily.

Keep Track

- Percent correct. (Divide the number of questions you answered correctly by the total number of questions you answered.) _____

- Number of questions you missed due to a reading error: _____

- Number of questions you missed due to errors in analysis: _____

- Number of assessment questions you missed: _____

- Number of lab value questions you missed: _____

- Number of drug/treatment questions you missed: _____

Nugget List

Chapter number _____ Topic _____

Chapter 20

Practice Test: Nursing Management of Childbearing Women and Newborns

Karen S. March

PRACTICE TEST

General

1. During a prenatal visit, a woman who is at 12 weeks gestation asks the nurse what might cause her indigestion and heartburn. The best reply by the nurse is that:
   A. increased pancreatic activity results in fat intolerance.
   B. elevated levels of estrogen cause gastric hyperacidity.
   C. pressure from the growing uterus increases gastric motility.
   D. progesterone causes decreased motility of smooth muscle.

2. A nurse on a busy postpartum unit has three patients in need of attention. A nursing assistant volunteers to recheck vital signs on a hypertensive patient. Which of the following is the best response by the nurse?
   A. Ask the nursing assistant to give a sitz bath to a patient.
   B. Allow the nursing assistant to obtain the vital signs and report back.
   C. Decline any assistance by the nursing assistant at this time.
   D. Ask the nursing assistant to deliver a stool softener to a patient.

3. A postpartum nurse is providing care for a 15-year-old patient who intends to give her baby up for adoption. The nurse understands that which of the following is an essential aspect of care for this patient?
   A. communication between a social worker and the patient
   B. permission from the patient's parents for the adoption
   C. presence of a physician at time of patient discharge
   D. no mother–baby interaction during hospitalization

4. The nurse is providing care for a patient who delivered 30 minutes ago. The patient has an IV of lactated Ringer's with 25 units of Pitocin infusing. Upon evaluation, the nurse finds that the patient's lochia is excessive. Vital signs are BP 156/98; P 84; R 20; T 98°F. The nurse informs the healthcare provider of the findings, and the following order is received: methylergonovine (Methergine) 0.2 mg IM now. The most appropriate response by the nurse is which of the following?
   A. Question the order because the medication is contraindicated for this patient.
   B. Do not administer the medication but increase the rate of the IV fluids.
   C. Request an order for IV administration of the medication in this emergency.
   D. Administer the medication and reevaluate the bleeding within 30 minutes.

5. The nurse is teaching a class about fetal development to expectant mothers. Which of the following facts should the nurse be certain to include?
   A. The fetal heartbeat is audible by doppler at 12 weeks of pregnancy.
   B. The sex of the fetus is determined by week 10 of pregnancy.
   C. Lanugo will begin to cover the entire body of the fetus by week 36 of pregnancy.
   D. It is common to feel the fetus move for the first time by week 24 of pregnancy.

6. The nurse is caring for a patient whose last menstrual period began on October 1, 2009. Using Nägele's rule, the estimated date of birth is which of the following?
   A. January 1, 2010
   B. April 8, 2010
   C. June 1, 2010
   D. July 8, 2010

7. The nurse is caring for a patient in the early stages of labor who is using pattern-paced breathing. The patient states that she feels lightheaded and that her fingers tingle. The best response by the nurse is to do which of the following?
   A. Administer oxygen via nasal cannula.
   B. Encourage the patient to breathe into a paper bag.
   C. Notify the patient's physician of the symptoms.
   D. Tell the patient to slow down her breathing.

8. The nurse is caring for a patient with an electronic fetal monitor. The nurse notices that the fetal heart rate declines after each contraction begins and that the lowest heart rate occurs just after the peak of each contraction. The first priority for the nurse should be to do which of the following?
   A. Change the patient's position.
   B. Document the findings as benign decelerations.
   C. Insert a scalp electrode.
   D. Prepare for an amnioinfusion.

9. The nurse is caring for a patient who is in labor. Which of the following nursing actions reflects application of the gate control theory during labor?
   A. Administer pain medication when the patient is dilated 4 cm.
   B. Encourage the client to save strength by resting between contractions.
   C. Massage the patient's back.
   D. Turn the patient onto her left side.

ALTERNATE FORMAT

10. Place in order the seven cardinal movements of labor that occur in a vertex presentation.
    A. restitution
    B. descent
    C. flexion
    D. expulsion
    E. extension
    F. external rotation
    G. internal rotation

11. The nurse is providing care for a patient with worsening preeclampsia who is admitted to the labor and birth unit. The physician explains the plan of care for the patient, including induction of labor, to both the patient and her husband. The nurse determines that the couple needs further information based on which of the following comments from the husband?
    A. "I will help my wife to use the breathing techniques we learned in childbirth class."
    B. "I will give my wife clear liquids to drink during labor."
    C. "I'm going to have a friend come in to watch the football game with us on TV."
    D. "I will stay with my wife during her labor just like we planned."

12. The nurse is providing education about signs and symptoms of preeclampsia and warning signs of possible complications to a pregnant woman at 30 weeks gestation. The nurse determines that the patient needs further instruction when she makes which of the following statements?
    A. "If I notice changes in my vision, I will notify my physician immediately."
    B. "I will weigh myself every morning and call my doctor if I gain 0.5 kg or more in 1 week."
    C. "I will count my baby's movements twice a day, in the morning and in the evening after I eat."
    D. "If I have a headache, I will take acetaminophen (Tylenol)."

13. The nurse is providing care for a pregnant woman who was diagnosed with gestational diabetes mellitus (GDM) following screening at 24 weeks gestation. The nurse realizes that the fetus is at greatest risk for which of the following?
    A. macrosomia
    B. congenital anomalies of the nervous system
    C. preterm birth
    D. low birth weight

14. The nurse is caring for a patient who has developed HELLP syndrome. The nurse knows that definitive treatment for HELLP requires which of the following?
    A. replacement of platelets and clotting factors
    B. magnesium sulfate infusion
    C. induction of labor and delivery of the infant
    D. intensive steroid therapy

15. The nurse is providing care for a patient who has recently been diagnosed with oligohydramnios. The nurse knows that this condition is associated with which of the following types of fetal abnormality?
    A. renal
    B. cardiac
    C. gastrointestinal
    D. neurologic

16. The nurse is providing education to a pregnant woman about presumptive, probable, and positive signs of pregnancy. The patient demonstrates understanding of the information when she states that which of the following is a positive sign of pregnancy?
    A. elevated hCG levels
    B. fetal movement palpated by a nurse–midwife
    C. Braxton Hicks contractions
    D. quickening

17. The nurse is providing education to a pregnant woman who has been experiencing nausea and vomiting. The patient demonstrates understanding of ways to reduce the nausea and vomiting when she states which of the following?
    A. "I will ask my husband to bring me eggs and bacon in bed every day."
    B. "I will limit my eating to a small breakfast with a large lunch and dinner daily."
    C. "I will have less nausea if I eat small, frequent meals throughout the day."
    D. "If something makes me sick, I will try eating it again another day."

18. A woman who is at 16 weeks gestation informs the nurse that she always had a glass of wine with dinner before she became pregnant; however, she has abstained from alcohol during her first trimester. The woman wonders if it is safe for her to have a glass of wine with dinner now. The best response by the nurse is which of the following?
    A. "Because you are in your second trimester, there is no problem with having a glass of wine with dinner."
    B. "Because you are past the first trimester, you may have a glass of wine on occasion but not more than three times per week."
    C. "Because you are in your second trimester, it is safe for you to have a glass of wine with dinner."
    D. "Because there are no data about how much alcohol is problematic, abstinence throughout the entire pregnancy is recommended."

19. Which of the following positions would be least effective when gravity is desired to assist in fetal descent?
    A. lithotomy
    B. kneeling
    C. sitting
    D. walking

20. The nurse is providing care for a laboring woman whose membranes have ruptured. The nurse realizes that the patient's risk for which of the following has increased with rupture of the membranes?
    A. intrauterine infection
    B. hemorrhage
    C. precipitous labor
    D. supine hypertension

21. A nulliparous woman is late in the transition phase of the first stage of labor. She becomes restless and very irritable and tells her partner to stop touching her and to leave her alone. The best response by the nurse is which of the following?
    A. Tell the partner that this is a good time to leave the room and take a break.
    B. Explain to the partner that the patient's behavior is normal, and help the partner continue to coach the patient.
    C. Inform the partner that a nurse would be more effective to coach at this time.
    D. Reassure the partner that the patient does not mean what has been said and encourage the partner to ignore it.

22. The most critical action for the nurse to take when caring for a newborn immediately after birth is which of the following?
    A. keeping the newborn's airway open
    B. getting the baby to breast immediately
    C. fostering mother–infant bonding
    D. administering eye drops and vitamin K

23. Presumptive signs of pregnancy may include which of the following?
    A. uterine contractions
    B. quickening
    C. audible fetal heart tones
    D. softening of the cervical tip

24. The nurse working in a prenatal clinic becomes concerned that a patient may be a battered woman based on which of the following statements made by the patient?
    A. "We are really having trouble with money right now because my husband is laid off."
    B. "My boyfriend says I could never make it without him because I'm not too smart."
    C. "I only get to do things with my friends about once a month now that we're married."
    D. "I don't get out much for fun and I am exhausted because all I ever do is work."

25. The nurse is caring for a patient who arrived at the emergency department with a very supportive significant other for treatment of injuries to the face, head, and neck. Upon assessment, the nurse notes that the patient has multiple ecchymotic areas with abrasions, contusions, and a hematoma near the right eye. Which of the following would the nurse suspect as a plausible explanation for the injuries?
    A. falling down a flight of stairs
    B. running into a door in the dark
    C. falling off a trampoline during exercise
    D. being a victim of domestic violence

26. The nurse understands that it is prudent to begin depression assessments for pregnant women at what point in the pregnancy?
    A. during the first trimester
    B. during the second trimester
    C. during the early stages of labor
    D. after delivery and prior to discharge

27. During prenatal care, a patient who has had a previous cesarean birth asks the nurse about the possibility of having a vaginal birth after cesarean (VBAC). Which of the following factors from the patient's history would the nurse cite as a contraindication for VBAC?
    A. previous cesarean for breech presentation
    B. classic or T uterine incision with previous cesarean
    C. vertical abdominal incision with previous cesarean
    D. induction of labor is planned for this delivery

28. After birth, the nurse immediately dries off the newborn with a sterile towel. This action prevents heat loss through which of the following mechanisms?
    A. conduction
    B. convection
    C. evaporation
    D. radiation

29. The nurse is providing care for a patient who was moved to the intensive care unit shortly after giving birth because of severe anemia and DIC related to a bleeding episode. The infant remains in the nursery. Which nursing intervention would be most helpful for this family during the first 24 hours?
   A. Bring the infant for regular visits to the mother's bedside as her condition allows.
   B. Allow only the father to feed the infant in the newborn nursery.
   C. Discharge the infant to relatives as soon as possible.
   D. Assign the infant to one nurse in the nursery who can provide primary care.

Physical Assessment

1. Using Leopold's maneuvers, the nurse palpates a round, firm, movable body part in the fundal portion of the uterus and a long, smooth surface on the mother's right side. Based on these findings, the nurse expects to auscultate fetal heart tones in which maternal quadrant?
   A. lower left
   B. lower right
   C. upper left
   D. upper right

2. The nurse is caring for an infant just admitted to the newborn nursery following an emergency cesarean section. Upon initial assessment, the nurse notes that the skin of the infant has a slightly yellow tint. Based on this assessment, the nurse will review the maternal history for which of the following?
   A. hepatic insufficiency
   B. history of recreational drug use
   C. ABO incompatibility
   D. thyroid disease

3. The nurse working in an obstetrical office is providing care for a woman who suspects that she is pregnant. Upon completion of physical assessment, the physician reports the presence of Chadwick's sign. The nurse understands that the patient has which of the following clinical indications of pregnancy?
   A. softening of the cervix
   B. bluish–purple discoloration of cervical mucous membranes
   C. softening of the isthmus of the uterus
   D. quickening

4. The nurse is caring for a primigravida in a prenatal clinic. The patient is being monitored closely for pregnancy-induced hypertension (PIH). Which of the following assessments would be cause for concern for the nurse?
   A. blood pressure = 134/84 mm Hg
   B. weight gain of 0.5 kg during the past 2 weeks
   C. a dipstick value of 3+ for protein in the urine
   D. pitting pedal edema at the end of the day

5. When assessing a pregnant woman who is in the first stage of labor, the nurse recognizes which of the following as the most conclusive sign that uterine contractions are effective?
    A. dilation of the cervix
    B. descent of the fetus
    C. rupture of the amniotic membranes
    D. increase in bloody show

6. A woman gave birth to a healthy baby 2 days ago. What type of lochia would the nurse expect to find when assessing this patient?
    A. lochia rubra
    B. lochia sangra
    C. lochia alba
    D. lochia serosa

7. The nurse is caring for a newborn immediately following delivery. At 1 minute, the infant has a heart rate of 120, has good respiratory effort with a strong cry, has some flexion of all extremities, grimaces to flicking on the soles of the feet, and is completely pink. Based on this assessment, the nurse must document the 1 minute Apgar as which of the following?
    A. 6
    B. 7
    C. 8
    D. 9

8. The nurse is providing care for a patient who gave birth vaginally 1 hour ago. Estimated blood loss was less than 500 mL. When assessing this patient's vital signs, the nurse would expect to find which of the following?
    A. T = 97.8°F; P = 88; R = 20; BP = 110/66
    B. T = 97.5°F; P = 120; R = 34; BP = 88/50
    C. T = 101.2°F; P = 78; R = 18; BP = 112/64
    D. T = 97.0°F; P = 58; R = 28; BP = 144/92

9. The nurse is caring for a woman during the immediate postpartum period. During assessment, the nurse notes that the patient is experiencing profuse bleeding. The most likely cause of the bleeding is which of the following?
    A. uterine atony
    B. uterine inversion
    C. vaginal hematoma
    D. vaginal laceration

10. The nurse suspects a uterine infection in the postpartum patient. Which of the following assessments is most likely to validate the presence of infection?
    A. elevated pulse and blood pressure
    B. odor of the lochia
    C. appearance of the episiotomy site
    D. distention of the abdomen

11. A newborn is placed under a radiant heat warmer after birth. The nurse evaluates the newborn's body temperature every hour. This nursing action is taken to prevent which of the following?
   A. cold stress
   B. respiratory depression
   C. tachycardia
   D. thermogenesis

Interpretation of Lab Values

1. The nurse is caring for a pregnant woman with preeclampsia whose labor is to be induced. Prior to initiating the Pitocin infusion, the nurse reviews the patient's latest laboratory test results, which reveal a platelet count of 90,000; an elevated AST level; and a falling hematocrit. The nurse notifies the physician because the lab results are indicative of which of the following abnormalities?
   A. eclampsia
   B. disseminated intravascular coagulation
   C. HELLP syndrome
   D. idiopathic thrombocytopenia purpura

2. The nurse is providing education about desirable glucose levels to a patient with pregestational diabetes. The nurse explains that a normal fasting blood glucose level should fall within which of the following ranges?
   A. 45 to 65 mg/dL
   B. 60 to 110 mg/dL
   C. 120 to 150 mg/dL
   D. 150 to 180 mg/dL

3. The nurse is monitoring pregnancy progress in an insulin dependent pregnant adolescent. Which of the following laboratory tests would provide the best information about ongoing control of the patient's diabetes during pregnancy?
   A. fasting blood glucose
   B. glycosylated hemoglobin
   C. oral glucose tolerance test
   D. postprandial glucose

4. The nurse is providing care for an insulin dependent patient with diabetes in labor and delivery. The nurse anticipates that the patient's need for insulin in the first 24 hours after delivery will do which of the following?
   A. drop significantly
   B. gradually return to normal
   C. increase slightly
   D. stay the same as predelivery

5. The nurse is providing care for a patient with preeclampsia. In a review of the patient's laboratory test results, which of the following should be of concern to the nurse?
   A. WBC = 10,000/mm^3
   B. platelet count = 125,000/mm^3
   C. plasma fibrinogen = 195 mg/dL
   D. fibrin degradation products = 4 μg/mL

ALTERNATE FORMAT

6. Which of the following lab values should be monitored when providing care for an infant of a diabetic mother (IDM)? SELECT ALL THAT APPLY.
   A. blood glucose
   B. direct Coombs test
   C. red blood cell count
   D. serum bilirubin
   E. serum calcium
   F. white blood cell count

7. Alpha-fetoprotein (AFP) testing is used primarily to screen for which of the following conditions?
   A. urological defects
   B. neural tube defects
   C. cystic fibrosis
   D. trisomy 21

Drugs and Treatments

1. The nurse is providing care to a patient with preterm labor who is prescribed terbutaline sulfate (Brethine). Which of the following interventions would identify side effects of this drug?
   A. Assess deep tendon reflexes.
   B. Assess breath sounds.
   C. Assess for bradycardia.
   D. Assess for hypoglycemia.

2. The nurse is caring for a patient in preterm labor at 30 weeks gestation. The nurse receives orders to administer two doses of betamethasone 12 mg intramuscularly. The nurse knows that the purpose of administering this drug to the patient is which of the following?
   A. to stimulate fetal surfactant production
   B. to suppress uterine contractions
   C. to reduce tachycardia associated with terbutaline administration
   D. to stimulate maternal respiratory status

3. The nurse is providing care for a patient with severe preeclampsia who is receiving magnesium sulfate by intravenous infusion. The nurse assesses the patient and documents the following findings: T = 98.6 °F; P = 96; R = 24; BP = 190/114; 3+ DTRs; no ankle clonus. The nurse places a call to the physician, anticipating an order for which of the following drugs?
   A. hydralazine
   B. magnesium sulfate bolus
   C. diazepam
   D. calcium gluconate

4. The nurse is caring for a patient with severe preeclampsia who is receiving an infusion of magnesium sulfate. The nurse becomes concerned upon assessing which of the following conditions with this patient?
   A. a sleepy sedated affect
   B. respirations at 8 breaths per minute
   C. deep tendon reflexes of 2+
   D. absent ankle clonus

5. Dinoprostone (Cervidil) is ordered for a pregnant woman at 43 weeks gestation. The nurse recognizes that this medication will be administered to:
   A. enhance uteroplacental perfusion for the aging placenta.
   B. increase the volume of amniotic fluid in a late-term pregnancy.
   C. ripen the cervix in preparation for induction of labor.
   D. stimulate the amniotic membranes to rupture.

6. A pregnant patient who is at 36 weeks gestation is scheduled for an amniocentesis. The nurse explains to the patient that an ultrasound will be performed prior to the amniocentesis. The nurse realizes that teaching has been effective when the patient states which of the following as rationale for the amniocentesis?
   A. "It will help to tell if there is more than one baby."
   B. "It will be done to determine the age of my baby."
   C. "It will be done to see where the placenta and baby are."
   D. "It will identify if my baby has any congenital defects."

7. The nurse has received orders to administer a dose of vitamin K (AquaMEPHYTON) intramuscularly. The time frame for administering this drug should be which of the following?
   A. within 1 hour of birth or after the first breastfeeding
   B. within 6 hours of birth or after the first dextrose water
   C. within 12 hours of birth or after the first meconium stool
   D. within 24 hours of birth or after the first formula is given

ANSWERS

General

1. **(D)**; Progesterone exerts effects on the GI tract by causing relaxation of the cardiac sphincter and delayed gastric emptying, which results in decreased GI motility. Because GI motility is decreased, there is no increased peristaltic activity during pregnancy. Estrogen production actually causes decreased secretion of hydrochloric acid. The growing uterus puts pressure on the stomach and intestines, resulting in constipation.

2. **(A)**; The nurse should utilize the nursing assistant within the appropriate practice capacity, which could include providing comfort measures. The nursing assistant should not perform vital signs that are part of a diagnostic assessment, which would be the case for the patient with known hypertension. The nursing assistant may not legally dispense medications within the hospital setting.

3. **(A)**; This is a complex clinical situation that requires input from social services and activation of necessary resources. Permission from the patient's parents is not required.

There is no requirement for physician presence at discharge. Mother–baby interaction during hospitalization is not barred.

4. **(A)**; Methylergonovine (Methergine) is contraindicated in patients with blood pressure greater than 140/90, so the nurse should question this order.

5. **(A)**; Fetal heart beats are heard by doppler at 12 weeks. The sex of the fetus is determined at conception. It is common for lanugo to cover the body of the fetus at week 20 and to disappear by week 36. It is common for mothers to begin feeling the fetus move between weeks 16 and 20.

6. **(D)**; Using Nägele's rule, the calculation would occur as follows: Begin with the first day of the last menstrual period and subtract 3 months (October 1 − 3 months = July 1). Add 7 days (July 1 + 7 days = July 8, 2010).

7. **(B)**; The nurse should encourage the patient to breathe into a paper bag because the symptoms described are classic signs of hyperventilation (blowing off too much CO_2), which could result in respiratory alkalosis if it is not addressed.

8. **(A)**; The changes in fetal heart rate are late decelerations, which indicate that there is inadequate placental perfusion. This is considered an ominous sign. Although a scalp electrode may be required, the first priority should be to shift the patient's weight off of the vena cava to allow for better circulation to the placenta.

9. **(C)**; According to the gate control theory, pain sensations travel along nerve pathways to the brain. Only a limited number of sensations can travel along these pathways at one time. Therefore, distraction techniques, such as massage, reduce or block transmission of pain along the nerve pathways. Although the other nursing actions are appropriate for a laboring client, they do not address the gate control theory.

10. **(B, C, G, E, A, F, D)**; The cardinal movements of labor in order are descent, flexion, internal rotation, extension, restitution, external rotation, and expulsion.

11. **(C)**; Development of worsening preeclampsia is a cause for concern for the patient and her family. Upon admission to the hospital, the patient should be maintained in a quiet, low-stimulus environment. Typically, the patient is admitted to a private room in a quiet location where she can be monitored closely. Visitors are limited to close family members or a significant other. The patient should be encouraged to maintain the left lateral recumbent position most of the time. Bright lights and sudden loud noises may precipitate seizure activity in patients with severe preeclampsia.

12. **(D)**; The patient should be aware that onset of a headache beyond 30 weeks in the pregnancy may be a sign of elevated blood pressure, which should be reported to the physician promptly.

13. **(A)**; Infants of mothers with diabetes are at risk for macrosomia (excessive growth) related to high maternal blood glucose levels, which result in elevated glucose levels in the fetus. Consequently, the fetal islets of Langerhans are continually stimulated to produce insulin. A chronic hyperinsulin state in the fetus leads to excessive growth.

14. **(C)**; The nurse knows that when HELLP syndrome is diagnosed and the patient's condition is stabilized, definitive treatment requires delivery of the infant as soon as possible regardless of gestational age.

15. **(A)**; Oligohydramnios (decreased volume of amniotic fluid) is associated with fetal urinary tract defects.

16. **(B)**; Positive signs of pregnancy are those that are completely objective and cannot be confused with any other pathologic state. They include audible fetal heartbeat, *palpation of fetal movement by a trained examiner*, and visualization of the fetus by ultrasound. Presumptive signs of pregnancy are symptoms that are experienced and reported by the pregnant woman. Because they can be caused by other conditions, they are not considered proof of pregnancy. Presumptive signs include amenorrhea, nausea and vomiting in pregnancy (morning sickness), excessive fatigue, urinary frequency, changes in the breast, and quickening. Probable changes are objective changes that can be assessed by an examiner but that can also have other causes. Therefore, they are not considered confirmation of pregnancy. These include changes in the pelvic organs (Goodell's sign, Chadwick's sign, Hegar's sign, and McDonald's sign), enlargement of the abdomen, Braxton Hicks contractions, uterine souffle, changes in skin pigmentation, ballottement, and elevated hCG levels.

17. **(C)**; The patient can limit nausea and vomiting by eating small, frequent meals throughout the day and by avoiding odors or causative factors as well as greasy or highly seasoned foods. The patient should also consider drinking carbonated beverages. Patients also should be encouraged to eat some dry crackers or toast before arising in the morning—as opposed to a full meal of bacon and eggs. Large meals should be discouraged.

18. **(D)**; There are no concrete data about the volume of alcohol intake related to fetal abnormalities. Maternal abstinence from alcohol is recommended throughout the entire pregnancy.

19. **(A)**; A woman who is kneeling, sitting, or walking derives some benefit from gravity to facilitate fetal descent. A patient who is in a lithotomy position does not reap the same benefit.

20. **(A)**; When the membranes rupture, the open pathway to the uterus increases the woman's risk of intrauterine infection.

21. **(B)**; Late in the transition phase of the first stage of labor, it is normal for the laboring patient to feel out of control and to become irritable. However, patients in this phase do not want to be left alone. The best response by the nurse is to explain to the partner that the patient's behavior is normal and to help the partner continue to coach the patient.

22. **(A)**; Physiological needs always take priority, so the most important action for the nurse immediately after a birth is to keep the newborn's airway open.

23. **(B)**; Presumptive signs include amenorrhea, nausea and vomiting in pregnancy (morning sickness), excessive fatigue, urinary frequency, changes in the breast, and *quickening*. Probable changes are objective changes that can be assessed by an examiner but that can also have other causes. Therefore, they are not considered confirmation of pregnancy. These include changes in the pelvic organs (Goodell's sign, Chadwick's sign, Hegar's sign, and McDonald's sign), enlargement of the abdomen, Braxton Hicks contractions, uterine souffle, changes in skin pigmentation, ballottement, and elevated hCG levels. Positive signs of pregnancy are those that are completely objective and cannot be confused with any other pathologic state. They include

audible fetal heartbeat, palpation of fetal movement by a trained examiner, and visualization of the fetus by ultrasound. Presumptive signs of pregnancy are symptoms that are experienced and reported by the pregnant woman. Because they can be caused by other conditions, they are not considered proof of pregnancy.

24. **(B)**; This statement affirms that the woman does not have much self-esteem. Battered women often are submissive, passive, and dependent. With a need to seek approval from men in their lives, many battered women do not work outside the home, are isolated from family and friends, and are totally dependent on their partner.

25. **(D)**; Given the physical findings, the most plausible explanation for the injuries is that the patient has been a victim of domestic violence. However, the nurse should ask the patient what happened. If the patient fell down a flight of stairs, it would have been likely for the patient to suffer multiple bruises all over the arms and legs in addition to the head. The injuries described seem too severe for running into a door. If falling off of a trampoline during exercise caused the injuries, it is at least as likely that the patient would have suffered a spinal cord injury in addition to those noted.

26. **(A)**; Knowing that between 3 and 30% of all postpartum women will experience postpartum depression, experts indicate that prenatal assessment for depression should begin as early as the first trimester and should be completed each trimester to update a woman's risk status.

27. **(B)**; The American College of Obstetricians and Gynecologists (ACOG, 2004) guidelines state that a classic or T uterine incision is a contraindication for VBAC.

28. **(C)**; Evaporation is the loss of heat that occurs when a liquid is converted to a vapor. The newborn's skin is moist with amniotic fluid and blood from delivery. The skin must be dried immediately to prevent heat loss due to evaporation.

29. **(A)**; It is important to connect the mother with her infant as soon as possible.

Physical Assessment

1. **(D)**; Fetal heart tones are best heard directly over the fetal back. The long, smooth surface palpated on the mother's right side is the back of the fetus. The round, firm, movable fetal body part palpated in the upper portion of the uterus is the head of the fetus. Therefore, the fetus is in breech position, and fetal heart tones would be auscultated in the maternal upper quadrant.

2. **(C)**; ABO incompatibility (mother with blood type O and baby with blood type A or B) can result in jaundice of the newborn.

3. **(B)**; Chadwick's sign is a bluish–purple discoloration of the mucous membranes of the cervix, vagina, and vulva. Goodell's sign is a softening of the cervix. Hegar's sign is a softening of the isthmus of the uterus. Quickening is when the mother perceives fetal movement.

4. **(C)**; Close monitoring and careful management are indicated when the patient develops proteinuria. Other assessment findings noted are expected during pregnancy.

5. **(A)**; During the active phase of the first stage of labor, the cervix dilates from about 4 cm to 7 cm.

6. **(A)**; Lochia rubra is dark red discharge that occurs for the first 2 to 3 days following a birth. Lochia serosa is a pinkish discharge that follows from about day 3 to day 10. Lochia alba, a creamy or yellowish discharge, persists for another week or two after lochia serosa subsides.

7. **(C)**; The infant's 1 minute Apgar should be rated as an 8 based on the following scoring system: HR >100 = 2; good respiratory effort with a strong cry = 2; some flexion of extremities = 1; grimacing to flicking on the soles of the feet = 1; and completely pink skin color = 2 for a total of 8.

8. **(A)**; One hour after a normal vaginal delivery, the nurse expects the patient to have normal vital signs.

9. **(A)**; Uterine atony is a very common cause of early postpartum hemorrhage.

10. **(B)**; Normally, the lochia flow has a musty, stale odor that is not offensive. Any foul odor to the lochia is suggestive of infection, and additional laboratory assessment and follow-up are required promptly.

11. **(A)**; Maintenance of the newborn's body temperature is critical to survival. Measures are taken to prevent cold stress, which forces metabolic and physiologic demands.

Interpretation of Lab Values

1. **(C)**; The patient's laboratory results reflect HELLP syndrome, which stands for *h*emolysis, *e*levated *l*iver enzymes, and *l*ow *p*latelet count (less than 100,000/mm³).

2. **(B)**; Normal fasting blood glucose should fall within the range of 60 to 110 mg/dL.

3. **(B)**; Glycosylated hemoglobin (Hgb A1c) provides the best information to the nurse about ongoing control of the patient's diabetes during pregnancy.

4. **(A)**; During the first 24 hours postpartum, women with preexisting diabetes typically require very little insulin and are usually managed with sliding scale coverage.

5. **(B)**; The patient's platelet count is low (normal 150,000–400,000/μL), which is a concern because the patient could be at risk for development of disseminated intravascular coagulation (DIC). WBC is normal (normal = 4500–11,000/μL), as is plasma fibrinogen (normal = 150–400 mg/dL) and fibrin degradation products (normal = 2–10 μg/mL). When the patient develops thrombocytopenia (low platelet count), the nurse should be concerned that the patient could be developing DIC.

6. **(A, C, D, E)**; The infant of a diabetic mother is at risk for hypoglycemia, hypocalcemia, hyperbilirubinemia, and polycythemia. A direct Coombs test measures the presence of antibodies against the newborn's red blood cells, which is associated with Rh and ABO incompatibility. The measurement of white blood cell count in newborns is usually performed to determine presence of infection.

7. **(B)**; Alpha-fetoprotein (AFP) levels are elevated in cases of infants with open neural tube defects, anencephaly, omphalocele, or gastroschisis.

Drugs and Treatments

1. **(B)**; Terbutaline (Brethine) is a sympathomimetic drug that can produce wheezing as a side effect for patients. Drugs in this category tend to cause tachycardia, palpitations, angina, cough, and dyspnea. They are not known to affect deep tendon reflexes or blood glucose levels.

2. **(A)**; Betamethasone is a glucocorticoid that is administered to this patient to stimulate fetal surfactant production.

3. **(A)**; The nurse anticipates an order for hydralazine, an antihypertensive drug, to treat the BP of 190/114.

4. **(B)**; Magnesium sulfate acts as a CNS depressant, so a sleepy sedated affect is considered normal. The nurse should be concerned upon assessing a respiratory rate of only 8 breaths per minute because respiratory depression is a sign of developing toxicity.

5. **(C)**; Dinoprostone is an abortifacient drug that can be used to *ripen the cervix in preparation for induction of labor in a woman who has passed her estimated date of birth (EDB)*. It can also be used to evacuate the uterus in case of a missed abortion or intrauterine fetal death up to 28 weeks gestation; management of benign hydatidiform mole; or to terminate pregnancy from 12–20 weeks gestation.

6. **(C)**; The ultrasound prior to an amniocentesis is performed to identify placement of the placenta and the fetus to avoid accidental injury to either with the amnio needle. Although the ultrasound may provide further information about the fetus, that is not the purpose when it is performed just before an amniocentesis.

7. **(A)**; Vitamin K (AquaMEPHYTON) is administered prophylactically to prevent hemorrhage and should be administered within 1 hour of birth, or the dose may be delayed until after the first breastfeeding. Current recommendations strongly highlight the need for treatment for infants who will be exclusively breastfed.

Keep Track

- Percent correct. (Divide the number of questions you answered correctly by the total number of questions you answered.) _____

- Number of questions you missed due to a reading error: _____

- Number of questions you missed due to errors in analysis: _____

- Number of assessment questions you missed: _____

- Number of lab value questions you missed: _____

- Number of drug/treatment questions you missed: _____

Nugget List

Chapter number _____   Topic _____

Chapter 21

Practice Test: Nursing Management of Patients Undergoing Surgery

Karen S. March

PRACTICE TEST

General

1. A diabetic patient will go to surgery for a mid-thigh amputation of the left leg. An amputation puts this patient at high risk for which of the following nursing diagnoses?
   A. spiritual distress
   B. body image disturbance
   C. ineffective denial
   D. impaired social interaction

ALTERNATE FORMAT

2. The perianesthesia nurse recognizes which of the following patient conditions as contributing to a more complex surgical experience? SELECT ALL THAT APPLY.
   A. diabetes
   B. cancer
   C. age
   D. anemia
   E. obesity

3. The nurse is providing care for a preoperative patient who has smoked 2.5 packs per day for 35 years. This patient has a lifetime history of how many pack-years?
   A. 70 pack-years
   B. 75 pack-years
   C. 82 pack-years
   D. 87 pack-years

4. The nurse is performing an admission assessment on a patient who is scheduled for surgery later in the day. The patient asks the nurse, "What was the big deal about no smoking before surgery?" The nurse's best reply is which of the following?
   A. "Smoking puts you at higher risk for postoperative nausea and vomiting."
   B. "Smoking increases your risk of postoperative atelectasis and pneumonia."
   C. "Smoking decreases the effectiveness of some anesthetic agents."
   D. "Smoking causes vasodilation, which causes very low blood pressure in surgery."

5. According to guidelines released by the American Society of Anesthesiologists, patients should fast:
   A. 8 or more hours from food and fluids prior to surgery.
   B. 6 hours from food and 2 hours from clear liquids.
   C. completely for at least 12 hours prior to major surgery.
   D. from food and clear liquids for 4 hours prior to surgery.

ALTERNATE FORMAT

6. Early ambulation postoperatively provides many benefits to the patient, including which of the following? **SELECT ALL THAT APPLY.**
   A. increases heart rate
   B. increases cardiac output
   C. stimulates peristalsis
   D. decreases venous return
   E. supports wound healing

7. The nurse is preparing a patient for surgery and is checking the medical record to verify the existence of a valid surgical consent. Which of the following aspects must be present for consent to be valid?
   A. The information has been explained by the nurse.
   B. The patient has unanswered questions about the procedure.
   C. The patient signed with an X in the presence of two witnesses.
   D. The patient's insurability has been fully disclosed.

8. Which of the following are critical points of the surgical time-out as defined by the Association of Perioperative Registered Nurses (AORN)?
   A. takes place in the preop holding area
   B. involves the patient, a nurse, and the surgeon
   C. requires verification of site by the patient and surgeon
   D. all team members verbally agree to patient, site, and procedure

ALTERNATE FORMAT

9. The nurse should be considerate of which of the following cultural considerations when caring for patients during the postoperative phase? **SELECT ALL THAT APPLY.**
   A. Numerical pain rating scales are appropriate for all patients.
   B. Modesty dictates minimal exposure for assessment only.
   C. Same sex care providers are preferred when possible.
   D. Expression of pain may vary according to cultural background.

10. The nurse is providing care for a patient who will undergo a total hip replacement surgery today. The nurse knows that preoperative teaching about DVT prophylaxis has been effective when the patient makes which of the following statements?
    A. "I will have to take warfarin (Coumadin) for about 4 weeks after discharge."
    B. "I will need to wear compression devices at night for at least 2 weeks after surgery."
    C. "If I ambulate within 24 hours after surgery, my risk of DVT will be significantly lower."
    D. "I will need to give myself injections of enoxaparin (Lovenox) for about 2 weeks."

Physical Assessment

1. A patient who will undergo planned surgery, such as a hip replacement, must have a preoperative health evaluation done within 30 days prior to surgery to be in compliance with which of the following?
   A. Medicare requirements
   B. insurance regulatory standards
   C. American Medical Association standards
   D. Joint Commission requirements

ALTERNATE FORMAT

2. The nurse is providing care for a patient in the postanesthesia care unit where the Aldrete system is used to identify patients who are ready for discharge. Which of the following parameters are indicators used in assessing readiness for discharge from PACU? SELECT ALL THAT APPLY.
   A. respirations
   B. temperature
   C. color
   D. consciousness
   E. circulation
   F. activity

3. The postanesthesia nurse is providing care for a patient who returned from surgery within the past 30 minutes and has been arousable. Upon assessment, the nurse finds that the patient has snoring respirations with inspiratory stridor, retractions, and a pulse oximetry of 88%. Which of the following actions should the nurse take immediately?
   A. Stimulate the patient and increase the oxygen.
   B. Place the patient in full supine position.
   C. Place the patient supine and provide rescue breaths.
   D. Call a code and bring the crash cart to the bedside.

ALTERNATE FORMAT

4. The nurse is working on an acute care surgical floor. Which of the following patients would the nurse expect to have considerable pain? SELECT ALL THAT APPLY.
   A. a patient who had cardiac surgery two days ago and must cough and deep breathe
   B. a patient who had a bowel resection with temporary colostomy earlier today
   C. a patient who had a laparoscopic cholecystectomy five days ago
   D. a patient who had a total hip replacement three days ago

Interpretation of Lab Values

1. Which of the following are considered early signs of malignant hyperthermia?
   A. T >100.4°F postoperatively; tachycardia
   B. T > 102.5°F postoperatively; chills
   C. masseter spasm; ↑'d levels of expired CO_2
   D. metabolic alkalosis; hypotension

Drugs and Treatments

1. The nurse is providing care for a preoperative patient who normally takes quinapril (Accupril). The nurse will verify with the physician whether or not to hold the drug prior to surgery because it is likely to cause which of the following during surgery?
   A. hypotension
   B. impaired cardiac function
   C. respiratory depression
   D. bronchospasm

2. The nurse at an outpatient surgical center is providing preoperative teaching for a patient with diabetes who normally takes metformin (Glucophage) and glipizide (Glucotrol XL) daily. When the nurse informs the patient about the likelihood of having sliding scale regular insulin coverage during the postoperative period, the patient is alarmed and asks why that is necessary when the pills have worked well. The best response by the nurse is which of the following?
   A. "Your pancreatic function will be impaired postop because of anesthesia."
   B. "The stress of surgery will cause your blood glucose to elevate considerably."
   C. "We have always managed blood glucose levels this way after surgery."
   D. "You will be right back on your pills within 24 hours after surgery."

ALTERNATE FORMAT

3. The nurse understands that the following medications should be stopped prior to surgery because they increase risk of bleeding. SELECT ALL THAT APPLY.
   A. amiodarone
   B. aspirin
   C. amlodipine (Norvasc)
   D. metoprolol (Lopressor)
   E. clopidogrel (Plavix)
   F. prednisone
   G. ibuprofen

4. Which of the following medications may be given during cardiac surgery to reduce the risk of atrial fibrillation?
   A. atropine
   B. atenolol
   C. enalapril
   D. verapamil

5. Which of the following drugs may be administered to reduce pain and discomfort or to reduce anesthesia requirements?
   A. fentanyl
   B. midazolam (Versed)
   C. ondansetron (Zofran)
   D. glycopyrrolate

6. Prophylactic antibiotics should be administered within which of the following time frames for optimal protection against surgical site infection?
   A. within 4 hours prior to surgery
   B. within 2 hours prior to surgery
   C. before the patient leaves the inpatient unit
   D. within 60 minutes prior to the initial incision

ANSWERS

General

1. **(B)**; The patient is at risk for body image disturbance postoperatively related to amputation of an extremity.

2. **(A, B, D, E)**; Patients with Type I diabetes present complex challenges for surgery related to implications for controlling blood glucose. They also experience slower wound healing and a greater potential for infection. Immunocompromised patients (cancer, chemotherapy, post-organ-transplant, HIV) present significant challenges for hypothermia, infection, and adrenal dysfunction. Patients with anemia, blood disorders, and obesity also risk less than optimal surgical outcomes.

3. **(D)**; The patient has smoked $2.5 \times 35 = 87.5$ pack-years.

4. **(B)**; Smoking increases the individual's risk for postoperative atelectasis and pneumonia by damaging the mucociliary system. Nonsmokers are at a higher risk for postoperative nausea and vomiting. Smoking has no effect on individual anesthetic agents. Smoking causes vasoconstriction, which is especially a concern for patients who undergo cardiac or vascular surgery.

5. **(B)**; The American Society of Anesthesiologists released guidelines in 1999 indicating that patients should fast from food for 6 or more hours and from clear liquids for at least 2 hours prior to surgery. Longer periods of fasting can cause dehydration, hypovolemia, and hypoglycemia in addition to excessive thirst and hunger.

6. **(A, B, C, E)**; Early ambulation promotes increased heart rate and cardiac output, which increases tissue perfusion and wound healing. Ambulation also stimulates peristalsis and increases venous return.

7. **(C)**; The physician is responsible for providing a thorough explanation of the need for surgery, what is involved in the required procedure, and anticipated risks and recovery time. The physician should ensure that all of the patient's questions about the procedure have been answered in a manner that is understandable and satisfactory to the patient. The nurse may witness the patient's signature. Patients who are unable to sign their name may use a mark (perhaps an X), providing that there are two witnesses.

8. **(D)**; According to the AORN *Guidelines for Implementing the Joint Commission Universal Protocol to Promote Correct Site Surgery*, a time-out takes place in the procedure or operating room after the patient is prepped and draped. Specific documentation of the time-out must include the following: *identification of the patient, agreement about the correct site* and side, *agreement about the procedure* to be performed, correct patient position, and availability of implants or special equipment as required.

9. **(B, C, D)**; Modesty is extremely important in some cultures (i.e., Hispanic, Arab, Muslim, etc.). Care should be taken to maintain modesty for females. Exposure of the body should occur only when necessary for examination or treatment. The head should be covered for female patients who request it. Same sex care providers are preferred when possible. It is also critical to remember that expression of pain may vary considerably depending upon cultural background. The nurse should explain to the patient the importance of treating pain and should exercise sensitivity about alternative pain therapies.

10. **(A)**; Patients who have total hip or knee replacement surgery, repair of hip fracture, and major gynecologic surgeries are at higher risk for development of venous thromboembolism and should remain on antithrombotic drug therapy (warfarin or enoxaparin) for 2 to 4 weeks following surgery.

Physical Assessment

1. **(D)**; A preoperative health evaluation must be completed within 30 days prior to a planned surgery. The evaluation may be completed by an internist, the surgeon, or an anesthesia provider.

2. **(A, C, D, E, F)**; The Aldrete system requires assessment of activity (Is the patient able to move limbs voluntarily on command?); respirations (Is the patient able to deep breathe and cough freely?); circulation (Is the blood pressure within 20% of preprocedure readings?); consciousness (Is the patient fully awake?); and color (Is skin color normal and is pulse oximetry >92% on room air?).

3. **(A)**; An arousable postoperative patient who experiences acute airway obstruction should be stimulated by speaking to the patient, encouraging the patient to take some deep breaths, and turning up the oxygen. If the patient were not arousable, an oral airway could be placed to maintain an open airway. Airway obstruction/occlusion should be less of a problem as the patient becomes more awake and responsive.

4. **(A, B)**; Incisional pain is most significant within the first 24 to 48 hours. Research has indicated that cardiac patients report that coughing is the most painful activity. Patients with abdominal surgery also suffer significant pain. The patient who had a total hip replacement three days ago is likely to have less pain postoperatively than preoperatively. The patient who had a laparoscopic cholecystectomy five days ago would have had significant pain related to CO_2 insufflation during surgery, but the pain should be significantly less 5 days later following ambulation.

Interpretation of Lab Values

1. **(C)**; Early signs of malignant hyperthermia include masseter spasm (jaw contracture), sinus tachycardia, and an increase in end tidal (expiratory) CO_2 levels. The anesthesia provider is often the first person to suspect malignant hyperthermia because of the rise in end tidal CO_2. A level 2 to 3 times normal is considered to be a diagnostic indicator of malignant hyperthermia. Other signs include rigor, hypoxemia, and tea-colored urine. Hyperthermia is a *late* sign.

Drugs and Treatments

1. **(A)**; Quinapril (Accupril) is an ACE inhibitor that can cause hypotension. Unless it is prescribed to treat heart failure, the surgeon may elect to hold the drug on the morning of surgery.

2. **(B)**; The nurse should inform the patient that the stress of acute illness or surgery will cause elevation of blood glucose levels and that sliding scale insulin coverage provides control of glucose during the postoperative phase that is superior to oral hypoglycemic agents. Pancreatic function is not affected by anesthesia. The nurse should not guarantee return to oral agents within 24 hours because it may not occur within that time frame.

3. **(B, E, F, G)**; Aspirin and ibuprofen both increase the risk of perioperative bleeding. Aspirin should be stopped 7 to 10 days before surgery, and ibuprofen should be stopped 2 weeks before surgery. Plavix inhibits platelet aggregation, and the surgeon

may want the patient to stop taking it 2 weeks prior to surgery. Prednisone is a steroid that increases risk for postoperative bleeding.

4. **(B)**; Beta blockers may be administered during cardiac surgery to reduce the likelihood of atrial fibrillation. Atropine increases heart rate. Enalapril is an ACE inhibitor. Verapamil is a calcium channel blocker.

5. **(A)**; Fentanyl may be administered to reduce pain and discomfort or to reduce anesthesia requirements.

6. **(D)**; Research has indicated that prophylactic antibiotics should be administered within 60 minutes prior to the initial incision to ensure adequate antimicrobial levels in the tissues and to maintain them for the entire surgery.

Keep Track

- Percent correct. (Divide the number of questions you answered correctly by the total number of questions you answered.) _____

- Number of questions you missed due to a reading error: _____

- Number of questions you missed due to errors in analysis: _____

- Number of assessment questions you missed: _____

- Number of lab value questions you missed: _____

- Number of drug/treatment questions you missed: _____

Nugget List

Chapter number _____ Topic _____

Chapter 22

Practice Test: Nursing Management of Patients Being Treated for Cancer

Karen S. March

PRACTICE TEST

General

1. The nurse is caring for a patient who was informed by a physician following surgery that a malignant neoplasm in the colon has invaded nearby tissues. Which of the following statements by the patient indicates understanding of this information?
   A. "I have cancer of the colon that has begun to spread."
   B. "I have growths in my bowel that can be easily treated."
   C. "I have growths in my bowel that will have to be watched."
   D. "The doctor said there is really nothing to worry about."

2. The nurse is caring for a patient who was seen by a dermatologist for a lump at the base of the skull. Following examination of the lump, the physician described it as a benign neoplasm. Based on this information, the nurse expects what type of follow-up?
   A. The patient will be scheduled for admission to the hospital.
   B. The patient will be scheduled for removal by inpatient surgery.
   C. The patient will be scheduled for removal by outpatient surgery.
   D. The patient will have the lump removed in the office.

3. The nurse understands that patients older than the age of 65 years are at higher risk for cancer because of:
   A. enhanced resistance.
   B. declining free radicals.
   C. living in warm environments.
   D. altered immune responses.

4. The nurse knows that which of the following types of cancer typically demonstrate a familial tendency?
   A. brain
   B. lung
   C. lymph
   D. bladder

ALTERNATE FORMAT

5. The nurse is caring for a female patient who is concerned that she may be at higher than normal risk of breast cancer. Which of the following factors identified by the patient place her at higher than normal risk? SELECT ALL THAT APPLY.
   A. 60 years of age
   B. works night shift
   C. breastfed two children
   D. used birth control pills for 25 years
   E. drinks a few Manhattans each evening

6. Which of the following are non-modifiable risk factors for breast cancer?
   A. hormone replacement therapy
   B. alcohol consumption
   C. age at menarche
   D. sedentary lifestyle

ALTERNATE FORMAT

7. The nurse is caring for a patient who has had chemotherapy and now is experiencing myelosuppression. Which of the following interventions would be appropriate during the care of this patient? SELECT ALL THAT APPLY.
   A. Perform hand hygiene before and after patient care.
   B. Monitor and record vital signs.
   C. Encourage ample family visiting.
   D. Offer frequent turning and repositioning.

8. The nurse is caring for a patient who asks about the current recommendations for monthly breast self-examination. The best response by the nurse is that:
   A. "Women older than age 30 should perform monthly breast self-examination."
   B. "Women aged 20–39 years should perform monthly breast self-examination."
   C. "Women older than 40 years of age should have a yearly mammogram."
   D. "Women older than 50 years of age should have a yearly mammogram."

9. The nurse understands that the American Cancer Society classifies all of the following as warning signs of cancer *except*:
   A. unintentional weight loss.
   B. a sore that does not heal.
   C. unusual bleeding or discharge.
   D. nagging cough or hoarseness.

10. The nurse understands that the process known as angiogenesis is problematic for patients who have cancer because:
    A. it serves no real purpose in treatment of cancer.
    B. new vessels supply the tumor with nutrients and oxygen.
    C. it delivers tumor necrosis factor to the nucleus of the tumor.
    D. it facilitates development of the tumor nucleus.

11. The nurse is caring for a patient with breast cancer who asks about sites of metastasis for this cancer. The best reply by the nurse is:
    A. "Breast cancer does not normally metastasize."
    B. "Breast cancer normally metastasizes to the kidneys."
    C. "Breast cancer normally metastasizes to the bowel."
    D. "Breast cancer normally metastasizes to the bone."

12. The nurse is caring for a patient who has esophageal cancer with metastasis. The nurse understands that metastasis implies which of the following?
    A. The patient will not survive more than one week.
    B. The patient will have to receive radiation therapy.
    C. The patient will probably die from the disease.
    D. The patient must agree to a regimen of chemotherapy.

13. A 45-year-old female received news that mammography has identified a mass in the right breast. The patient asks the nurse what this means. The best response by the nurse is:
    A. "The doctor will have to talk to you about the results."
    B. "The doctor will come to discuss chemotherapy with you."
    C. "The results of this test are very specific for breast cancer."
    D. "More testing must be done to determine what the mass is."

14. When the nurse teaches a group of youths about the dangerous effects of tobacco use, the nurse is practicing what level of cancer prevention?
    A. primary
    B. secondary
    C. tertiary

15. The nurse understands that a patient with colon or rectal cancer is likely to have which of the following clinical manifestations?
    A. hematuria
    B. flatulence
    C. weight gain
    D. vomiting

16. The nurse is teaching a patient about external radiation for cancer. Which of the following statements by the patient indicates understanding about the frequency of this form of treatment?
    A. "External radiation is like an X-ray focused on the cancer in my body."
    B. "It is likely that I will have a treatment every day for about 4 months."
    C. "It is likely that I will have treatments 5 days a week for several weeks."
    D. "It is likely that I will have treatments 7 days a week for several weeks."

17. The patient is having preoperative external radiation. When the patient asks why this will happen before surgery, the best response by the nurse is:
    A. "The radiation will help to shrink the size of your tumor."
    B. "Radiation before surgery is the preferred method of your doctor."
    C. "Radiation may kill the cancer, and then surgery won't be needed."
    D. "You will need to ask your doctor about his treatment goals."

18. The nurse is caring for a patient with leukemia who is being prepared for bone marrow transplant. The nurse understands that this patient will:
    A. receive both chemotherapy and external radiation therapy.
    B. receive total body irradiation.
    C. receive chemotherapy only.
    D. receive targeted external radiation only.

19. The nurse is assigned to care for a client who will receive brachytherapy. The nurse understands this means that:
    A. the patient will receive chemotherapy via venous access device.
    B. the patient will receive intensive chemotherapy as an inpatient.
    C. low-dose radiation and chemotherapy will be administered jointly.
    D. radioactive implants will be inserted into tissue adjacent to the tumor.

20. The nurse is providing care for a patient receiving brachytherapy. In planning care for this patient, the nurse must:
    A. plan to spend extra time with the patient to provide emotional support.
    B. ensure that chemotherapy drugs do not extravasate into the patient's tissues.
    C. organize care so that patient contact is limited to one-half hour per shift.
    D. encourage visitation from family and friends to support the patient.

21. The nurse is caring for a patient who is experiencing extreme fatigue related to radiotherapy. When planning this patient's care, the nurse should do which of the following to aid in conservation of energy for the patient?
    A. Avoid entering the room unless absolutely necessary.
    B. Cluster patient care activities to allow for long rest periods.
    C. Ask the patient to ring the bell if he or she needs anything.
    D. Turn and reposition the patient every 2 hours for comfort.

22. The nurse is admitting a patient diagnosed with leukopenia. Which of the following is the most important nursing intervention for this patient?
    A. Wash hands before and after each patient contact.
    B. Encourage the patient to use an electric razor.
    C. Monitor blood pressure and pulse every 4 hours.
    D. Allow ample visitation to keep the patient's spirits up.

23. The nurse is caring for a patient who will undergo bone marrow harvesting. The nurse informs the patient that the harvest will occur:
    A. under local anesthetic at the bedside.
    B. under conscious sedation at the bedside.
    C. under local anesthetic in same-day surgery.
    D. in the operating room under general anesthesia.

24. The nurse understands that patient consequences related to graft rejection following bone marrow transplant include which of the following?
    A. The patient will die without another transplant.
    B. The patient will have relapse of cancer symptoms.
    C. The patient must remain in the hospital.
    D. The patient must receive continuous chemotherapy.

25. The nurse is caring for a cachexic cancer patient near the end of life. As a patient advocate, it is most important for the nurse to:
    A. discuss plans for enteral nutrition with the physician.
    B. encourage the patient and family to consider a PEG tube.
    C. ask about the patient's personal goals for end-of-life care.
    D. provide adequate amounts of artificial nutrition and fluids.

26. The nurse recalls that some of the most common early signs of leukemia are which of the following?
    A. pallor, joint pain, fever
    B. lethargy, petechia, splenomegaly
    C. fatigue, alopecia, hemorrhage
    D. jaundice, mouth lesions, hepatomegaly

27. The nurse understands that myelosuppression associated with chemotherapy can cause bleeding tendencies as a result of which of the following alterations?
    A. leukocytopenia
    B. lymphocytosis
    C. vitamin C deficiency
    D. thrombocytopenia

Physical Assessment

1. The nurse is assigned to care for a patient who is receiving brachytherapy. Which of the following system assessments, if performed consistently, can help to decrease patient suffering?
   A. gastrointestinal
   B. renal
   C. skin
   D. lymphatic

2. The nurse who is caring for a patient undergoing chemotherapy must be particularly attentive to monitoring for which of the following signs and symptoms of toxicity?
   A. crackles
   B. increased urine output
   C. increased capillary refill
   D. bradycardia

3. The nurse understands that a vital component of post-bone-marrow transplantation care involves:
   A. administration of analgesics for postprocedural pain.
   B. astute monitoring for signs of infection and bleeding.
   C. emotional support of the patient during recovery.
   D. continual marrow surveillance for signs of acceptance.

4. The nurse is caring for a patient who has developed stomatitis during chemotherapy. Which of the following clinical manifestations should the nurse anticipate finding upon physical examination?
   A. an inflamed erythematous stoma on the anterior abdomen
   B. burning pain with swallowing and open lesions on the lips
   C. erythematous mucous membranes across the entire body
   D. inflammation and purulent drainage from the stoma

Interpretation of Lab Values

1. The nurse is monitoring lab results for a patient who will receive chemotherapy. The nurse determines that the WBC is normal if it is:
   A. less than 3500 mm^3.
   B. 4000 to 9000 mm^3.
   C. 7000 to 11,000 mm^3.
   D. greater than 11,500 mm^3.

2. The nurse is reviewing results of tests done on a patient with multiple myeloma. Which of the following results is diagnostic for this type of cancer?
   A. impaired cognitive functioning
   B. peripheral neuropathy
   C. excessive melanocytes in the bone marrow
   D. excessive Bence Jones proteins by serum electrophoresis

3. The nurse is caring for a patient who is undergoing chemotherapy. The nurse understands that the patient's risk of infection is related to results from which of the following laboratory tests?
   A. CEA
   B. PSA
   C. ANC
   D. RBC

Drugs and Treatments

1. Ondansetron (Zofran) is administered to the patient receiving chemotherapy to:
   A. prevent nausea and vomiting.
   B. promote a feeling of well-being.
   C. increase effectiveness of therapy.
   D. improve renal function.

2. The nurse is caring for a patient who will receive external radiation therapy. The patient asks the nurse why the ugly ink marks and tattoos over the area to be radiated are necessary. The best response by the nurse is:
   A. "The markings indicate where the technician should focus treatments."
   B. "The markings let you know the exact location of your cancer."
   C. "Exact markings are critical to limit damage to healthy tissues."
   D. "Exact markings indicate potentially salvageable tissue."

3. The nurse is caring for a patient who is receiving interleukins for treatment of renal cell carcinoma. For which of the following conditions must the nurse monitor the patient during treatment?
   A. capillary leak syndrome
   B. acute respiratory distress syndrome
   C. hypertension
   D. decreased cardiac output

4. The nurse is caring for a patient who receives filgrastim (Neupogen) following a bone marrow transplant. Throughout treatment, the nurse should monitor:
   A. red blood cell count and transfuse as necessary.
   B. hemoglobin and hematocrit and signs of dehydration.
   C. for bone pain and administer analgesics as needed.
   D. bleeding time and avoid the use of sharp objects.

5. The nurse is caring for a patient who receives interferon alfa-2a for treatment of hairy cell leukemia. Throughout treatment, the nurse must closely monitor the patient for:
   A. depression.
   B. weight gain.
   C. elevated WBCs.
   D. elevated RBCs.

6. A 25-year-old male patient will soon be starting chemotherapy. Pretreatment counseling for this patient should include discussion about:
   A. mutation of sperm cells during chemotherapy.
   B. the possibility of temporary impotence following treatment.
   C. banking sperm in case permanent sterility results.
   D. possible development of breast enlargement during treatment.

7. The nurse is caring for a patient who is undergoing chemotherapy. Administration of which of the following drugs will help to reduce the duration of anemia related to therapy?
   A. filgrastim (Neupogen)
   B. erythropoietin (Procrit)
   C. interleukin-2
   D. cetuximab (Erbitux)

ANSWERS

General

1. **(A)**; The patient should understand that "malignant neoplasm that has invaded nearby tissues" means that cancer of the colon has begun to spread.

2. **(D)**; Benign neoplasms, by definition, are slow-growing, localized growths that are not malignant. They are usually easily removed—often in the physician's office with local anesthetic applied to the area. There is usually no tissue damage or other complications associated with these growths.

3. **(D)**; People older than age 65 years are at higher risk for cancer due to hormonal changes, altered immune responses, and accumulation of free radicals. Additionally, age has been cited as a factor related to development of cancer.

4. **(B)**; Cancers that typically demonstrate familial tendency include breast, colon, *lung*, ovarian, and prostate.

5. **(B, D, E)**; Hormonal risks for development of breast cancer include *use of birth control pills* or hormone replacement therapy, early menarche (before 12 years of age), late menopause (after 55 years of age), and first pregnancy after 30 years of age. Nonhormonal risk factors include family history, lack of regular exercise, postmenopausal obesity, *increased use of alcohol, working the night shift*, older than 65 years of age, no full-term pregnancies, never breastfed, higher socioeconomic status, Jewish heritage, and two or more first-degree relatives with breast cancer at an early age.

6. **(C)**; Age at menarche is a non-modifiable risk factor for breast cancer. A woman makes choices about hormone replacement therapy, consumption of alcohol, and type of lifestyle.

7. **(A, B)**; Myelosuppression is bone marrow depression related to chemotherapy. Neutropenia ($\downarrow$ neutrophils), thrombocytopenia ($\downarrow$ platelets), and anemia ($\downarrow$ Hgb and $\downarrow$ Hct) are limiting factors for chemotherapy. Within 7–10 days after a treatment, the patient is extremely susceptible to infection. Therefore, the nurse must perform hand hygiene before and after patient care (to prevent spread of infection) and monitor and record vital signs (temperature elevation and $\uparrow$ heart rate may indicate infection).

8. **(C)**; Women should begin performing monthly breast self-exam at age 20 years. From age 20 to 39 years, women should have a breast examination by a healthcare provider every three years. Women older than age 40 years should have annual breast examinations by a healthcare provider and an annual mammogram.

9. **(A)**; The seven warning signs of cancer acknowledged by the American Cancer Society are change in bowel or bladder habits; *a sore that does not heal; unusual bleeding or discharge*; thickening or lump in the breast or elsewhere; indigestion or difficulty in swallowing; obvious change in wart or mole; and *nagging cough or hoarseness*.

10. **(B)**; Angiogenesis is problematic in relation to metastasis because new vessels supply the tumor with nutrients and oxygen.

11. **(D)**; The nurse should tell the patient that breast cancer commonly metastasizes to the bone. If that occurs, the patient may suffer pathological fractures.

12. **(C)**; Metastasis implies a worsened prognosis with increased mortality. The patient with esophageal cancer with metastasis is likely to die from the disease.

13. **(D)**; Mammography is a cancer screening tool. A positive screening test does not imply a definitive diagnosis of cancer. The nurse should provide objective information, such as "more tests are required."

14. **(A)**; The nurse who teaches youths about the dangers of tobacco use is practicing primary prevention of cancer by trying to reduce the risk of occurrence of cancer.

15. **(B)**; Patients with colon or rectal cancer are likely to have changes in bowel habits, occult blood in the stool, *flatulence*, indigestion, weight loss, and fatigue.

16. **(C)**; The patient expresses understanding of the usual frequency of treatments by stating that treatments will be administered 5 days a week for about 5 minutes each day.

17. **(A)**; Preoperative radiation may decrease the size of the tumor, which should increase the chances of successful surgical removal. It can also kill tumor cells beyond the surgical site.

18. **(B)**; The patient with leukemia will receive total body irradiation during preparation for bone marrow transplantation to ensure treatment to all areas that might be harboring leukemic cells.

19. **(D)**; Brachytherapy or internal radiation therapy utilizes sealed radioactive sources (implants) inserted into or near a tumor. This directed therapy allows a relatively high dose of radiation to be administered over a relatively short period of time. With this type of therapy, a high dose of radiation is directed at the tumor, and surrounding tissues receive minimal radiation and consequently suffer less damage as a result of the radiation.

20. **(C)**; In planning care for the patient undergoing brachytherapy, the nurse should organize care so that a maximum of 30 minutes per shift is spent in the patient's room. At all times during care, the nurse must keep in mind principles of minimizing radiation exposure: time, distance, and shielding. Exposure is directly related to time spent in close proximity to the source. Current recommendations are that nurses should spend no more than 30 minutes per shift in the patient's room. All staff caring for the patient must wear radiation badges, and nursing staff should be rotated to keep individual radiation exposure as low as possible. Distance is also important in reducing exposure to radiation. The nurse should encourage patient self-care activities as much as possible and should perform duties as far away from the patient as possible. The final principle for minimizing radiation exposure is shielding. If necessary, a shield can be placed at the patient's bedside, and most nursing care should be done from behind the shield. Lead aprons are not recommended.

21. **(B)**; The nurse should cluster patient care activities to allow for long rest periods. This is the most effective means to help conserve the patient's energy. The nurse must be attentive to the patient's needs but should not constantly enter the patient's room because it would be exhausting for the patient.

22. **(A)**; The patient with leucopenia may be at risk for infection. Therefore, it is critically important for nurses to wash their hands before and after each patient contact.

23. **(D)**; Bone marrow harvesting occurs in the operating room under general anesthesia. It generally involves multiple punctures into the anterior or posterior iliac crest to obtain 500 to 700 mL of marrow.

24. **(A)**; If a patient suffers graft rejection following bone marrow transplant, another transplant must be done or the patient will die.

25. **(C)**; As a patient advocate, the nurse's most important job in caring for one who is near end of life is to ascertain the patient's goals for end-of-life care. This is important because the patient may or may not wish to have artificial nutrition or hydration. It is the patient's right to choose.

26. **(A)**; Early signs of leukemia include pallor, joint pain, fever, and anorexia.

27. **(D)**; Bleeding tendency occurs as a result of thrombocytopenia ($\downarrow$ platelets).

Physical Assessment

1. **(C)**; It is critically important for the nurse to consistently assess the patient's skin for signs of reaction to the radiotherapy. These might include redness, erythema, and desquamation. The nurse should pay particular attention to areas with skin folds (axilla and groin) and should notify the physician of any signs of skin breakdown as early as possible. Prompt recognition and treatment will help to decrease patient suffering.

2. **(A)**; The nurse who is caring for a patient undergoing chemotherapy must monitor the patient for signs and symptoms of heart failure and signs of decreased cardiac output. These might include *crackles* in the lungs, cough, decreased urine output, restlessness, delayed capillary refill, etc. Patients who have undergone long-term chemotherapy experience decreased pulmonary function as a lifelong effect associated with treatment.

3. **(B)**; Following a bone marrow transplant, the nurse must be especially vigilant about monitoring for signs and symptoms of infection and bleeding.

4. **(B)**; The patient who has developed stomatitis is likely to have burning in the mouth, pain with swallowing, and open lesions on the lips.

Interpretation of Lab Values

1. **(B)**; The WBC is normal if it is 4000 to 9000 mm^3.

2. **(D)**; Serum electrophoresis reveals excessive Bence Jones proteins.

3. **(C)**; For the patient undergoing chemotherapy, the nurse must assess the risk of infection in relation to the ANC (absolute neutrophil count). An ANC of less than 500 is considered an indicator of serious risk for infection. The ANC is calculated by multiplying the WBC by the total percentage of neutrophils (polys and bands).

Drugs and Treatments

1. **(A)**; Ondansetron (Zofran) is an antiemetic medication used in conjunction with chemotherapy to prevent nausea and vomiting.

2. **(C)**; The nurse understands that external radiation provides targeted treatment to the area of the body affected by cancer. Exact markings are critical to limit damage to healthy tissues during treatment.

3. **(A)**; The nurse must monitor the patient for capillary leak syndrome related to interleukin therapy for cancer. Capillary leak syndrome is manifested by generalized edema, decreased urine output, and hypotension.

4. **(C)**; Patients will experience skeletal pain as the drug works to stimulate the bone marrow to produce white blood cells.

5. **(A)**; Interferon may cause fatal or life-threatening neuropsychiatric disorders. The patient must be closely monitored for depression. If depression occurs, the drug should be stopped. Usually depression resolves when the drug is discontinued.

6. **(C)**; It is very likely that males will experience either temporary or permanent sterility following chemotherapy. These patients should be aware of that prior to treatment and should be offered the opportunity to bank sperm for future use.

7. **(B)**; Administration of erythropoietin (Procrit) helps to reduce anemia-associated symptoms of chemotherapy by stimulating red blood cell production. Filgrastim (Neupogen) stimulates white blood cell production to decrease risk of infection. Interleukins stimulate the production of T lymphocytes as part of cancer treatment. Cetuximab (Erbitux) is a monoclonal antibody that can be useful in treatment of non-Hodgkin's lymphoma, metastatic breast cancer, leukemia, and metastatic colorectal cancer.

Keep Track

- Percent correct. (Divide the number of questions you answered correctly by the total number of questions you answered.) _____

- Number of questions you missed due to a reading error: _____

- Number of questions you missed due to errors in analysis: _____

- Number of assessment questions you missed: _____

- Number of lab value questions you missed: _____

- Number of drug/treatment questions you missed: _____

Nugget List

Chapter number _____ Topic _____

Chapter 23

Practice Test: Leadership

Marian C. Condon

PRACTICE TEST

General

1. Two newly-licensed nurses have been hired for staff positions on a medical–surgical unit. In reviewing the competencies they will need, the nurses properly assume that:
   A. there will be no managerial responsibilities.
   B. managerial responsibilities will be handled by the nurse manager.
   C. all nurses have some degree of managerial responsibility.
   D. there will be additional reimbursement for managerial tasks.

2. When formulating healthcare policy recommendations, nurse leaders in organizations such as the American Nurses Association (ANA) and National League for Nursing (NLN) consider the fact that the United States:
   A. spends less money on health care than other developed nations.
   B. has a record of better national healthcare outcomes than other developed nations.
   C. spends more money on health care than other developed nations.
   D. provides quality health care to all its citizens.

3. In planning to provide for patient safety on their units, nurse managers consider the fact that incidents that fall into the category of *preventable medical errors* are:
   A. relatively rare.
   B. mostly the fault of individuals.
   C. made by physicians.
   D. a significant cause of patient morbidity and mortality.

ALTERNATE FORMAT

4. Which of the following behaviors or physical symptoms justify the nurse's concern that a colleague may be dependent on alcohol or drugs? SELECT ALL THAT APPLY.
   A. decreased attention to personal appearance
   B. drinking alcohol at staff social events
   C. frequent absences from work without adequate explanation
   D. a persistent runny nose

ALTERNATE FORMAT

5. The nurse has been confronted by management concerning elements of dress and personal adornment seen as inconsistent with agency guidelines. Based on a federal court ruling, management may legally require the nurse to remove or cover which of the following? SELECT ALL THAT APPLY.
   A. a religious head covering
   B. body piercings
   C. tattoos
   D. artificial hair coloring

6. A new nurse manager is being oriented to the managerial role by a nurse educator. The nurse educator knows that orientation is going well when the new nurse manager states that which of the following actions is not permissible?
   A. reminding an individual staff member, but not all staff members, of a selected agency policy
   B. applying agency policies to some, but not all, staff members
   C. reporting a staff member's behavior without the staff member's permission
   D. documenting a staff member's behavior without the staff member's permission

7. Proper initial actions on the part of a nurse manager who believes that a staff nurse may have a substance abuse problem include all *except*:
   A. becoming familiar with the organizational policies concerning substance abuse.
   B. becoming familiar with the requirements of the State Board of Nursing.
   C. beginning the process of terminating the employee.
   D. collecting and recording all evidence that points to the existence of an abuse problem.

ALTERNATE FORMAT

8. A nurse wishes to act as a change agent. Nurses are more likely to promote change effectively if they act on which of the following assumptions about change? SELECT ALL THAT APPLY.
   A. Change needs to be dealt with only occasionally.
   B. Change can evoke feelings of fear, grief, and loss.
   C. Change is necessary for growth.
   D. Change is a process rather than an event.

9. Nurses who wish to be successful change agents on their units follow the steps of the change process, which are:
   A. unfreezing, moving, and refreezing.
   B. building teams, diagnosing the problem, acquiring resources, and gaining acceptance.
   C. knowing, persuading, deciding, implementing, and confirming.
   D. assessing, planning, implementing, and evaluating.

ALTERNATE FORMAT

10. **A nurse who wishes to act as a change agent knows that all of the following steps are essential if change is to be implemented successfully. Indicate the order in which the steps should be carried out:**
    1. Prepare to handle resistance.
    2. Build a coalition of supporters.
    3. Collect necessary data and information.
    4. Help the staff prepare for change.
        A. 4, 2, 3, 1
        B. 3, 4, 2, 1
        C. 4, 3, 1, 2
        D. 3, 2, 4, 1

11. **A nurse who is considering several offers of employment understands that working on a unit that utilizes the primary care system of care delivery will involve:**
    A. starting IVs as needed throughout the unit.
    B. working with other RNs to provide total care to assigned patients.
    C. delegating various responsibilities to unlicensed assistive personnel (UAP).
    D. working on a team that will likely include LPNs and UAP.

12. **A staff nurse is somewhat anxious about delegating appropriately to UAP. The charge nurse properly assures the staff nurse that delegation is safe if all but which of the following criteria are met?**
    A. The task is within the scope of practice of the delegating nurse.
    B. The delegatee possesses the knowledge, skills, and abilities necessary for the task.
    C. The delegating nurse does not have enough time to complete the task personally.
    D. The delegatee will be appropriately supervised.

13. **Which of the following tasks would the nurse delegate appropriately to an unlicensed staff member?**
    A. teaching a cardiac patient about MI risk factors
    B. assessing distal circulation in an orthopedic patient's casted extremity
    C. measuring and recording hourly urinary output in a surgical patient
    D. discussing end-of-life comfort measures with a dying patient's family

14. **The nurse would properly assign which of the following clients to an unlicensed staff member?**
    A. a surgical patient who has just returned from the postanesthesia unit
    B. a thoracotomy patient whose chest tube was removed an hour ago
    C. a lung cancer patient receiving the first of 4 rounds of chemotherapy
    D. a patient 3 days post-CVA who needs assistance with activity

ALTERNATE FORMAT

15. **A newly-hired nurse is unsure about from whom verbal orders may be accepted. A more experienced nurse properly states that nurses may accept verbal orders conveyed via telephone by which of the following providers? SELECT ALL THAT APPLY.**
    A. nurses who work in a physician's office
    B. licensed physicians
    C. certified registered nurse practitioners
    D. physician assistants

16. The nurse knows that certain records will be needed for the agency's next accreditation visit. Guidelines published by which of the following organizations should be utilized in deciding which records to retain?
    A. AMA
    B. The Joint Commission
    C. ANA
    D. CCNE

17. When considering the need for life-long learning in light of increasing globalization, the nurse decides to become more knowledgeable about which of the following?
    A. changes to which U.S. nurses who emigrate to other countries will have to adjust
    B. the French language
    C. unfamiliar diseases
    D. the effects of shift work on health

18. A nurse is considering whether a specific nursing intervention would be appropriate for a patient in renal failure. The best source of guidance would be which of the following?
    A. the advice of a more experienced nurse
    B. the advice of a urologist
    C. a relevant research article in a recent peer-reviewed nursing journal
    D. information found in the renal section of a nursing textbook

19. The nurse knows that which of the following factors is not a component of evidence-based care?
    A. patient preference
    B. source of cost reimbursement
    C. research evidence
    D. clinical expertise

ALTERNATIVE FORMAT

20. A group of staff nurses is preparing a report on what they learned at a conference about evidence-based practice (EBP). They will state that which of the following resources or organizations are related to EBP? SELECT ALL THAT APPLY.
    A. research studies
    B. The Cochrane Collaboration
    C. clinical practice guidelines
    D. The American Association of Colleges of Nursing

21. The nurse is preparing to teach a surgical patient how to care for the dressing at home. The nurse will base decisions about what information to present and how best to present the information on all but which of the following?
    A. the patient's age
    B. the patient's learning style
    C. the patient's developmental stage
    D. the patient's existing knowledge

22. The nurse is about to provide dietary teaching for a patient recovering from surgery for diverticulitis. Which of the following patient statements would cause the nurse to postpone the teaching session?
    A. "I know I should not eat foods that contain small seeds."
    B. "My discomfort has returned."
    C. "I want to know how to take care of my dressing when I get home."
    D. "I've had attacks before; I know how to prevent them."

23. The nurse is preparing to provide educational materials about Type I diabetes to an 18-year-old patient. In choosing materials, the nurse will take into consideration all but which of the following factors?
    A. grade level in school
    B. developmental level
    C. patient preference
    D. reading level

24. The nurse is preparing to delegate tasks to an LPN and an unlicensed staff member on a surgical floor. Which of the following tasks should be delegated to the LPN?
    A. administering an IV antibiotic to a 1-day postop bowel resection patient
    B. calculating and recording oral intake and output in a renal surgery patient
    C. counseling the family of an elderly hip replacement patient who is disoriented
    D. administering a unit of blood to a postsplenectomy patient

25. The nurse enters the room of a post-knee-replacement patient for the purpose of providing discharge teaching. Which of the following patient statements would cause the nurse to postpone the session?
    A. "I hope I'll be able to ride my bike again."
    B. "The physical therapist is coming soon, and I know she's going to hurt me again."
    C. "I don't know how I'll manage when I go home."
    D. "My surgeon will be in later to see me."

ALTERNATE FORMAT

26. The nurse is about to provide dietary education to a diabetic patient who does not hear well. Which of the following behaviors on the part of the nurse are appropriate? SELECT ALL THAT APPLY.
    A. asking the patient for permission to turn the television off
    B. speaking very loudly
    C. facing the patient directly
    D. speaking very slowly

27. The nurse has just taught a patient how to change his colostomy bag. Which of the following is the best indication that the teaching has been successful?
    A. The patient states that he understands how to change the bag.
    B. The patient correctly identifies the steps in the procedure.
    C. The patient demonstrates how to apply a new bag.
    D. The nurse knows the patient to be highly intelligent and cooperative.

ALTERNATE FORMAT

28. **The nurse wishes to carry out an admission assessment on a patient whose language the nurse does not speak. Which of the following behaviors on the part of the nurse is appropriate in this situation? SELECT ALL THAT APPLY.**
    A. asking the patient's son to translate the nurse's questions and the patient's answers
    B. obtaining the services of a qualified interpreter and addressing questions to her
    C. arranging for use of an electronic interpreter service
    D. interpreting the patient's smile as a sign of agreement and consent

ALTERNATE FORMAT

29. **In planning health education for patients from ethnically diverse backgrounds, the nurse keeps which of the following in mind? SELECT ALL THAT APPLY.**
    A. Cancer incidence is higher for African Americans than any other group.
    B. Among ethnic groups, Asian American women have the lowest cervical cancer rate.
    C. Alcoholism is a major problem in many Native American groups.
    D. Stomach cancer rates are comparatively higher in Asian and Pacific Islander groups.

30. **A Muslim patient's husband has requested that his wife be cared for by a female nursing technician. The nurse's best response to this request is:**
    A. to ascertain the wishes of the patient.
    B. to assign a female nursing technician to care for the patient.
    C. to assure both spouses that male technicians are fully qualified to provide care.
    D. to consult the patient's physician.

31. **The nurse wishes to provide culturally sensitive and competent care to patients. The nurse knows that acceptance:**
    A. means that the nurse agrees with the patient's viewpoint.
    B. is nonjudgmental.
    C. is conveyed mostly through words.
    D. means that the nurse understands the patient's viewpoint.

32. **To provide culturally competent care to patients, the nurse must know which of the following about eye contact?**
    A. Maintaining eye contact is a sign of respect.
    B. Patients who do not maintain eye contact are not comfortable with the provider.
    C. Gender may influence a patient's behavior in terms of eye contact.
    D. It may be necessary for the nurse to invite the patient to make eye contact.

33. **A nurse working on a medical–surgical unit is attempting to encourage a quiet patient to verbalize. Which of the following statements is likely to be most effective?**
    A. "It's hard to get to know you because you're so quiet."
    B. "You don't have to be afraid. It's okay to talk to me."
    C. "I have some time to spend with you. I'm interested in how you are doing."
    D. "Do you have any questions you'd like to ask?"

34. A nurse employed in an outpatient clinic knows that which of the following actions would constitute a violation of the Health Insurance Portability and Accountability Act (HIPAA)?
    A. reading a note made by another healthcare provider in a patient's chart
    B. telling a patient that a biopsy came back positive for cancer
    C. leaving test results on a patient's home answering machine without written consent
    D. failing to change the paper on an exam room table between patients

35. The nurse becomes aware that a patient has been found to be HIV positive. The patient refuses to convey this information to his wife, who is pregnant. The nurse has a duty to:
    A. tell the patient's wife.
    B. tell the wife's obstetrician.
    C. report the patient to the health department.
    D. keep the information confidential.

36. The nurse has asked the nurse manager to adjust the schedule so that the nurse can have a 3-day vacation over a specific time period. A day later, the nurse manager informs the nurse that it will not be possible to grant this request. The most appropriate statement for the nurse to make is:
    A. "You are treating me unfairly."
    B. "If I were one of your favorites, you'd give me the time off."
    C. "I don't understand why my request can't be granted."
    D. "You gave Mary (another nurse) time off just last month."

37. When interacting with physicians, the nurse keeps which of the following statements in mind?
    A. Nurse–physician conflict is unavoidable.
    B. Nurse–physician conflict has been shown to adversely affect patient care.
    C. Nurse–physician conflict has not been shown to affect patient care.
    D. Nurse–physician conflict is mainly the fault of physicians.

ALTERNATE FORMAT

38. A patient's family member approaches the nurse in the corridor and states loudly that the patient is "a mess" and receiving "horrible care" from the nursing staff. Which of the following behaviors on the part of the nurse is appropriate? SELECT ALL THAT APPLY.
    A. accompanying the family member to a conference room or other private area
    B. assuring the family member that the patient is receiving excellent care
    C. acknowledging that the family member is angry and upset
    D. asking the family member for more details about the situation

39. A patient in the preoperative area who has breast cancer and is about to undergo a mastectomy states, "I can't believe this horrible thing is happening to me." The nurse's best response is:
    A. "I know it seems awful now, but you're going to be fine."
    B. "Breast reconstruction is very successful nowadays."
    C. "Tell me more about how you are feeling."
    D. "Tell me about your family."

40. The nurse has just returned from a seminar on the importance of self-care. An important principle for the nurse to remember is that a warning sign of job-related stress is:

    A. smiling and laughing a lot.
    B. being absent from work more frequently.
    C. managing time more effectively.
    D. being tardy less often.

41. A principle that the nurse manager will keep in mind is that objectives used in staff performance appraisals should be:

    A. written in measurable terms.
    B. applicable to staff at all levels.
    C. based on the manager's personal preferences.
    D. approved by physicians.

42. The nurse manager must make a decision and has chosen to involve the nursing staff in the process. The staff nurse recognizes that in this instance, the manager is demonstrating the leadership style known as:

    A. authoritarian.
    B. laissez-faire.
    C. democratic.
    D. directive.

43. The nurse has been asked to participate in a hiring decision. A principle that must be kept in mind is that equal opportunity laws prohibit:

    A. checking applicants' references.
    B. rejecting an otherwise qualified older applicant.
    C. hiring an applicant who will require accommodation for a disability.
    D. advising an applicant that removal of a nose ring is a condition of employment.

44. The nurse has been floated to the oncology unit and asked to administer chemotherapeutic drugs. The nurse bases his or her refusal on the principle of:

    A. justice.
    B. beneficence.
    C. autonomy.
    D. nonmalfeasance.

45. In considering whether to pursue professional growth in leadership or management, the staff nurse takes into consideration the fact that leadership skills include:

    A. the ability to utilize resources effectively.
    B. the ability to utilize staff effectively.
    C. the ability to influence the views and actions of others.
    D. the ability to function as a contributing team member.

46. The nurse manager wishes to help a staff nurse who has been employed on the unit for 1 year to improve the staff nurse's performance in certain areas. The manager's best strategy is to:

    A. review the nurse's orientation materials and identify anything that was left out.
    B. review the staff nurse's job description and point out areas of weakness.
    C. notify the nurse via e-mail of areas in which improvement is expected.
    D. collaboratively agree upon target behaviors and dates for reevaluation.

47. The nurse manager is preparing for a performance appraisal conference with a staff member. Which of the following actions are appropriate?
    A. Interview other staff members about the employee's performance.
    B. Begin the conference with an open-ended question.
    C. Include personal feelings in the comments section of the evaluation form.
    D. Interview physicians about the employee's performance.

48. The nurse leader wishes to apply principles of Total Quality Management (TQM). Which of the following terms is relevant?
    A. unitwide
    B. reactive
    C. participative
    D. coercive

49. The nurse manager is aware that a conflict has developed between administration and the staff. The most appropriate view of conflict is that it is:
    A. divisive and harmful.
    B. likely detrimental.
    C. potentially useful.
    D. to be avoided.

50. The nurse manager is determining staffing needs and will take into consideration all the following factors *except*:
    A. patient census.
    B. area population data.
    C. patient acuity.
    D. staff skill level.

ANSWERS

General

1. **(C)**; In the modern healthcare environment, all professional nurses have some degree of managerial responsibility. Nurse managers handle managerial responsibilities on the unit level; staff nurses must employ managerial skills in supervising LPNs and UAP. There is no additional reimbursement for the managerial tasks carried out by staff nurses.

2. **(C)**; The United States spends more on health care than other developed countries. U.S. national healthcare outcomes lag behind those of most other developed countries. The United States has poorer overall outcomes than other developed countries. In the United States, underserved populations have poorer health than populations that are better served.

3. **(D)**; Preventable medical errors are a significant cause of patient mortality and morbidity. Errors involve healthcare providers in all categories. Errors have been found to be related to flaws in agency procedures and protocols as well as individual error.

4. **(A, C, D)**; A noticeably decreased attention to personal appearance can signal increasing disorganization and poor self-care related to substance abuse. Frequent absences

from work may be related to a hung-over state. Cocaine abuse can cause a runny nose unrelated to allergy or viral infection. Drinking alcohol in moderation at social events is a normal behavior for many people.

5. **(B, C, D)**; Body piercings, tattoos, and artificial hair colors are not protected under the right to freedom of expression. Religious head coverings are protected.

6. **(B)**; Agency policies must be applied consistently to all employees. Managers may remind employees who are violating policy about the nature of the policy. Managers may report behaviors without employees' permission. Managers may document behavior without employees' permission.

7. **(C)**; Termination is a last resort in most agencies. Because substance abuse is properly seen as an illness, the initial goal is usually to obtain treatment for the employee. The manager must become familiar with organizational policies. The manager must be familiar with state board policies.

8. **(B, C, D)**; Change often evokes feelings of fear, grief, and loss; change is necessary for growth and is a process rather than an event. The need to deal with change, on some level, is a frequent rather than an occasional phenomenon.

9. **(D)**; Assessment, planning, implementation, and evaluation are steps in the change process as in the nursing process. Unfreezing, moving, and refreezing comprise steps in Lewin's model of change. Building teams, diagnosing the problem, acquiring resources, and gaining acceptance are steps in Havelock's model. Knowing, persuading, deciding, implementing, and confirming are steps in Rogers's model.

10. **(D)**; Necessary data or information is collected first (assessment and planning) to determine what sort of change is needed. The implementation steps include building a coalition that will support the proposed change. The next step is helping the staff prepare for change. Developing strategies for handling resistance is the last step in the change process.

11. **(B)**; Primary care involves all-RN staffing. Having one RN start all the IVs on the unit is consistent with the functional model of care delivery. Delegating responsibilities to UAP is consistent with team nursing. Organizing RNs, LPNs, and UAP into teams is consistent with team nursing.

12. **(C)**; RNs delegate tasks to LPNs and UAP for a variety of reasons, such as increased efficiency as well as reasons having to do with time. Delegated tasks must be within the scope of practice of the delegating nurse. The delegatee must possess the knowledge, skills, and abilities necessary for the task. The delegatee must be appropriately supervised.

13. **(C)**; Measuring and recording urinary output is an appropriate task for UAP. Assessment and patient and family teaching are RN responsibilities that cannot be delegated.

14. **(D)**; The care of stable patients may be delegated to UAP. Patients who have just returned from the postanesthesia unit, patients who have recently had a chest tube removed (and are at risk for pneumothorax), and patients whose response to chemotherapy is unknown all require careful assessment and should be cared for by a nurse.

15. **(B, C, D)**; Licensed physicians, nurse practitioners, and physician assistants all have prescriptive authority and may convey verbal orders in person and over the phone.

RNs, LPNs, and UAP who work in physicians' offices may not convey verbal orders on behalf of providers who have prescriptive authority.

16. **(B)**; The Joint Commission is the accrediting agency for hospitals and other types of healthcare agencies. The American Medical Association (AMA) is a professional organization that advocates for physicians. The American Nurses Association (ANA) is a professional organization that advocates for the nursing profession. The Commission on Collegiate Nursing Education (CCNE) accredits baccalaureate and graduate degree nursing education programs.

17. **(C)**; As U.S. culture becomes more diverse, immigrants from different countries will present with diseases common in their homeland. Relatively few U.S. nurses choose to seek employment in foreign countries. French is spoken by relatively few immigrants. Globalization is unrelated to shift work.

18. **(C)**; Current research articles in peer-reviewed journals constitute the evidence upon which clinical practice guidelines and, ultimately, decisions about nursing practice should be based. The advice of a more experienced nurse may or may not be based on evidence. Physicians may be considered experts on medical practice but not nursing practice. Although the information found in nursing texts is increasingly based on evidence, texts may contain some information based on convention rather than evidence.

19. **(B)**; The source of cost reimbursement is not one of the three components of evidence-based practice. Patient preference, research evidence, and clinical expertise are components.

20. **(A, B, C)**; Research studies are the building blocks of EBP. The Cochrane Collaboration is a global collective that conducts systematic reviews of research studies and generates evidence summaries from which the clinical practice guidelines used by healthcare professionals are derived. The American Association of Colleges of Nursing (AACN) is a consortium of baccalaureate nursing programs and is not related to EBP.

21. **(A)**; A patient's actual age does not necessarily correlate with her or his developmental age. Information presented in a manner congruent with a patient's learning style will be better understood. The information and method of presentation should be tailored to the patient's developmental age.

22. **(B)**; The patient's discomfort should be treated. Discomfort interferes with learning. That a patient has some knowledge does not imply sufficient knowledge. The nurse should alter the teaching plan and address the learning need the patient is currently expressing. Patients may overestimate their knowledge.

23. **(A)**; Grade level does not accurately predict reading level. Many students read at a level below their grade level. Teaching materials must be appropriate for the patient's developmental level. Patient preference should be taken into consideration. The patient's actual reading level should be determined before educational materials are chosen.

24. **(A)**; Administering IV antibiotics is within the LPN, but not the UAP, scope of practice. Calculating and recording oral intake is a task suitable for an unlicensed staff member. Counseling and teaching are RN responsibilities. Blood administration is within only the RN's scope of practice.

25. **(B)**; Patients who are experiencing fear or anxiety that will not be assuaged by information included in the teaching session are unable to focus on instruction. The other comments are irrelevant.

26. **(A, C)**; Competing background noise should be eliminated, with the patient's permission. Facing the patient directly facilitates lip-reading. Speaking in a very loud voice can be perceived as aggressive and does not improve hearing. Speaking slowly is not helpful, but using short sentences and easily understood words is helpful.

27. **(C)**; A return demonstration done correctly is the best indicator of patient learning. Patients can believe incorrectly that they have mastered a procedure. Knowing the steps in a procedure (declarative learning) does not guarantee that the patient can carry the steps out (procedural learning). Procedures can be difficult for anyone to master.

28. **(C)**; Electronic interpreter services can be very effective and preserve patient confidentiality. Asking relatives to translate violates confidentiality and may result in withholding of information. Addressing questions to the interpreter instead of the patient is insulting and inappropriate. In some cultures, smiling indicates a desire to be polite rather than approval, agreement, or consent.

29. **(A, C, D)**; Among ethnic groups, Asian American women have a relatively *high* rate of cervical cancer because modesty may prevent them from having regular GYN exams.

30. **(B)**; Modesty is extremely important to Muslim women. In Muslim culture, men often speak for their wives. Competence is not the issue; Muslim patients prefer that personal care be provided by same-sex staff members. Nursing problems are solved by nurses.

31. **(B)**; To accept a patient's views and beliefs, the nurse must suspend judgment. The nurse can accept the patient's viewpoint without agreeing with it. Acceptance must be conveyed both verbally and nonverbally; body language that conveys disapproval, shock, dislike, or anger will be perceived by the patient. It is not necessary for the nurse to understand the patient's viewpoint to accept it.

32. **(C)**; In some cultures, it is considered inappropriate for a man or woman to make eye contact with a person of the opposite sex who is unrelated by blood or marriage. Maintaining eye contact is a sign of respect in *some* cultures and subcultures but by no means in all. Failure to maintain eye contact may have to do with gender or constitute a sign of respect for a person perceived to be of higher status. The nurse must accept the patient's behavior; an invitation to alter it would likely be interpreted by the patient as nonacceptance and criticism.

33. **(C)**; The nurse conveys a desire to spend time with the patient, an interest in the patient's experience, and willingness to let the patient guide the conversation. The nurse is expressing dissatisfaction and judgment. The nurse is assuming the patient is being quiet due to fear. The nurse is placing a limit on what the patient can say by inviting questions specifically.

34. **(C)**; Leaving a message containing sensitive medical information where others might hear it constitutes a violation of the part of HIPAA that concerns patient confidentiality. It is often necessary for staff members to read notes written by others. Conveying diagnoses to patients is a medical responsibility unless the nurse is a CRNP. HIPAA does not address patient safety.

35. **(D)**; The nurse's obligation is to respect the patient's privacy and keep the information confidential. HIV is not a reportable communicable disease.

36. **(C)**; Making an I statement that expresses the nurse's lack of understanding is both respectful and productive because the manager will likely provide an explanation. Accusations do not contribute to successful conflict resolution because they generally cause managers to become defensive.

37. **(B)**; Nurse–physician conflict does affect patient care negatively. Nurse–physician conflict can be avoided if nurses and physicians respect each other and adhere to principles of good communication. Both nurses and physicians sometimes behave disrespectfully, communicate poorly, and lack conflict resolution skills.

38. **(A, C, D)**; Walking to a different area gives the angry person time to calm down. Conflicts should not be witnessed by patients, visitors, etc. Acknowledging expressed emotions is an important step in conflict resolution. The nurse must obtain information about the situation before a judgment about the provided care can be made. The nurse should not react in a defensive manner.

39. **(C)**; It is not clear whether the horrible thing to which the patient is referring is the cancer, the surgery, or both. The nurse should invite the patient to provide more information. The nurse cannot be certain about what the outcome for the patient will be. The nurse should not assume that the patient is upset about issues related to breast reconstruction. The nurse must not ignore the patient's concerns and switch to a more comfortable topic.

40. **(B)**; Missing work more often is a classic sign of stress. The other choices reflect the presence of little stress or very manageable levels of stress.

41. **(A)**; Performance objectives must be measurable. Objectives must be specific to the level (RN, LPN, UAP) of the staff member being evaluated. Performance objectives must be based on recognized, broadly accepted standards. Nurses, not physicians, set the performance standards for their profession.

42. **(C)**; In terms of decision making, the democratic style involves shared decision making. The authoritarian style involves unilateral decision making on the part of the manager. The term "laissez-faire" is applied to leaders who provide little structure or direction. The term "directive" is sometimes used in place of the term "authoritarian." It describes leaders who provide high structure and expect obedience from subordinates.

43. **(B)**; Age discrimination is not permissible. Checking applicants' references is permissible and important. The need to accommodate a disability is not an acceptable reason for rejecting a qualified applicant. Employers have the right to insist that employees adhere to institutional guidelines regarding dress and personal adornment.

44. **(D)**; Only qualified oncology nurses can safely administer chemotherapy. Nonmalfeasance refers to the nurse's ethical duty to do no harm. Justice refers to the nurse's duty to act in a manner that is fair to all involved. Beneficence refers to the nurse's duty to do good. Autonomy refers to the nurse's duty to refrain from interfering with the rights of others.

45. **(C)**; Influence is a component of leadership. Effective resource utilization is a management skill. Effective staff utilization is a management skill. The ability to function as a contributing team member is not related to leadership or management.

46. **(D)**; Staff members who are allowed to participate in the goal-setting process and who are provided with a time frame are more likely to be successful in reaching goals. Solutions to performance problems should focus on improving performance in areas of deficiency. Performance counseling must be done in person.

47. **(B)**; Open-ended questions (How would you evaluate your performance over the past year?) yield more information than closed-ended questions (Do you think you've done a good job over the past year?), which can be answered yes or no. Interviewing other staff members about the employee's performance is inappropriate; the nurse manager is responsible for monitoring and evaluating employees' performance. Evaluations must be based on objective data regarding performance, not on personal feelings. Nurses evaluate nurses.

48. **(C)**; TQM involves a participative rather than an autocratic process. TQM is organization-wide. TQM is proactive (acting in a way designed to head off problems), not reactive (waiting for problems to develop and then attempting to deal with them). In TQM, employees are motivated, not coerced, into good performance.

49. **(C)**; Conflict is potentially useful because it can reveal areas of dysfunction, miscommunication, or unfairness that may damage the organization unless it is remedied.

50. **(B)**; Area population data do not predict patient care needs on a given unit. The patient census, patient acuity, and skill level of current staff members are all relevant.

Keep Track

- Percent correct. (Divide the number of questions you answered correctly by the total number of questions you answered.) _____

- Number of questions you missed due to a reading error: _____

- Number of questions you missed due to errors in analysis: _____

- Number of assessment questions you missed: _____

- Number of lab value questions you missed: _____

- Number of drug/treatment questions you missed: _____

Nugget List

Chapter number _____ Topic _____

Chapter 24

Comprehensive Practice Exam 2

Karen S. March

COMPREHENSIVE PRACTICE EXAM

1. The patient is prescribed digoxin (Lanoxin) 125 micrograms PO every day. The nurse finds digoxin (Lanoxin) 0.250 milligram tablets in the Pyxis. Which of the following is the appropriate action for the nurse?
   A. Call the pharmacy to request delivery of the correct dose.
   B. Administer 4 tablets from the Pyxis to deliver the full dose.
   C. Administer ½ tablet for the dose and waste the remainder.
   D. Notify the physician for a clarification of the order.

2. The nurse is caring for a patient admitted with digoxin toxicity. During a review of the patient's medical record, the nurse realizes that which of the following findings provides some explanation for the patient's condition?
   A. Mg^{++} 2.2 mEq/dL
   B. K^+ 2.8 mEq/dL
   C. Ca^{++} 8.8 mg/dL
   D. Na^+ 138 mEq/L

ALTERNATE FORMAT

3. The nurse is preparing to administer Lanoxin 0.125 mg IV to the patient as ordered. The drug is available in ampules labeled "digoxin 500 mcg/2 mL." Which of the following actions will be performed by the nurse prior to and during administration of this drug? SELECT ALL THAT APPLY.
   A. Take an apical heart rate for a full minute prior to administration.
   B. Draw up 1 mL of drug from the ampule with a filter needle.
   C. Dilute the drug in 4 mL D_5W and administer over 5 minutes.
   D. Review the patient's lab work for serum sodium levels.

4. The nurse is caring for a patient who is receiving thrombolytic therapy. Which of the following actions by the nurse should be questioned?
   A. injecting an intravenous heparin bolus into an existing line
   B. performing a femoral artery stick for arterial blood gas
   C. shaving the patient with an electric razor
   D. performing mouth care with swabs and mouthwash

5. The nurse is caring for a patient who will undergo synchronized cardioversion for treatment of a dysrhythmia. Which of the following equipment items must be at the bedside prior to delivering the cardioversion?
   A. an IV infusion pump
   B. a mechanical ventilator
   C. an intubation box
   D. a bag–valve–mask device

ALTERNATE FORMAT

6. A patient collapses in a department store and is pulseless. An automatic external defibrillator (AED) is immediately available. Prioritize the steps that the nurse should take to ensure safe use of the equipment.
   A. Attach the AED pads to the victim's chest.
   B. Turn the power on.
   C. Announce, "Stand clear."
   D. Wait for the shock to be delivered.
   E. Push the "Analyze" button.
   F. Deliver up to three shocks if indicated.

7. The nurse is assisting with insertion of a pulmonary artery catheter. When attempting to place the catheter on the sterile field, the tip of the catheter touches the nurse's arm. The best response by the nurse is to:
   A. obtain another sterile pulmonary artery catheter.
   B. soak the tip of the catheter in povidone iodine for 5 minutes.
   C. wipe the full length of the catheter in an alcohol-soaked 4 × 4.
   D. wipe the tip of the catheter with alcohol and flush with iodine.

8. The nurse would expect that a patient who is admitted with known atrial fibrillation would be taking which of the following medications?
   A. furosemide (Lasix)
   B. metformin (Glucophage)
   C. warfarin (Coumadin)
   D. metoprolol (Lopressor)

9. The patient is ordered dopamine by infusion at 5 μg/kg/min. The IV bag contains 400 mg of dopamine in 250 mL of 0.9% NaCl. The patient weighs 220 lb. Based on this information, the infusion pump must be set at what rate to ensure that the medication is infused correctly?
   A. 1.9 mL/hr
   B. 3.8 mL/hr
   C. 9.4 mL/hr
   D. 18.8 mL/hr

10. The patient is ordered dobutamine by infusion at 5 mcg/kg/min. The IV bag contains 250 mg of dobutamine in 250 mL D_5W. The patient weighs 198 lb. Based on this information, the infusion pump must be set at what rate to infuse the medication correctly?
    A. 24 mL/hr
    B. 27 mL/hr
    C. 30 mL/hr
    D. 40 mL/hr

11. An IV of 1000 mL lactated Ringer's (LR) with 20 grams magnesium sulfate arrives from the pharmacy. The nurse is to deliver a bolus of 3 grams magnesium sulfate over 30 minutes followed by a maintenance infusion of 1.5 grams/hr. The nurse knows that the correct rates for the bolus and the maintenance infusion are:
    A. 30 mL/hr for the bolus, then 15 mL/hr for the maintenance infusion.
    B. 150 mL/hr for the bolus, then 75 mL/hr for the maintenance infusion.
    C. 150 mL/hr for the bolus, then 50 mL/hr for the maintenance infusion.
    D. 300 mL/hr for the bolus, then 75 mL/hr for the maintenance infusion.

12. The nurse is caring for an ICU patient following carotid endarterectomy. The patient's blood pressure is 188/116 mm Hg according to an arterial line. The nurse has the following treatment options available. Which should be employed first?
    A. Level the arterial line transducer to the phlebostatic axis.
    B. Obtain a cuff BP for correlation with the arterial line.
    C. Initiate and titrate IV nitroprusside (Nipride) to maintain BP <150/85.
    D. Initiate and titrate IV nitroprusside (Nipride) to maintain BP <130/80.

13. Sequential compression devices are used as prophylaxis against which of the following postoperative complications?
    A. pneumonia
    B. atelectasis
    C. infection
    D. venous thrombosis

14. The nurse is teaching a patient about warfarin (Coumadin) therapy in preparation for discharge. As part of the instruction, the nurse informs the patient that it will be necessary to have which of the following lab tests monitored on a weekly basis?
    A. aPTT
    B. serum warfarin level
    C. INR
    D. clotting studies

15. The COPD patient is ordered ipratropium bromide and albuterol sulfate (Combivent) one puff and fluticasone propionate (Flovent) two puffs at 6 p.m. Place in order the sequence that should be used for proper administration of these drugs.
    A. Administer two puffs of Flovent.
    B. Identify the patient by two identifiers.
    C. Administer one puff of Combivent.
    D. Verify that both drugs are correct as ordered.
    E. Encourage the patient to gargle.

ALTERNATE FORMAT

16. The patient is prescribed hydrocortisone sodium succinate (Solu-Cortef) 60 mg IV now. The drug is available in vials of "Solu-Cortef 100 mg/2mL." What volume of drug will the nurse withdraw from the vial to administer the correct dose?

_____

17. The nurse is providing care for a ventilated patient on a telemetry floor. When the patient begins to cough forcefully, the ventilator alarms. The nurse expects to find which of the following alarms active on the ventilator?
    A. minute volume
    B. high pressure
    C. low pressure
    D. tidal volume

ALTERNATE FORMAT

18. The nurse is providing care for a mechanically ventilated patient on a telemetry unit. During report, the nurse is informed that the patient is being ventilated on the assist control (AC) mode. Based on this information, the nurse understands which of the following implications? SELECT ALL THAT APPLY.
    A. The patient can initiate a breath any time.
    B. Ventilator-initiated breaths will be full tidal volume.
    C. Patient-initiated breaths may or may not be full tidal volume.
    D. Metabolic acidosis is not an uncommon outcome.
    E. Respiratory alkalosis is not an uncommon outcome.

ALTERNATE FORMAT

19. The nurse is providing care for a mechanically ventilated patient on a telemetry unit. During report, the nurse is informed that the patient is being ventilated on the synchronized intermittent mandatory ventilation (SIMV) mode. Based on this information, the nurse understands which of the following implications? SELECT ALL THAT APPLY.
    A. The patient can initiate a breath any time.
    B. Ventilator-initiated breaths will be full tidal volume.
    C. Patient-initiated breaths are at full tidal volume.
    D. Metabolic acidosis is not an uncommon outcome.
    E. Respiratory alkalosis is not an uncommon outcome.

ALTERNATE FORMAT

20. The nurse is providing care for a mechanically ventilated patient on a telemetry unit. During report, the nurse is informed that the patient is being prepared for weaning and will have a pressure support trial during the shift. Based on this information, the nurse understands which of the following implications? SELECT ALL THAT APPLY.
    A. The patient shows some indication of preparedness to wean.
    B. The ventilator rate will be set low, and the patient will do most of the work.
    C. The tidal volume will be set low, and the patient must breathe deeply.
    D. The nurse must monitor the patient very closely for signs of respiratory compromise.
    E. The ventilator will alarm if the patient experiences difficulty with breathing.

ALTERNATE FORMAT

21. The nurse is providing care for a mechanically ventilated patient on a telemetry unit. During report, the nurse is informed that the patient is being ventilated on the synchronized intermittent mandatory ventilation (SIMV) mode. Because of some changes in respiratory status, positive end expiratory pressure (PEEP) of 10 cm H_2O will be added within the next hour. Based on this information, the nurse understands which of the following implications? SELECT ALL THAT APPLY.
    A. The patient can initiate a breath any time.
    B. Ventilator-initiated breaths will be full tidal volume.
    C. Patient-initiated breaths are at full tidal volume.
    D. Blood pressure should be monitored because hypotension may occur.
    E. Blood pressure should be monitored because hypertension may require treatment.

22. A patient on a telemetry floor is intubated and on a mechanical ventilator. When the ventilator high pressure alarm sounds, the nurse begins to troubleshoot the ventilator. Which of the following is most likely to result in a high pressure alarm?
    A. The patient has become disconnected from the ventilator tubing.
    B. The patient has adventitious breath sounds and requires suctioning.
    C. Water has collected within the tubing between the patient and ventilator.
    D. The tubing on the pressure circuit of the ventilator is disconnected.

23. The gold standard test for diagnosis of pulmonary embolus is which of the following?
    A. arterial blood gas
    B. bronchoscopy
    C. spiral CT
    D. pulmonary angiogram

ALTERNATE FORMAT

24. The nurse receives the following arterial blood gas results from the laboratory:

pH	7.30
pCO_2	48
HCO_3^-	24
pO_2	90

Which of the following terms should the nurse use to properly interpret these results? SELECT ALL THAT APPLY.
    A. partially compensated
    B. uncompensated
    C. compensated
    D. respiratory
    E. metabolic
    F. acidosis
    G. alkalosis
    H. hypoxia
    I. normal ABG

25. When receiving report on a patient, the nurse is informed that the patient has a flaccid right side. The nurse expects to find which of the following upon assessment of the patient?
    A. increased resistance to passive stretch
    B. decreased or absent muscle tone
    C. localized spasms of muscle groups
    D. temporary loss of sensation

26. The nurse is assigned to care for a patient who was admitted with a diagnosis of myasthenia gravis. The nurse understands that common early symptoms of myasthenia gravis include:
    A. weakness, fatigue, and ptosis.
    B. nausea, dizziness, and dysphagia.
    C. numbness, tingling, and burning in the extremities.
    D. significant muscular weakness unilaterally.

27. During report, the nurse is told that a patient has ptosis. The nurse expects to find which of the following upon assessing the patient?
    A. facial droop
    B. drooping of the eyelids
    C. paresthesia of the face
    D. arm weakness

28. The nurse is caring for a patient who sustained a spinal cord injury at the level of C5. The patient has been placed on a mechanical ventilator. When planning care, the nurse should anticipate that the patient:
    A. will remain dependent on mechanical ventilation.
    B. should be taught to use intercostal muscles for breathing.
    C. may breathe on his or her own after spinal cord edema subsides.
    D. is more likely to develop chronic airway limitation.

29. The nurse is providing care for a patient who suffered rupture of a cerebral aneurysm. The nurse understands that bleeding from an aneurysm most often occurs into which space in the brain?
    A. subdural
    B. epidural
    C. subarachnoid
    D. intracerebral

30. The nurse is assessing a patient who is admitted with a cerebral aneurysm. The nurse understands that the leading cause of death in patients with cerebral aneurysms is which of the following?
    A. rebleeding
    B. herniation
    C. vasospasm
    D. dysrhythmia

31. The nurse is caring for a patient with increased intracranial pressure. During physical assessment, the nurse will observe for signs of which of the following critical indicators?
    A. decreased level of consciousness
    B. decreased visual acuity
    C. widened pulse pressure
    D. blurred vision

32. The nurse caring for a patient with increased intracranial pressure understands that the patient will not have a lumbar puncture performed for which of the following reasons?
    A. The patient may not be able to tolerate the test.
    B. Lumbar puncture may cause brain herniation.
    C. The patient cannot lie flat for the test.
    D. Lumbar puncture is not a conclusive test.

33. The nurse is assigned to care for a patient with arteriovenous malformation (AVM) prior to treatment. The patient asks the nurse what the physician will be able to do to fix the problem. The best response by the nurse is:
    A. "You will have to ask the physician about that directly."
    B. "The treatment will depend upon the extent of your AVM."
    C. "The only treatment for an AVM is a frontal craniotomy."
    D. "I don't know. We will have to ask the physician about it."

34. The patient with a history of seizures indicates understanding of discharge instructions by articulating that medication should be stopped when:
    A. side effects occur.
    B. blood levels are therapeutic.
    C. seizure activity ceases.
    D. ordered by the physician.

35. Which of the following patients is at highest risk for suicide?
    A. a 24-year-old female who lives with her parents and recently broke up with a boyfriend
    B. a 66-year-old widower with liver cancer who talks about saving his pain pills
    C. a 45-year-old married female with a stressful job and significant financial stress
    D. a 35-year-old religious, married man with children who has testicular cancer

36. Electroconvulsive therapy (ECT) may be used for treatment of which of the following patient conditions?
    A. severe anorexia
    B. histrionic personality disorder
    C. lithium-resistant mania
    D. antisocial personality disorder

37. The nurse is caring for a young adult patient admitted to the mental health unit with major depression and suicidal ideation. The patient has a history of cutting the wrists intermittently for more than 2 years. Upon admission, the patient stays in the room and eats only about 20% of each meal. On day three of hospitalization, the patient eats about 80% of each meal and is talking with others in group. The nurse realizes that the patient is:
   A. showing improvement.
   B. highly suicidal.
   C. exhibiting mood swings.
   D. in need of electroshock therapy.

38. You are the nurse responsible for assessing a patient who has been on chlorpromazine (Thorazine) for extrapyramidal side effects (EPSEs). The nurse knows that extrapyramidal side effects include which of the following?
   A. acute dystonia
   B. sexual dysfunction
   C. amenorrhea
   D. breast secretion

39. The nurse is caring for a patient who is prescribed lithium carbonate for control of bipolar disorder. The patient has been taking the drug for approximately 18 months. A serum lithium level drawn during this hospitalization is 1.0 mEq/L. The nurse interprets this drug level as which of the following?
   A. within normal limits
   B. borderline subtherapeutic
   C. slightly above normal
   D. within the toxic range

40. Which of the following physical manifestations is related to side effects of anticholinergic medications?
   A. diarrhea
   B. vomiting
   C. blurred vision
   D. polyuria

41. The nurse is assigned to care for a patient with the diagnosis of pyelonephritis. The nurse provides teaching about prevention of future episodes of pyelonephritis based on the knowledge that:
   A. the disorder occurs more normally in men.
   B. it occurs with greater frequency in women.
   C. large amounts of fluid intake can prevent it.
   D. each episode causes prerenal azotemia.

42. The nurse is caring for a patient in renal failure who has developed anasarca. Based on this information, the nurse understands that a priority nursing diagnosis for the patient is which of the following?
   A. risk for infection
   B. risk for impaired skin integrity
   C. altered comfort
   D. pain

43. The nurse is caring for a patient who has just been diagnosed with acute postrenal failure. The nurse understands that which of the following is a likely cause?
    A. hemorrhage
    B. ureteral calculi
    C. sepsis
    D. acute pyelonephritis

44. The nurse understands that which of the following are examples of possible etiologic factors in the development of prerenal azotemia?
    A. heart failure
    B. acute tubular necrosis
    C. glomerulonephritis
    D. occluded Foley

45. The nurse understands that which of the following medications are considered among highly nephrotoxic drugs?
    A. digoxin (Lanoxin)
    B. furosemide (Lasix)
    C. prednisone
    D. gentamicin

46. The nurse providing care for a patient diagnosed with pyelonephritis recognizes which of the following medications as common therapy for the disease?
    A. furosemide (Lasix)
    B. ciprofloxacin (Cipro)
    C. methylprednisolone (Solu-Medrol)
    D. piperacillin and tazobactam (Zosyn)

47. The nurse is caring for a patient who is diagnosed with acute glomerulonephritis. Upon review of laboratory results and assessment of the patient, the nurse would expect to find which of the following?
    A. anuria and +4 pitting edema of the lower extremities
    B. proteinuria, hematuria, and azotemia
    C. BP 190/110; serum creatinine 1.0; U/O 1620 mL/day
    D. urine cultures positive with *Pseudomonas* or *Streptococcus*

48. The nurse should identify which of the following expected outcomes for the hospitalized toddler with nephrotic syndrome?
    A. The child will have decreased albuminemia.
    B. The child will have decreased proteinuria.
    C. The child will have increased urine specific gravity.
    D. The child will have increased blood urea nitrogen.

49. The nurse understands that which of the following factors provides a stimulus for the production of red blood cells (RBCs)?
    A. low Hgb and Hct
    B. filgrastim (Neupogen)
    C. decline of B_{12} levels
    D. epoetin alfa (Epogen)

50. The nurse is providing education to the patient with pernicious anemia. Which of the following statements by the patient indicates comprehension of the information?
    A. "I will need to take vitamin B_{12} replacement for the rest of my life."
    B. "When I get over this episode, I will not have to take the medicine regularly."
    C. "If I add vitamin B_{12} foods to my diet consistently, I don't need medication."
    D. "I have a higher chance of developing Alzheimer's because of B_{12} deficiency."

51. The nurse who is caring for a patient with disseminated intravascular coagulation (DIC) would anticipate the need for which of the following factors and/or blood products?
    A. packed red blood cells
    B. whole blood
    C. fresh frozen plasma
    D. immune globulins

52. The nurse is caring for a patient with disseminated intravascular coagulation (DIC). The nurse would expect which of the following laboratory findings?
    A. low D-dimer
    B. prolonged partial thromboplastin time
    C. decreased prothrombin time
    D. increased platelet count

53. The nurse is caring for a patient with leukemia. Which of the following clinical manifestations would the nurse expect to find upon physical assessment of the patient?
    A. angina, dyspnea, fatigue
    B. petechiae, muscle aching, splenomegaly
    C. insomnia, shortness of breath, hematuria
    D. night sweats, splenomegaly, ecchymoses

54. The nurse is caring for a patient with neutropenia. A priority nursing diagnosis for this patient would be:
    A. risk for infection.
    B. impaired tissue perfusion.
    C. impaired gas exchange.
    D. decreased cardiac output.

55. The nurse is working in a same-day procedure unit with patients scheduled for different types of procedures. Which of the following patients would be a candidate for an MRI?
    A. a patient with a history of hip replacement
    B. a patient who has a tibial fracture repaired with screws
    C. a patient who has a biologic tissue mitral valve
    D. a patient who has an automated internal defibrillator

56. The nurse is caring for a patient postlaminectomy. The nurse will include which of the following in the patient's plan of care?
    A. Encourage early ambulation to decrease risk for DVT.
    B. Provide ample fluids for oral intake to promote dye excretion.
    C. Logroll the patient with the assistance of at least two others.
    D. Report any tingling of extremities to the physician.

57. The nurse is providing discharge teaching for a patient who has undergone total hip replacement. Which of the following statements by the patient indicate a need for more teaching?
    A. "I will notify my doctor if I notice any foul-smelling drainage from my incision."
    B. "I will have to go to an outpatient laboratory for weekly testing of my PT."
    C. "When I can walk without a walker, I can stop attending physical therapy."
    D. "I will need to use a reacher to get things I drop on the floor."

58. The nurse is providing education about medications to a patient with gout. The nurse explains that probenecid (Benemid) acts by:
    A. inhibiting uric acid production.
    B. increasing excretion of uric acid.
    C. decreasing excretion of purines.
    D. raising the serum level of purines.

59. A patient with rheumatoid arthritis is likely to be on all of the following medications for control of the condition *except*:
    A. aspirin.
    B. methotrexate.
    C. prednisone.
    D. furosemide (Lasix).

60. The nurse is caring for a patient who has had lab work done during a hospital admission. The patient's erythrocyte sedimentation rate (ESR) is 45 mm/hr. Which of the following interpretations by the nurse is correct?
    A. The value is within the normal range.
    B. The value indicates the presence of inflammation.
    C. The test result is inconclusive.
    D. The result indicates a red blood cell problem.

61. The nurse is caring for a patient with acute diverticulitis. Prior to discharge the nurse should instruct the patient to increase which of the following foods in the diet?
    A. cucumbers, popcorn, cantaloupe
    B. oat bran muffin, broccoli, apples
    C. peas, strawberries, corn
    D. tomatoes, peas, corn

62. The nurse is caring for a patient with acute diverticulitis. Prior to discharge the nurse should instruct the patient to avoid which of the following foods in the diet?
    A. squash, potatoes, brown rice
    B. chicken, hamburger, peanut butter
    C. roasted peanuts, sesame seed bread, grapes
    D. salmon, grilled vegetables, pears

63. The physician has ordered insertion of a nasogastric tube. Which of the following actions by the nurse would facilitate insertion?
    A. lubricating the tube with petroleum jelly
    B. asking the patient to swallow while the tube is passed
    C. placing the coiled tube in warm water prior to insertion
    D. asking the patient to turn the head during insertion

64. The nurse working in a primary care office sees a patient who came in for evaluation of gastroesophageal reflux disease (GERD). When documenting the patient's history, the nurse expects the patient to report that symptoms are worse when:
    A. exercising.
    B. straining.
    C. sitting.
    D. walking.

65. The nurse is providing teaching about dietary modifications to a patient with gastroesophageal reflux disease (GERD). The nurse should suggest elimination of which of the following foods or substances for this patient?
    A. caffeine, onions, peppermint
    B. lettuce, carrots, whole wheat
    C. potatoes, grapes, squash
    D. juices, ice cream, asparagus

66. The nurse is providing care for a patient who is receiving total parenteral nutrition (TPN) via a single-lumen central catheter. An intravenous antibiotic dose is due, and the nurse finds that the peripheral site is no longer functional. Which of the following independent nursing interventions provides the best option for infusion of the antibiotic?
    A. Administer the intravenous antibiotic through the TPN line.
    B. Insert a multilumen catheter over a guide wire.
    C. Identify a new site and insert another peripheral line.
    D. Insert a peripherally inserted central catheter.

67. The nurse working in the emergency department realizes that which of the following patients with acute abdominal pain is most likely to have acute appendicitis?
    A. an 8-month-old female
    B. a 13-year-old male
    C. an 80-year-old woman
    D. a 46-year-old male

68. The nurse is caring for a patient with an acute exacerbation of Crohn's disease. Which of the following nursing interventions is least appropriate for this patient?
    A. Encourage bed rest with bathroom privileges.
    B. Encourage strict NPO status.
    C. Administer prescribed cathartics.
    D. Place a deodorizer in the patient's room.

69. Assessment of the patient's gag response is a priority nursing intervention following which of the following procedures?
    A. colon biopsy
    B. bronchoscopy
    C. barium enema
    D. colonoscopy

70. The nurse has been providing teaching to a pregnant woman with Type I diabetes. Which of the following statements by the patient indicates an understanding of the impact of pregnancy on insulin needs?
    A. "Because pregnancy increases my metabolism, I'll need less insulin."
    B. "During my pregnancy, I will need more insulin to have stable glucose levels."
    C. "Because my blood glucose levels are stable, I'll check them only once per day."
    D. "My placenta continually produces insulin, which decreases my blood glucose."

71. The nurse is caring for a patient with Type II diabetes. Which of the following statements by the patient indicates understanding of predisposing factors for the disease?
    A. "Both of my parents and one grandparent had diabetes."
    B. "My youngest child was diagnosed with Type I diabetes."
    C. "I got diabetes because I've eaten too many sweets over the years."
    D. "My pancreas stopped making insulin, which caused my disease."

72. The nurse is providing teaching to a patient who has been diagnosed with Type I diabetes. Which statement by the patient indicates an understanding of key characteristics of the disease?
    A. "I may be able to decide if I take insulin or oral medications."
    B. "I probably developed this disease because I am overweight."
    C. "My pancreas has completely stopped producing insulin."
    D. "My body has developed insulin resistance over time."

73. The nurse is caring for a patient in the emergency department who was admitted with a serum glucose level of 857 mg/dL. The patient is nauseated, vomiting, lethargic, and polyuric. Vital signs are BP 78/50; P 125; R 28. A priority nursing intervention for this patient would be:
    A. monitor vital signs every 4 hours.
    B. encourage small sips of water to increase fluid status.
    C. administer fluid resuscitation as ordered.
    D. admit to a medical–surgical floor for follow-up.

74. The nurse is providing education about hypoglycemia to a patient who was newly diagnosed with Type II diabetes. The nurse realizes that teaching has been effective when the patient makes which of the following statements?
    A. "I should always carry some sugar-free candy or Life Savers with me."
    B. "I will know when my blood glucose is low because I will be nauseous."
    C. "My blood glucose is likely to be very low because I have started medication."
    D. "It is not extremely likely that I will experience hypoglycemia."

75. The nurse is providing education about treatment for hypoglycemia to a patient with diabetes. Which of the following treatments should the nurse advise for the patient?
    A. graham crackers and peanut butter; recheck glucose in 4 hours
    B. 4 oz of orange juice; recheck glucose in 1 hour
    C. 8 oz of orange juice with sugar; recheck glucose in 1 hour
    D. 8 oz skim milk; recheck glucose in 2 hours

76. The nurse is caring for a patient with a disorder of calcium metabolism. The nurse recognizes that which of the following glands is most likely responsible for this problem?
    A. adrenal cortex
    B. thyroid gland
    C. parathyroid gland
    D. posterior pituitary

ALTERNATE FORMAT

77. The nurse must calculate intake and output for the patient with continuous bladder irrigation. At the beginning of the shift, the patient had 2000 mL of irrigation fluid in the bag. By the end of the shift, 1250 mL remains. The total catheter output throughout the shift was 1000 mL. How much urine output did the patient have throughout the shift?

    _____

78. The nurse is providing care for a patient with benign prostatic hypertrophy. Clinical manifestations, as described by the patient, include:
    A. urinary frequency with strong stream.
    B. urinary frequency and dribbling.
    C. daytime urinary frequency with incontinence.
    D. fever, chills, nausea, and vomiting.

79. Which of the following diagnostics are used as markers to monitor therapeutic response to treatment for testicular cancer?
    A. alpha fetoprotein and hCG
    B. scrotal ultrasound and PSA
    C. prostate-specific antigen
    D. serum testosterone

80. The nurse is providing education about medications for a patient with erectile dysfunction. Which of the following statements by the patient indicates understanding of the instructions?
    A. "I can't use sildenafil (Viagra) because I take ACE inhibitors for my blood pressure."
    B. "Sildenafil (Viagra) could cause severe hypertension in conjunction with nitrates."
    C. "Because I have multiple sclerosis, sildenafil (Viagra) may cause priapism."
    D. "Sildenafil (Viagra) is a drug that must be self-administered by penile injection."

81. The nurse is caring for a patient whose last menstrual period began on November 1, 2009. Using Nägele's rule, the estimated date of birth is which of the following?
    A. February 1, 2010
    B. May 8, 2010
    C. July 1, 2010
    D. August 8, 2010

82. The nurse is providing care for a patient with worsening preeclampsia who is admitted to the labor and birth unit. The physician explains the plan of care for the patient, including induction of labor, to the patient and her husband. The nurse determines that the couple needs further information based on which of the following comments from the husband?
    A. "I will help my wife use the breathing techniques from childbirth class."
    B. "I will give my wife clear liquids to drink during labor."
    C. "We're going to watch the boxing match on TV with our toddlers."
    D. "I will stay with my wife during her labor just like we planned."

83. The nurse is providing care for a patient who has recently been diagnosed with oligohydramnios. The nurse knows that this condition is associated with which of the following types of fetal abnormality?
    A. renal
    B. cardiac
    C. gastrointestinal
    D. neurologic

84. The nurse is providing education to a pregnant woman about presumptive, probable, and positive signs of pregnancy. The patient demonstrates understanding of the information when she states that which of the following is a positive sign of pregnancy?
    A. elevated hCG levels
    B. audible fetal heartbeat
    C. Braxton-Hicks contractions
    D. quickening

85. The nurse is providing care for a laboring woman whose membranes have ruptured. The nurse realizes that the patient's risk for which of the following has increased with rupture of the membranes?
    A. intrauterine infection
    B. hemorrhage
    C. precipitous labor
    D. supine hypertension

86. Presumptive signs of pregnancy may include which of the following?
    A. uterine contractions
    B. amenorrhea
    C. audible fetal heart tones
    D. softening of the cervical tip

87. The nurse working in an obstetrical office is providing care for a woman who suspects that she is pregnant. Upon completion of physical assessment, the physician reports the presence of Goodell's sign. The nurse understands that the patient has which of the following clinical indications of pregnancy?
    A. softening of the cervix
    B. bluish–purple discoloration of cervical mucous membranes
    C. softening of the isthmus of the uterus
    D. quickening

88. Which of the following are critical points of the surgical "time-out" as defined by the Association of Perioperative Registered Nurses (AORN)?
    A. takes place in the preoperative holding area
    B. involves the patient, a nurse, and the surgeon
    C. requires verification of site by the patient and surgeon
    D. all team members verbally agree to patient, site, and procedure

89. The nurse at an outpatient surgical center is providing preoperative teaching for a patient with diabetes who normally takes metformin (Glucophage) and glipizide (Glucotrol XL) daily. When the nurse informs the patient about the likelihood of having sliding scale regular insulin coverage during the postoperative period, the patient is alarmed and asks why that is necessary when the pills have worked well. The best response by the nurse is which of the following?
    A. "Your pancreatic function will be impaired postop because of anesthesia."
    B. "Sliding scale coverage provides better glucose control early postop."
    C. "We have always managed blood glucose levels this way after surgery."
    D. "You will be right back on your pills within 24 hours after surgery."

90. The nurse knows that which of the following types of cancer typically demonstrate a familial tendency?
    A. brain
    B. colon
    C. lymph
    D. bladder

91. The nurse is caring for a female patient who is concerned that she may be at higher than normal risk of breast cancer. Which of the following factors identified by the patient place her at higher than normal risk for development of breast cancer?
    A. 60 years of age
    B. works night shift
    C. breast fed two children
    D. menopause at 48 years of age

92. The nurse is providing care for a patient receiving brachytherapy. In planning her care for this patient, the nurse must:
    A. plan to spend extra time with the patient to provide emotional support.
    B. assist the patient with self-care activities and implant manipulation.
    C. encourage patient self-care activities as much as possible.
    D. encourage visitation from family and friends to support the patient.

93. The nurse is admitting a patient diagnosed with thrombocytopenia. Which of the following is the most important nursing intervention for this patient?
    A. Wash hands before and after each patient contact.
    B. Encourage use of mouth swabs instead of a toothbrush.
    C. Monitor blood pressure and pulse every 4 hours.
    D. Allow ample visitation to keep the patient's spirits up.

94. The nurse is caring for a patient who is undergoing chemotherapy. The nurse understands that the patient's risk of infection is related to results from which of the following laboratory tests?
    A. CEA
    B. PSA
    C. ANC
    D. RBC

95. The nurse is caring for a patient who will receive external radiation therapy. The patient asks the nurse why the ugly ink marks and tattoos over the area to be radiated are necessary. The best response by the nurse is:
    A. "The markings indicate where the technician should focus treatments."
    B. "The markings let you know the exact location of your cancer."
    C. "Exact markings are critical to limit damage to healthy tissues."
    D. "Exact markings indicate potentially salvageable tissue."

96. Which of the following behaviors justifies a nurse's concern that a colleague may be dependent upon alcohol or drugs?
    A. meticulous about one's outward appearance
    B. frequently disappears for periods during the shift
    C. enjoys drinking alcohol at staff social events
    D. infrequently absent from work without cause

97. The nurse knows that certain records will be needed for the agency's next accreditation visit. Guidelines published by which of the following organizations should be utilized in deciding which records to retain?
    A. The Joint Commission
    B. AMA
    C. ANA
    D. CCNE

98. The nurse has just taught a patient how to change his colostomy bag. Which of the following is the best indication that the teaching has been successful?
    A. The patient states that he understands how to change the bag.
    B. The patient correctly identifies the steps in the procedure.
    C. The patient demonstrates how to apply a new bag.
    D. The nurse knows the patient to be highly intelligent and cooperative.

99. A nurse employed in an outpatient clinic knows that which of the following actions would constitute a violation of the Health Insurance Portability and Accountability Act (HIPAA)?
    A. reading a note made by another healthcare provider in a patient's chart
    B. telling a patient that a biopsy came back positive for cancer
    C. leaving test results on a patient's home answering machine without written consent
    D. failing to change the paper on an exam room table between patients

100. The nurse has just returned from a seminar on the importance of self-care. An important principle for the nurse to remember is that a warning sign of job-related stress is:
    A. smiling and laughing a lot.
    B. being absent from work more frequently.
    C. managing time more effectively.
    D. being tardy less often.

ANSWERS

1. **(C)**; The nurse must translate micrograms into milligrams: $\dfrac{0.125\ \mu g}{1000\ \frac{\mu g}{mg}} = 0.125$ mg

   Then, mathematically, $\dfrac{0.250\ \frac{mg}{dose}}{0.125\ \frac{mg}{tablet}} = 2\ \dfrac{tablets}{dose}$.

2. **(B)**; The patient has hypokalemia, which can potentiate digoxin toxicity.

3. **(A, C)**; Digoxin (Lanoxin) may be given undiluted or diluted in 4 mL NSS. There is more risk of precipitation with undiluted administration. Digoxin must be administered over a minimum of 5 minutes. Low serum potassium levels may potentiate digoxin toxicity.

4. **(B)**; Thrombolytic drugs break down existing clots and predispose the patient to bleeding. Typically, patients receiving thrombolytic drugs also receive heparin infusion to impair the clotting ability of the blood. The thrombolytic drug breaks down existing clots while heparin helps to prevent formation of new clots. Therefore, once thrombolytic therapy has been initiated, it is not prudent to perform either venipuncture or arterial puncture. The femoral arterial site is especially dangerous in that it is a very large artery that is deep. In patients *without* thrombolytics, the nurse would hold pressure for 20 to 30 minutes on a femoral artery to reestablish a seal. That time would be significantly prolonged if the patient had received thrombolytic therapy.

5. **(D)**; When the nurse is involved with bedside synchronized cardioversion, it is critical to consider the ABCs—airway, breathing, and circulation. It is possible that the patient may suffer respiratory or cardiac arrest during this procedure, so it is essential for the nurse to have a bag–valve–mask device available in case it is needed.

6. **(B, A, E, C, D, F)**; According to basic life support protocols, the first step in the application of an AED is to turn the power on. The second step is to attach the pads to the victim's chest, followed by pushing the "Analyze" button. The device will often announce "Stand clear," and the equipment operator should also ensure that all bystanders are clear of the patient. If indicated, a shock will be delivered. If indicated, a total of three shocks are delivered before the patient is assessed for presence of a pulse.

7. **(A)**; When working with invasive catheters or tubes, it is critical to maintain sterility of the equipment prior to insertion. This helps to decrease the risk of introducing infectious organisms into the patient's bloodstream. If equipment is contaminated prior to insertion, a new tube or catheter must be obtained.

8. **(C)**; The nurse would suspect that any patient with known atrial fibrillation would be treated with warfarin (Coumadin) to decrease risk of stroke. Patients with atrial fibrillation are at risk of clot formation because of lack of contractions within the atria. Coumadin does not break down established clots, but it does prevent enlargement of existing clots. In conjunction with the body's fibrinolytic system, Coumadin helps to reduce the chance of thromboembolism.

9. **(D)**; First, convert the patient's weight to kg by dividing 220 by 2.2, which equals 100 kg. Next, figure out how many mLs = 1 mcg by dividing the total volume (250 mL) by

the number of micrograms of dopamine (400,000) to equal 0.000625 mL/mcg. Then apply the information to the following equation:

$$\frac{5 \, \mu g \times 100 \, kg}{minute} \times \frac{60 \, minutes}{1 \, hour} \times 0.000625 \, \frac{mL}{\mu g} = 18.75 \, \frac{mL}{hr}$$

Because most IV pumps will allow fractions only to the 10th, you would round this to 18.8 mL/hr.

10. **(B)**; First, convert the patient's weight to kg by dividing 198 by 2.2, which equals 90 kg. Next, figure out how many mLs = 1 mcg by dividing the total volume (250 mL) by the number of micrograms of dobutamine (250,000) to equal 0.001 mL/mcg. Then apply the information to the following equation:

$$\frac{5 \, \mu g \times 90 \, kg}{minute} \times \frac{60 \, minutes}{1 \, hour} \times 0.001 \, \frac{mL}{\mu g} = 27 \, \frac{mL}{hr}$$

11. **(D)**; First, calculate the bolus using the following ratio method:

$$\frac{1000 \, mL}{20 \, grams} = \frac{x \, mL}{3 \, grams} \; ; \text{where } 3000 = 20x. \text{ Therefore, } x = 150 \text{ mL to infuse over 30}$$

minutes (0.5 hr). 150 mL $\times$ 0.5 hour $= 300 \, \dfrac{mL}{hr}$ (BOLUS).

Next, calculate the maintenance infusion using the same ratio technique:

$$\frac{1000 \, mL}{20 \, grams} = \frac{x \, mL}{1.5 \, gram}; \text{where } 1500 = 20x. \text{ Therefore, } x = 75 \text{ mL to infuse each hour } or$$

75 mL/hr (maintenance).

12. **(A)**; The nurse should level the arterial line transducer to the phlebostatic axis. This will help ensure that the displayed blood pressure is accurate. Next, the nurse should initiate and titrate IV nitroprusside (Nipride) to maintain BP < 150/85. Carotid endarterectomy patients frequently return from the operating room with significant hypertension, but lowering the BP too dramatically all at once could lead to ischemic injury. Therefore, the higher BP parameters would be more appropriate for this patient.

13. **(D)**; Sequential compression devices are evidence-based interventions that are used, along with compression stockings, to prevent the development of venous thrombosis during the postoperative period.

14. **(C)**; Upon discharge, it is essential for the patient to have INR levels monitored a few times per week for at least a few weeks after surgery. This is necessary because the levels are affected by dietary intake and other factors. Warfarin dosage is adjusted as needed to maintain a therapeutic INR during the recovery period. The goal for INR during treatment with warfarin (Coumadin) is 2–3.

15. **(D, B, C, A, E)**; The nurse must first verify that the drugs are correct as ordered and then identify the patient by at least two means. Next, the Combivent (bronchodilator) should be administered followed in a few minutes by the Flovent (glucocorticoid). Finally, the patient should gargle to decrease the chances of developing oral candidiasis.

16. **(1.2 mL)**; Use the ratio method to solve $\dfrac{100 \, mg}{2 \, mL} = \dfrac{60 \, mg}{x}$; then $100x = 120$.
$\dfrac{120}{100} = x$, so $x = 1.2$ mL.

17. **(B)**; When a patient coughs forcefully during ventilation, the high pressure alarm will sound as an indicator that airway pressure exceeds what is expected based on settings on the ventilator.

18. **(A, B, E)**; Assist control is a mode of ventilation that is often used with patients who are postoperative or heavily sedated. It allows breaths to be administered to the patient at a set tidal volume for *every* breath—whether initiated by the ventilator or by the patient. As patients wake up from anesthesia, it is not uncommon for them to initiate more breaths per minute. With each effort, a full tidal volume breath is administered. Over time, this situation can produce respiratory alkalosis.

19. **(A, B)**; Synchronized intermittent mandatory ventilation (SIMV) is a mode in which a specific rate and tidal volume are set for ventilation. During each of the ventilator-initiated breaths, the patient receives the full tidal volume. The patient can initiate breaths at any time. Patient-initiated breaths will vary in tidal volume depending upon the inspiratory effort of the patient.

20. **(A, D)**; The mechanically ventilated patient who will undergo pressure support trials has demonstrated some indication of readiness to wean. When the patient is on a pressure support trial, it is critically important for the nurse to monitor the patient very closely because there is no set rate or tidal volume, and therefore no alarms indicate if the patient is compromised. As a stand-alone mode in stable ventilator patients, pressure support simply decreases the work of breathing by maintaining a continuous positive airway pressure, but the patient must still initiate all breaths with a tidal volume that provides effective respiration.

21. **(A, B, D)**; The patient can initiate a breath any time. All ventilated breaths will be full tidal volume. Patient-initiated breaths will have variable tidal volumes. The addition of positive end expiratory pressure (PEEP) results in increased intrathoracic pressure because PEEP causes the alveoli to remain expanded at the end of expiration. The increased intrathoracic pressure results in decreased ventricular filling and decreased cardiac output. Therefore, blood pressure assessments should be completed on patients who are having PEEP added during mechanical ventilation. If the patient becomes hypotensive, the nurse would contact the physician for further orders, which may include vasopressor drugs.

22. **(B)**; When the patient has adventitious breath sounds, it frequently prompts coughing. When the patient coughs against the ventilator, the high pressure alarm sounds. Frequently, patients require suctioning when the high pressure alarm sounds.

23. **(D)**; The gold standard test for diagnosis of pulmonary embolus is pulmonary angiogram, which is an expensive, invasive test with significant risks for the patient. Therefore, a spiral CT is performed more frequently and is highly accurate for diagnosing large emboli.

24. **(B, D, F)**; This ABG result reveals uncompensated respiratory acidosis.

ABG component	Value	What it reveals related to acid-base balance
pH	7.30	*Acidotic; uncompensated*
pCO_2	48	Elevated; contributes to acidotic pH; *primary problem*
HCO_3^-	24	Elevated; acting to buffer acidosis
pO_2	90	Within normal limits

25. **(B)**; Flaccidity implies that muscle tone is decreased or absent.

26. **(A)**; Myasthenia gravis is a chronic progressive disorder of the peripheral nervous system. Early common symptoms include weakness, fatigue, and unilateral ptosis.

27. **(B)**; Ptosis is drooping of the eyelids.

28. **(C)**; The diaphragm (which is responsible for inspiration, deep breathing, and effective cough) receives innervation from above C5. Injuries at or above C4 will result in diaphragmatic paralysis and necessitate life-long mechanical ventilation.

29. **(C)**; When cerebral aneurysms rupture, they bleed into the subarachnoid space in the brain.

30. **(A)**; The risk of rebleeding for patients with cerebral aneurysms is highest within the first 24–48 hours after the initial bleed. Nearly 75% of those who experience rebleeding will die.

31. **(A)**; The most significant sign of increased intracranial pressure is a change in level of consciousness.

32. **(B)**; The patient with increased intracranial pressure should not have a lumbar puncture because it is likely to result in brain herniation.

33. **(B)**; The nurse should realize that treatment options for AVM are dependent upon a number of factors—size, location, and pattern of venous drainage. Treatment options include (1) surgical resection at a major neurosurgical center; (2) coiling or embolization, which is performed by an interventional neuroradiologist; (3) gamma knife surgery; or (4) conservative treatment. Surgical resection involves surgical separation of the arteries and veins. Coiling or embolization involves insertion of tiny coils or glue into the arterial side of the AVM to obliterate blood flow. Gamma knife surgery can be used to treat AVMs that are not accessible for surgical resection because of their location. Conservative treatment involves symptom management and is used to treat AVMs that are unsafe for other treatment options.

34. **(D)**; The patient can indicate understanding of discharge instructions by articulating that medications will continue until the physician determines that they should be discontinued.

35. **(B)**; The 66-year-old (>65) widower (*male*) with liver cancer (*terminal illness*) who talks about saving his pain pills (*plan*) is the patient at highest risk for suicide of those presented. The 24-year-old female who lives with her parents and broke up with a boyfriend has one stress but no significant risks for suicide. The 45-year-old married female with a stressful job also has no significant risk for suicide. Although the 35-

year-old married man has a potentially terminal illness, he has social support and significant others, which results in reduced risk for suicide.

36. **(C)**; ECT is indicated for treatment of major depression, bipolar depressive disorder, lithium-resistant mania, and schizophrenia and schizoaffective disorders. ECT is not indicated for treating personality disorders or eating disorders.

37. **(A)**; The nurse recognizes that the patient is showing improvement because of both the increased appetite and increasing socialization.

38. **(A)**; Extrapyramidal side effects of the central nervous system are involved in the production and control of involuntary and gross motor movements producing *acute dystonia, akathisia, dyskinesia, and parkinsonism.* Amenorrhea, breast secretion, and sexual dysfunction are endocrine-related side effects of the drug.

39. **(A)**; A serum lithium level of 1.0 mEq/L is within normal limits. Lithium has a low therapeutic index, which means that toxicity can occur when levels rise only slightly above normal. For initial therapy of a manic episode, lithium levels may range from 0.8 to 1.4 mEq/L. However, when the therapeutic effect has been achieved, the dosage should be decreased to ensure maintenance serum levels of 0.4 to 1.0 mEq/L.

40. **(C)**; Common side effects of anticholinergics include dry mouth, *blurred vision*, urinary retention, and constipation.

41. **(B)**; Because normal GI bacteria typically causes the disorder, women are at greater risk for development than men because of their shorter urethra and the close proximity of the urethra to the rectum.

42. **(B)**; The nurse understands that a patient with anasarca has total body edema, which implies that skin integrity becomes a priority issue for continued care of the patient.

43. **(B)**; Of the choices listed, ureteral calculi is the likely cause of postrenal failure. By definition, conditions that cause postrenal failure cause obstruction to urine flow after the kidney.

44. **(A)**; The nurse understands that heart failure, hemorrhage, and shock are examples of possible etiologic factors in the development of prerenal azotemia.

45. **(D)**; Gentamicin is an aminoglycoside. This group of drugs is known to be highly nephrotoxic.

46. **(B)**; Antibiotics commonly used for treatment of pyelonephritis include sulfa drugs (Bactrim), cephalosporins (Maxipime, Ceclor), amoxicillin, levofloxacin, and *ciprofloxacin*.

47. **(B)**; The patient with acute glomerulonephritis will have symptoms that may include oliguria, *proteinuria, hematuria, azotemia*, and mild edema.

48. **(B)**; The nurse should expect that with treatment the child will have decreased proteinuria—loss of protein in the urine.

49. **(D)**; The drug epoetin alfa (Epogen) stimulates red blood cell production.

50. **(A)**; The patient's acknowledgment of the need to take replacement B_{12} for an entire lifetime indicates comprehension of the material that was taught.

51. **(C)**; The nurse who is caring for a patient with DIC should anticipate the need to administer cryoprecipitate to replace fibrinogen, platelets for thrombocytopenia, and *fresh frozen plasma* to replace all clotting factors except platelets.

52. **(B)**; The nurse who is caring for a patient with DIC would expect to find that partial thromboplastin time is prolonged, prothrombin time is prolonged, platelet count is decreased, and D-dimer is elevated.

53. **(D)**; Upon physical assessment of the patient with leukemia, the nurse would anticipate finding that the patient suffers from *night sweats*, gingival bleeding, *ecchymoses*, weakness, fatigue, anorexia, shortness of breath, decreased activity tolerance, epistaxis, pallor, and *splenomegaly* or hepatomegaly.

54. **(A)**; The patient with neutropenia is at significant risk for infection because normal phagocytic activity is lacking.

55. **(C)**; The only patient who would be a candidate for an MRI is the one with a biologic tissue mitral valve. Each of the other patients have contraindications. Patients with artificial joints, screws or plates, or automated internal defibrillators are not candidates because metal distorts the MRI image and can affect the magnetic field.

56. **(C)**; The nurse should logroll the patient with the assistance of at least two others because it is critical to maintain proper alignment of the spine at all times postoperatively.

57. **(C)**; The patient should be informed that the goal of physical therapy is to facilitate return to normal function. Typically patients use a walker first and then use a cane before final transition to ambulation without an assistive device.

58. **(B)**; Probenecid (Benemid) increases the excretion of uric acid by inhibiting tubular reabsorption.

59. **(D)**; The patient with rheumatoid arthritis is likely to be treated with aspirin and prednisone. Patients with severe rheumatoid arthritis are treated with methotrexate. Furosemide (Lasix) is not part of the treatment regimen for rheumatoid arthritis.

60. **(B)**; ESR is a test that indicates the rate at which red blood cells settle out of unclotted blood. Elevated levels indicate that an inflammatory process is present.

61. **(B)**; The patient should be instructed to increase foods that are high in fiber when the acute inflammation has subsided. These high-fiber foods include such things as wheat bran, *oat bran*, shredded wheat, oatmeal, whole wheat bread, multigrain bread, cooked asparagus, *broccoli*, squash, spinach, lettuce, carrots, peaches, *apples*, and oranges.

62. **(C)**; The patient with acute diverticulitis should be instructed to avoid foods with small seeds; *nuts* and foods with skins, like raisins, *grapes*, and corn; strawberries; raspberries; blueberries; figs; rye bread with caraway seeds; popcorn; *sesame seeds*; poppy seeds; sunflower seeds; nuts; cucumbers; and okra. Avoidance of these foods will help to decrease exacerbations of diverticulitis.

63. **(B)**; Asking the patient to swallow while the tube is passed will help to facilitate movement of the tube toward the stomach without causing significant irritation to the patient. Lubricating the tube with petroleum jelly, placing the coiled tube in warm water prior to insertion, and asking the patient to turn the head during insertion are maneuvers that would most certainly not facilitate easy tube insertion.

64. **(B)**; Gastroesophageal reflux symptoms are most pronounced with activities that increase intraabdominal pressure, such as bending, *straining*, lifting, and lying down.

65. **(A)**; The nurse should encourage the patient to eliminate chocolate, oranges, and tomatoes from the diet because they increase the risk of GERD symptoms. Patients experience symptoms of GERD following oral intake of substances that decrease lower esophageal stricture (LES) pressure. These substances include alcohol, *caffeine*, nicotine, chocolate, fatty foods, citrus fruits, *onions*, tomatoes, and *peppermint*.

66. **(C)**; The nurse should identify a new site and insert another peripheral line. It is not a good idea to administer the medication through the TPN line because protecting the patient from line sepsis is of the utmost importance. Insertion of a multi-lumen catheter over a guide wire is not a nursing intervention. Insertion of a peripherally-inserted central catheter requires a physician order.

67. **(B)**; The patient with acute abdominal pain who is most likely to have acute appendicitis is the 13-year-old male.

68. **(C)**; The patient with an exacerbation of Crohn's disease may be having 6–12 or more stools per day. It is absolutely not appropriate to administer cathartics to this patient.

69. **(B)**; A bronchoscopy involves insertion of a flexible scope through the trachea and into the larger airways. The patient's throat is anesthetized prior to insertion of this scope. Therefore, it is important for nurses to assess gag reflex when the patient returns to the nursing unit before administering any fluids by mouth.

70. **(B)**; During pregnancy, production of hormones increases a woman's insulin needs.

71. **(A)**; Family history of Type II diabetes is a strong predictor for diabetes in an individual. Patients do not get the disease as a result of intake of sweets. The pancreas typically still produces insulin with Type II diabetes.

72. **(C)**; Because there is absolutely no insulin production by the pancreas in Type I diabetes, patients with the disease become very ill very quickly. Patients must take insulin to survive.

73. **(C)**; This patient is severely dehydrated because of nausea, vomiting, and polyuria. Hemodynamic effects are highlighted by hypotension and tachycardia. The priority intervention for this patient must be to administer fluid resuscitation as ordered. Vital signs should be monitored at least hourly, and the patient should remain NPO and be admitted to a critical care monitored bed because the situation could be life-threatening.

74. **(D)**; It is not extremely likely that a patient with new onset Type II diabetes will experience hypoglycemia. Typically, physicians will prescribe conservative doses of medication to be used in conjunction with dietary modification and exercise. Also, patients will be instructed to test the blood glucose three to four times per day and to document the findings over a few weeks' time.

75. **(B)**; The nurse should advise the patient with hypoglycemia to drink 4 oz of orange juice (15 grams of carbohydrate) and recheck the glucose in 1 hour. Orange juice with sugar is not recommended. Neither is skim milk or graham crackers with peanut butter. Current recommendations are to administer the equivalent of 15 grams of carbohydrate and recheck the glucose within an hour.

76. **(C)**; The parathyroid gland is most responsible for calcium metabolism.

77. **(250 mL)**; 2000 − 1250 = 750 mL of irrigation infused during the shift. The total catheter output was 1000 mL, so 1000 mL total output − 750 mL irrigation = **250 mL urine**.

78. **(B)**; The patient with benign prostatic hypertrophy describes clinical manifestations of the disorder, which include *urinary frequency*, nocturia, weak stream, difficulty starting and stopping the stream, and *dribbling*.

79. **(A)**; Elevated levels of both alpha fetoprotein (AFP) and hCG provide strong evidence of testicular cancer. These levels are useful in monitoring the patient's response to therapy.

80. **(C)**; Patients with sickle cell anemia, leukemia, multiple sclerosis, and metastatic tumors may develop priapism following administration of phosphodiesterase type 5 inhibitors like sildenafil (Viagra). Patients should be cautioned about this potential side effect.

81. **(D)**; Using Nägele's rule, the calculation would occur as follows: Begin with the first day of the last menstrual period and subtract 3 months (November 1 − 3 months = August 1). Add 7 days (August 1 + 7 days = August 8, 2010).

82. **(C)**; Development of worsening preeclampsia is a cause for concern for the patient and her family. Upon admission to the hospital, the patient should be maintained in a quiet, low-stimulus environment. Typically, the patient is admitted to a private room in a quiet location where she can be monitored closely. Visitors are limited to close family members or a significant other. The patient should be encouraged to maintain the left lateral recumbent position most of the time. Bright lights and sudden loud noises may precipitate seizure activity in patients with severe preeclampsia.

83. **(A)**; Oligohydramnios, decreased volume of amniotic fluid, is associated with fetal urinary tract defects.

84. **(B)**; Positive signs of pregnancy are those that are completely objective and cannot be confused with any other pathologic state. They include *audible fetal heartbeat*, palpation of fetal movement by a trained examiner, and visualization of the fetus by ultrasound.

85. **(A)**; When the membranes rupture, the open pathway to the uterus increases the woman's risk of intrauterine infection.

86. **(B)**; Presumptive signs include amenorrhea, nausea and vomiting in pregnancy (morning sickness), excessive fatigue, urinary frequency, changes in the breast, and quickening.

87. **(A)**; Goodell's sign is a softening of the cervix. Chadwick's sign is a bluish–purple discoloration of the mucous membranes of the cervix, vagina, and vulva. Hegar's sign is a softening of the isthmus of the uterus. Quickening is when the mother perceives fetal movement.

88. **(D)**; According to the AORN *Guidelines for Implementing The Joint Commission Universal Protocol to Promote Correct Site Surgery*, a "time-out" takes place in the procedure or operating room after the patient is prepped and draped. Specific documentation of the "time-out" must include the following: *identification of the patient*, *agreement about the correct site* and side, *agreement about the procedure* to be performed, correct patient position, and availability of implants or special equipment as required.

89. **(B)**; The nurse should inform the patient that the stress of acute illness or surgery will cause elevation of blood glucose levels and that sliding scale insulin coverage provides control of glucose during the postoperative phase, which is superior to that provided by oral hypoglycemic agents. Pancreatic function is not affected by anesthesia. The nurse should not guarantee return to oral agents within 24 hours because it may not occur so quickly.

90. **(B)**; Cancers that typically demonstrate familial tendency include breast, *colon*, lung, ovarian, and prostate.

91. **(B)**; Hormonal risks for development of breast cancer include use of birth control pills or hormone replacement therapy; early menarche (before 12 years of age); late menopause (after 55 years of age); and first pregnancy after 30 years of age. Nonhormonal risk factors include family history; lack of regular exercise; postmenopausal obesity; increased use of alcohol; *working the night shift*; older than 65 years of age; no full-term pregnancies; never breast fed; higher socioeconomic status; Jewish heritage; and two or more first-degree relatives with breast cancer at an early age.

92. **(C)**; In planning care for the patient undergoing brachytherapy, the nurse should organize care so that a maximum of 30 minutes per shift is spent in the patient's room. At all times during care, the nurse must keep in mind the principles of minimizing radiation exposure: time, distance, and shielding. Exposure is directly related to time spent in close proximity to the source. All staff members caring for the patient must wear radiation badges, and nursing staff should be rotated to keep individual radiation exposure as low as possible. Distance is also important in reducing exposure to radiation. The nurse should *encourage patient self-care activities as much as possible* and perform duties as far away from the patient as possible. The final principle for minimizing radiation exposure is shielding. If necessary, a shield can be placed at the patient's bedside, and most nursing care should be done from behind the shield. Lead aprons are not recommended.

93. **(B)**; The patient with thrombocytopenia has a low platelet count and is therefore prone to bleeding. The nurse should encourage use of mouth swabs rather than a toothbrush to avoid bleeding in the mouth.

94. **(C)**; For the patient undergoing chemotherapy, the nurse must assess the risk of infection in relation to the ANC (absolute neutrophil count). An ANC of less than 500 is considered an indicator of serious risk for infection. The ANC is calculated by multiplying the WBC by the total percentage of neutrophils (polys and bands).

95. **(C)**; The nurse understands that external radiation provides targeted treatment to the area of the body affected by cancer. Exact markings are critical to limit damage to healthy tissues during treatment.

96. **(B)**; When a coworker frequently disappears for periods of time during a shift without adequate explanation, the nurse coworker is justified in having concerns about dependency on alcohol or drugs.

97. **(A)**; The Joint Commission is the accrediting agency for hospitals and other types of healthcare agencies. The American Medical Association (AMA) is a professional organization that advocates for physicians. The American Nurses Association (ANA) is a professional organization that advocates for the nursing profession. The Commission on Collegiate Nursing Education (CCNE) accredits baccalaureate and graduate degree nursing education programs.

98. **(C)**; A return demonstration done correctly is the best indicator of patient learning. Patients can incorrectly believe that they have mastered a procedure. Knowing the steps in a procedure (declarative learning) does not guarantee that the patient can carry the steps out (procedural learning). Procedures can be difficult for anyone to master.

99. **(C)**; Leaving a message containing sensitive medical information where others might hear it constitutes a violation of the part of HIPAA that concerns patient confidentiality. It is often necessary for staff members to read notes written by others. Conveying diagnoses to patients is a medical responsibility unless the nurse is a CRNP. HIPAA does not address patient safety.

100. **(B)**; Missing work more often is a classic sign of stress. The other choices reflect the presence of little stress or very manageable levels of stress.

Keep Track

- Percent correct. (Divide the number of questions you answered correctly by the total number of questions you answered.) _____

- Number of questions you missed due to a reading error: _____

- Number of questions you missed due to errors in analysis: _____

- Number of assessment questions you missed: _____

- Number of lab value questions you missed: _____

- Number of drug/treatment questions you missed: _____

Nugget List

Chapter number _____ Topic _____

Chapter 25

Comprehensive Practice Exam 3

Karen S. March

COMPREHENSIVE PRACTICE EXAM

1. The patient is prescribed digoxin (Lanoxin) 250 micrograms PO every day. The nurse finds digoxin (Lanoxin) 0.125 milligram tablets in the Pyxis. Which of the following is the appropriate action for the nurse?
   A. Call the pharmacy to request delivery of the correct dose.
   B. Administer 2 tablets from the Pyxis to deliver the full dose.
   C. Administer ½ tablet for the dose and waste the remainder.
   D. Notify the physician for a clarification of the order.

2. A patient who has been diagnosed with variant (Prinzmetal's) angina asks the nurse how this type of angina differs from unstable angina. The nurse's reply should include:
   A. "Variant angina is normally triggered by exertion."
   B. "The pain of variant angina is less than that of unstable angina."
   C. "Variant angina may be associated with EKG changes."
   D. "The chest discomfort of variant angina is worse."

ALTERNATE FORMAT

3. The nurse is preparing to administer Lanoxin 0.250 mg IV to the patient as ordered. The drug is available in ampules labeled "digoxin 500 mcg/2 mL." Which of the following actions will be performed by the nurse prior to and during administration of this drug? SELECT ALL THAT APPLY.
   A. Take an apical heart rate for a full minute prior to administration.
   B. Draw up 1 mL of drug from the ampule with a filter needle.
   C. Dilute the drug in 4 mL D_5W and administer over 5 minutes.
   D. Review the patient's lab work for serum sodium levels.

4. The nurse is caring for a patient who is receiving thrombolytic therapy. Which of the following actions by the nurse should be questioned?
   A. injecting an intravenous heparin bolus into an existing line
   B. performing venipuncture for labs after thrombolytics
   C. shaving the patient with an electric razor
   D. performing mouth care with swabs and mouthwash

5. The nurse articulates the difference between unstable angina and acute myocardial infarction (AMI) as demonstrated by which of the following explanations?
   A. "The pain of unstable angina is far less severe than the pain of AMI."
   B. "Unstable angina results from coronary artery occlusion for at least 1 hour."
   C. "Unstable angina and AMI can occur as a consequence of severe emotional stress."
   D. "Myocardial tissue dies as a result of acute myocardial infarction."

ALTERNATE FORMAT

6. The nurse is caring for a patient admitted with the following lab work:

Complete Blood Count	
Hematocrit (HCT)	42%
Hemoglobin (HGB)	14%
Red blood cells (RBC)	5.0 million/µL
Mean cell volume (MCV)	88 µ/m³
Mean cell hemoglobin (MCH)	29 pg
Mean cell hemoglobin concentration (MCHC)	36.2%
White blood cells (WBC)	6000/µL
Platelets (Plt)	280,000/µL
Serum Electrolytes	
Carbon dioxide	28 mEq/L
Chloride	99 mEq/L
Potassium	5.9 mEq/L
Sodium	138 mEq/L
Serum digoxin	0.8 ng/mL

Upon review, the nurse notes that the patient suffers from which of the following conditions?

   A. The patient is neutropenic.
   B. The patient is anemic.
   C. The patient is hyperkalemic.
   D. The patient is digoxin toxic.

ALTERNATE FORMAT

7. The nurse must defibrillate a patient who is in ventricular fibrillation. Place an X over areas of the torso to indicate correct paddle placement.

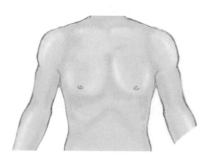

8. The nurse should be certain to mention which of the following teaching points about minimizing the adverse effects of nicotinic acid (Niacin) therapy?
   A. Take 325 mg of aspirin one-half hour before each dose to reduce flushing.
   B. Take with a full glass of water and keep your head elevated for 30 minutes.
   C. Take the drug on an empty stomach to ensure the full therapeutic effect.
   D. Monitor blood glucose levels at least monthly from the onset of therapy.

9. The patient is ordered dopamine by infusion at 5 µg/kg/min. The IV bag contains 400 mg of dopamine in 250 mL of 0.9% NaCl. The patient weighs 175 lb. Based on this information, the infusion pump must be set at what rate to ensure that the medication is infused correctly?
   A. 1.9 mL/hr
   B. 3.8 mL/hr
   C. 14.9 mL/hr
   D. 18.8 mL/hr

10. The patient is ordered dobutamine by infusion at 5 mcg/kg/min. The IV bag contains 250 mg of dobutamine in 250 mL D_5W. The patient weighs 250 lb. Based on this information, the infusion pump must be set at what rate to infuse the medication correctly?
    A. 24 mL/hr
    B. 27 mL/hr
    C. 34 mL/hr
    D. 40 mL/hr

11. An IV of 1000 mL lactated Ringer's (LR) with 20 grams magnesium sulfate arrives from the pharmacy. The nurse is to deliver a bolus of 4 grams magnesium sulfate over 30 minutes followed by a maintenance infusion of 2 grams/hr. The nurse knows that the correct rates for the bolus and the maintenance infusion are:
    A. 50 mL/hr for the bolus, then 100 mL/hr for the maintenance infusion.
    B. 200 mL/hr for the bolus, then 50 mL/hr for the maintenance infusion.
    C. 200 mL/hr for the bolus, then 100 mL/hr for the maintenance infusion.
    D. 400 mL/hr for the bolus, then 100 mL/hr for the maintenance infusion.

12. The nurse is providing discharge teaching for the patient with Buerger's disease. Which of the following instructions must be included?
    A. "You will need to attend physical therapy twice per week."
    B. "You will need to have a surgical revascularization procedure."
    C. "If you continue to smoke, you will probably require amputation."
    D. "If you maintain a cool environment, you will have fewer symptoms."

13. The nurse is providing care for a patient in the intensive care unit. Which of the following physical assessment findings would suggest the presence of a thoracic aneurysm?
    A. headache, fever, nonradiating chest pain
    B. tearing lower back pain with radiation to the abdomen
    C. substernal chest pain, dyspnea, stridor
    D. fleeting pulses, cool upper extremities

ALTERNATE FORMAT

14. The nurse is assigned to care for a 58-year-old patient in the ICU who underwent surgical repair of an abdominal aortic aneurysm 5 days ago. The patient remains on a mechanical ventilator because of failed extubation attempts. The nurse understands that this patient is at risk for development of venous thromboembolism because of which of the following factors? SELECT ALL THAT APPLY.
    A. age
    B. abdominal surgery
    C. admission to the ICU
    D. prolonged immobility >3 days

ALTERNATE FORMAT

15. The COPD patient is ordered ipratropium (Atrovent) one puff and fluticasone propionate (Flovent) two puffs at 6 p.m. Place in order the sequence that should be used for proper administration of these drugs. SELECT ALL THAT APPLY.
    A. Administer two puffs of Atrovent.
    B. Identify the patient by two identifiers.
    C. Administer one puff of Flovent.
    D. Verify that both drugs are correct as ordered.
    E. Encourage the patient to gargle.
    F. It does not matter whether the Atrovent or Flovent is given first.

ALTERNATE FORMAT

16. The patient is prescribed hydrocortisone sodium succinate (Solu-Cortef) 100 mg IV now. The drug is available in vials of "Solu-Cortef 40 mg/2mL." What volume of drug will the nurse withdraw from the vial to administer the correct dose?

_____

17. The nurse is providing care for a ventilated patient on a telemetry floor. When the low-pressure alarm sounds, the nurse should immediately perform which of the following interventions?
    A. Bag the patient until respiratory therapy arrives.
    B. Reconnect tubing that is disconnected from the ventilator.
    C. Sound the code-99 alarm for more assistance.
    D. Bag the patient and call out for assistance.

ALTERNATE FORMAT

18. The nurse is providing care for a mechanically ventilated patient on a telemetry unit. During report, the nurse is informed that the patient is being ventilated with the synchronized intermittent mandatory ventilation (SIMV) mode. Based on this information, the nurse understands which of the following implications? SELECT ALL THAT APPLY.
    A. The patient can initiate a breath any time.
    B. Ventilator-initiated breaths will be at full tidal volume.
    C. Patient-initiated breaths are at full tidal volume.
    D. Metabolic acidosis is not an uncommon outcome.
    E. Respiratory alkalosis is not an uncommon outcome.

ALTERNATE FORMAT

19. The nurse is providing care for a mechanically-ventilated patient who is being prepped as an organ donor. During report, the nurse is informed that the patient is being ventilated on controlled mandatory ventilation (CMV) mode. Based on this information, the nurse understands which of the following implications? SELECT ALL THAT APPLY.
    A. The patient can initiate a breath any time.
    B. Ventilator-initiated breaths will be at full tidal volume.
    C. Ventilator failure will require immediate bagging of the patient.
    D. This patient will make no efforts to initiate breaths.
    E. Respiratory alkalosis is not an uncommon outcome.

ALTERNATE FORMAT

20. The nurse is providing care for a mechanically-ventilated patient on a telemetry unit. During report, the nurse is informed that the patient is being prepared for weaning and will have a pressure support trial during the shift. Based on this information, the nurse understands which of the following implications? SELECT ALL THAT APPLY.
    A. The patient shows some indication of preparedness to wean.
    B. The ventilator rate will be set low, and the patient will do most of the work.
    C. The tidal volume will be set low, and the patient must breathe deeply.
    D. The nurse must monitor the patient very closely for signs of respiratory compromise.
    E. The ventilator will alarm if the patient experiences difficulty with breathing.

ALTERNATE FORMAT

21. The nurse is providing care for a mechanically-ventilated patient on a telemetry unit. During report, the nurse is informed that the patient is being ventilated on the synchronized intermittent mandatory ventilation (SIMV) mode. Because of some changes in respiratory status, positive end expiratory pressure (PEEP) of 10 cm H_2O will be added within the next hour. Based on this information, the nurse understands which of the following implications? SELECT ALL THAT APPLY.
    A. The ventilator dictates the rate and depth of breathing.
    B. Ventilator-initiated breaths will be at full tidal volume.
    C. The tidal volume of patient-initiated breaths will vary.
    D. Blood pressure should be monitored because hypotension may occur.
    E. Blood pressure should be monitored because hypertension may require attention.

22. A patient on a telemetry floor is intubated and on a mechanical ventilator. When the ventilator high-pressure alarm sounds, the nurse begins to troubleshoot. Which of the following is most likely to result in a high-pressure alarm?
    A. The patient has become disconnected from the ventilator tubing.
    B. The patient is coughing forcefully against the ventilator.
    C. Water has collected within the tubing between the patient and ventilator.
    D. The tubing on the pressure circuit of the ventilator is disconnected.

23. The most common test for diagnosis of pulmonary embolus is which of the following?
    A. arterial blood gas
    B. bronchoscopy
    C. spiral CT
    D. pulmonary angiogram

ALTERNATE FORMAT

24. The nurse receives the following arterial blood gas results from the laboratory:

pH	7.48
pCO_2	32
HCO_3^-	22
pO_2	90

Which of the following terms should the nurse use to properly interpret these results? SELECT ALL THAT APPLY.
    A. partially compensated
    B. uncompensated
    C. compensated
    D. respiratory
    E. metabolic
    F. acidosis
    G. alkalosis
    H. hypoxia
    I. normal ABG

25. The nurse is caring for a sedated patient in the intensive care unit. When the nurse applies nail bed pressure, the patient withdraws the hand. The response by the patient indicates which of the following?
    A. confusion
    B. arousal
    C. orientation
    D. attention

26. The nurse on a step-down unit must assess a patient's level of orientation. Which of the following patient responses indicates severe cerebral dysfunction?
    A. The patient identifies the state, city, and location of the hospital.
    B. The patient reports uncertainty about his or her location.
    C. The patient reports uncertainty about the time of day.
    D. The patient does not recognize an immediate family member.

27. To assess the patient's level of attention and concentration, the nurse should:
    A. tell the patient a story and then ask detailed questions.
    B. ask the patient to name the days of the week in reverse order.
    C. ask the patient to name the contenders in the last presidential election.
    D. ask the names, ages, and birth dates of the patient's children.

28. The nurse is caring for a patient who will undergo cerebral angiography. Following the procedure, it will be important for the nurse to encourage the patient to:
    A. ambulate as much as tolerated.
    B. lie in Trendelenburg position for 2 hours.
    C. increase fluid intake to at least 2 liters per day.
    D. remain on strict bed rest for at least 48 hours.

29. A patient is brought to the emergency department with a diagnosis of traumatic head injury following a motorcycle accident. Upon admission, vital signs are within normal limits, pupils are equal but react sluggishly, Glasgow Coma score = 6, and ICP is 35 mm Hg. The nurse is preparing to administer a dose of IV dexamethasone (Decadron) as ordered. The nurse understands that the expected outcome of this action is to:
    A. improve vital signs.
    B. reduce ICP.
    C. stabilize pupillary responses.
    D. improve renal function.

30. The nurse is providing care to a patient in the emergency department who has suffered an ischemic stroke. Which of the following medications provides the most advantage to the patient if administered within 3 hours of symptom onset?
    A. aspirin
    B. clopidogrel (Plavix)
    C. abciximab (ReoPro)
    D. tissue plasminogen activator (t-PA)

31. Which of the following medications is likely to be used to treat status epilepticus?
    A. phenytoin (Dilantin)
    B. valproic acid (Depakene)
    C. carbamazepine (Tegretol)
    D. lorazepam (Ativan)

32. The nurse is providing education to a young woman about phenytoin (Dilantin). During the education session, the patient indicates that she is taking birth control pills. Based on knowledge of drug interactions, which of the following teaching points must the nurse use to advise the patient?
    A. "When taking both medications, you are at risk for thrombophlebitis."
    B. "You should use an alternate form of birth control while taking Dilantin."
    C. "You can stop taking the Dilantin if you have severe GI distress."
    D. "You should not get pregnant while you are taking Dilantin."

33. The nurse is assigned to a patient who was admitted with a transient ischemic attack (TIA). Which of the following manifestations would the nurse anticipate finding upon admission of this patient?
    A. confusion
    B. lethargy
    C. unilateral vision loss
    D. restlessness

34. The emergency department nurse is assigned to care for a patient with suspected hemorrhagic stroke who has an estimated time of arrival of 5 minutes. Based upon this brief notification, the nurse should expect to assess which of the following manifestations upon admission of the patient?
    A. loss of consciousness with severe neurologic impairment
    B. visual field impairment and sensory deficits to lower extremities
    C. cranial deficits and contralateral hemiparesis
    D. eye movement disorders and decreased visual acuity

35. Which of the following patients is at highest risk for suicide?
    A. a 22-year-old female who lives with her parents and recently broke up with a boyfriend
    B. a 75-year-old widower with pancreatic cancer who talks about using insulin and pills
    C. a 45-year-old married female with a stressful job and significant financial stress
    D. a 35-year-old religious, married man with children who has testicular cancer

36. The nurse is evaluating the effectiveness of psychotropic medication on negative symptoms of psychosis in a patient by monitoring for a decrease in which of the following?
    A. alogia
    B. bizarre behavior
    C. illogicality
    D. somatic delusions

37. The nurse is assigned to care for a patient who laughs outrageously at slight provocation, craves attention, and always interacts in an exaggerated fashion to gain attention. Based on all of these factors, the nurse knows that this patient demonstrates which of the following types of personality disorder?
    A. paranoid
    B. histrionic
    C. narcissistic
    D. obsessive-compulsive

38. The nurse is providing care for a patient who admits to being preoccupied with perfection and control at home and at work. The patient also works 12- to 16-hour days, has low tolerance for imperfection, and admits to having difficulty relaxing. The nurse knows that this patient displays features of which of the following types of personality disorder?
    A. histrionic personality
    B. narcissistic personality
    C. obsessive-compulsive
    D. bipolar personality

39. You are the nurse responsible for assessing a patient who has been on chlorpromazine (Thorazine) for extrapyramidal side effects (EPSEs). The nurse knows that extrapyramidal side effects include which of the following?
    A. acute dystonia
    B. amenorrhea
    C. breast secretion
    D. sexual dysfunction

ALTERNATE FORMAT

40. The nurse is caring for a patient who takes antipsychotic medications. The patient has developed muscle rigidity, hyperpyrexia, tachypnea, diaphoresis, and drooling. The nurse recognizes these symptoms as indicative of a severe, life-threatening side effect of psychotropic therapy which is referred to as:

_____

41. The nurse is caring for a patient diagnosed with acute glomerulonephritis. In assessing this patient, which of the following questions should the nurse be sure to ask the patient?
    A. "Have you had itching or burning in the perineum?"
    B. "Have you recently experienced a sore throat?"
    C. "Have you been eating more protein than usual?"
    D. "Have you experienced painful urination?"

42. The nurse understands that the patient who has undergone a nephrectomy is most at risk for which of the following problems postoperatively?
    A. heart failure
    B. atelectasis
    C. infection
    D. venous thrombosis

43. The nurse is caring for a patient who has just been diagnosed with acute postrenal failure. The nurse understands that which of the following is a likely cause?
    A. hemorrhage
    B. prostatic hypertrophy
    C. sepsis
    D. acute pyelonephritis

44. The nurse understands that which of the following are possible etiologic factors in the development of prerenal azotemia?
    A. massive GI bleed
    B. acute tubular necrosis
    C. glomerulonephritis
    D. occluded Foley

45. The nurse understands that which of the following medications are considered among highly nephrotoxic drugs?
    A. digoxin (Lanoxin)
    B. furosemide (Lasix)
    C. prednisone
    D. amphotericin B

46. The nurse providing care for a patient diagnosed with pyelonephritis recognizes which of the following medications as common therapy for the disease?
    A. furosemide (Lasix)
    B. levofloxacin (Levaquin)
    C. methylprednisolone (Solu-Medrol)
    D. piperacillin and tazobactam (Zosyn)

47. The nurse is caring for a patient who is diagnosed with acute glomerulonephritis. Upon review of laboratory results and assessment of the patient, the nurse would expect to find which of the following?
    A. anuria and +4 pitting edema of the lower extremities
    B. proteinuria, BUN 65 mg/dL, urine output = 350 mL/24 hr
    C. BP 190/110; serum creatinine 1.0; U/O 1620 mL/day
    D. urine cultures positive with *Pseudomonas* or *Streptococcus*

48. The nurse is assigned to care for a 3-year-old child admitted with the tentative diagnosis of nephrotic syndrome. According to the child's mother, the child has not been feeling well for several weeks. The child has been irritable and withdrawn and has not eaten well for the past week. Which of the following clinical profiles would substantiate the tentative diagnosis?
    A. hyperlipidemia, hypertension, hyperthermia
    B. hematuria, hypertension, glycosuria
    C. hyperlipidemia, proteinuria, hypoalbuminemia
    D. proteinuria, polyuria, hyperalbuminemia

49. The nurse knows that red blood cell maturation is dependent upon which of the following vitamins or minerals?
    A. cyanocobalamin
    B. aquaMEPHYTON
    C. thiamine
    D. pyridoxine

50. The nurse is caring for a patient with deep vein thrombosis. The patient asks what will happen to the clot. The best response by the nurse is:
    A. "The body's fibrinolytic system will work to dissolve the clot eventually."
    B. "The body's hemostatic mechanism will stabilize the clot at its present location."
    C. "The clot will eventually break off in tiny fragments and float into the circulation."
    D. "Treatment with heparin will dissolve the clot and prevent future recurrence."

51. The nurse who is caring for a patient with disseminated intravascular coagulation (DIC) would anticipate the need for which of the following factors and/or blood products?
    A. packed red blood cells
    B. whole blood
    C. cryoprecipitate
    D. immune globulins

52. The nurse is caring for a patient with disseminated intravascular coagulation (DIC). The nurse would expect which of the following laboratory findings?
    A. low D-dimer
    B. prolonged prothrombin time
    C. decreased partial thromboplastin time
    D. increased platelet count

53. The nurse is caring for a patient with leukemia. Which of the following clinical manifestations would the nurse expect to find upon physical assessment of the patient?
    A. angina, dyspnea, fatigue
    B. petechiae, muscle aching, splenomegaly
    C. insomnia, hepatomegaly, hematuria
    D. shortness of breath, pallor, ecchymoses

54. The nurse is providing discharge education for the patient with sickle cell crisis. Which of the following statements by the patient indicates that teaching has been effective?
    A. "I will check my pulse oximetry reading at least twice per day."
    B. "I will be able to get back to work at the sawmill this winter."
    C. "Physical activity is good for me, but I need to avoid overexertion."
    D. "I will be sure to drink at least 2 to 3 liters of fluid per day."

55. The nurse is caring for a patient with hemophilia A who is admitted with hemi-arthrosis. The nurse anticipates that which of the following will be a priority in therapeutic management of this patient?
    A. monitor for signs of abnormal clotting
    B. administration of aspirin as an analgesic
    C. application of warm soaks for pain control
    D. immobilization of the affected joint

56. The nurse is caring for a patient who had a cast applied for treatment of a fractured tibia within the past 24 hours. Which of the following assessment findings should the nurse report immediately?
    A. temperature of 100.4°F
    B. uncontrolled pain
    C. mild edema
    D. itching under the cast

57. The nurse is caring for a patient who has a history of fractured tibia and fibula. Which of the following symptoms would suggest that a fat embolism is present?
    A. apprehension and truncal petechiae
    B. calf tenderness and swelling
    C. leg pain and tenderness
    D. bradycardia and hypertension

58. The nurse is providing education about medications to a patient with gout. The nurse explains that allopurinol (Zyloprim) acts by:
    A. inhibiting uric acid production.
    B. increasing excretion of uric acid.
    C. decreasing excretion of purines.
    D. raising the serum level of purines.

59. Treatment for compartment syndrome includes which of the following?
    A. elevation of the extremity
    B. acetaminophen
    C. nonsteroidal anti-inflammatory medications
    D. fasciotomy

60. The nurse is caring for a patient who has had lab work done during a hospital admission. The patient's erythrocyte sedimentation rate (ESR) is 45 mm/hr. Which of the following interpretations by the nurse is correct?
    A. The value is within the normal range.
    B. The value indicates the presence of inflammation.
    C. The test result is inconclusive.
    D. The result indicates a red blood cell problem.

61. The nurse is caring for a patient with acute diverticulitis. Prior to discharge the nurse should instruct the patient to increase which of the following foods in the diet?
    A. cucumbers, popcorn, cantaloupe
    B. multigrain bread, asparagus, spinach
    C. peas, strawberries, corn
    D. tomatoes, peas, corn

62. The nurse is caring for a patient with acute diverticulitis. Prior to discharge the nurse should instruct the patient to avoid which of the following foods in the diet?
    A. squash, potatoes, brown rice
    B. chicken, hamburger, peanut butter
    C. popcorn, sunflower seeds, blueberries
    D. salmon, grilled vegetables, pears

63. The nurse is assigned to care for a patient with achalasia. The nurse understands that the patient is likely to have which of the following clinical manifestations related to this diagnosis?
    A. frequent nausea and diarrhea
    B. dysphagia and chest pain
    C. slow peristalsis and constipation
    D. silent abdomen and lower quad pain

64. The nurse is caring for a patient with ulcerative colitis with orders for bed rest with bathroom privileges. The nurse understands the rationale for the activity restriction is:
    A. to conserve energy.
    B. to reduce intestinal peristalsis.
    C. to promote rest and comfort.
    D. to prevent injury.

65. Assessment of the patient's gag response is a priority nursing intervention following which of the following procedures?
    A. colon biopsy
    B. EGD
    C. barium enema
    D. colonoscopy

66. The nurse is providing care for a patient who is receiving total parenteral nutrition (TPN) via a single-lumen central catheter. An intravenous antibiotic dose is due, and the nurse finds that the peripheral site is no longer functional. Which of the following independent nursing interventions provides the best option for infusion of the antibiotic?
    A. Administer the intravenous antibiotic through the TPN line.
    B. Insert a multilumen catheter over a guide wire.
    C. Identify a new site and insert another peripheral line.
    D. Insert a peripherally inserted central catheter.

67. The nurse is caring for an 8-month-old admitted to the hospital with dehydration. The nurse knows that which of the following factors predisposes the infant to fluid imbalance?
    A. decreased body surface area in comparison with adult
    B. lower metabolic rate than in an adult
    C. inability of the kidneys to dilute or concentrate urine
    D. decreased daily exchange of extracellular fluid

68. The nurse is caring for a patient following a gastric resection and is monitoring the patient closely for signs of dumping syndrome. Which of the following symptoms is indicative of dumping syndrome?
    A. abdominal cramping and right lower quadrant pain
    B. bradycardia and indigestion
    C. double vision and chest pain
    D. tachycardia and diaphoresis

69. The nurse is caring for a 4-month-old infant with gastroesophageal reflux (GER). After feeding and burping the infant, the nurse should place the infant in which of the following positions?
    A. secured upright in an infant carrier
    B. supine with a pillow under the head
    C. on the right side with a blanket roll
    D. prone with head elevated 30 degrees

70. The nurse is caring for a patient following thyroidectomy. Which of the following symptoms, as reported by the patient, should alert the nurse to the development of postoperative complications?
    A. abdominal discomfort
    B. an odd sensation around the mouth
    C. loss of appetite
    D. increased thirst

71. Which of the following sets of laboratory results best reflects those anticipated in a patient with diabetic ketoacidosis?

pH	HCO$_3$	Blood glucose
A. 7.28	34 mEq/L	260 mg/dL
B. 7.18	13 mEq/L	120 mg/dL
C. 7.21	12 mEq/L	450 mg/dL
D. 7.38	24 mEq/L	620 mg/dL

ALTERNATE FORMAT

72. The nurse is caring for a patient who is being worked up for thyroid dysfunction and has the following lab results:

Test	Patient value	Normal value
Serum total thyroxine (T4)	14 µg/dL	4.5–12.0 µg/dL
Serum total triiodothyronine (T3)	220 ng/dL	70–190 ng/dL
Serum thyrotropin (TSH)	7.2 µU/mL	0.4–4.8 µU/mL

The nurse realizes which of the following? SELECT ALL THAT APPLY.
   A. anterior pituitary gland is working excessively
   B. anterior pituitary gland is working normally
   C. thyroid gland is producing excessively
   D. thyroid gland is producing normally

73. The following lab work for a patient with thyroid dysfunction is reviewed by the nurse:

Test	Patient value	Normal value
Serum total thyroxine (T4)	14 µg/dL	4.5–12.0 µg/dL
Serum total triiodothyronine (T3)	220 ng/dL	70–190 ng/dL
Serum thyrotropin (TSH)	1.2 µU/mL	0.4–4.8 µU/mL

Based on these results, the nurse realizes:
   A. the patient has primary hyperthyroidism.
   B. the patient has secondary hyperthyroidism.
   C. the dysfunction occurs in the thyroid gland.
   D. the patient has a pituitary adenoma.

74. The nurse must administer 10 units of regular insulin and 20 units of NPH insulin to a patient. Please place in order the steps that the nurse will take in preparing the injection.
A. Draw up the 10 units of regular insulin.
B. Draw up the 20 units of NPH insulin.
C. Wipe the top of each vial with alcohol.
D. Verify insulin order on medication administration record.
E. Verify the correct patient by using at least 2 forms of identification.
F. Administer insulin subcutaneously.

75. The nurse is providing discharge teaching for the patient with Type II diabetes who has been ordered the following medications prior to discharge:

Medication administration record
Atenolol (Tenormin) 25 mg PO daily
Metformin (Glucophage) 850 mg PO T.I.D.
Hydrochlorothiazide (HCTZ) 25 mg PO B.I.D.
Enteric coated aspirin 81 mg PO every day
Glipizide SR (Glucotrol XL) 10 mg PO B.I.D.

Which of the following statements by the patient indicates understanding of the implications of drug interactions among these medications?
- A. "I need to monitor my glucose levels at home so I know if the meds are working."
- B. "I need to monitor my glucose levels so I know if I am becoming hypoglycemic."
- C. "I need the HCTZ because the metformin and aspirin make my ankles swell."
- D. "I need the atenolol because the metformin and glipizide cause my heart to race."

76. A patient with Type II diabetes informs a nurse that he has not felt well since beginning therapy with metformin (Glucophage) about 2 weeks ago. When asked to provide more detail, the patient relates that he has been experiencing nausea and diarrhea consistently. The best reply by the nurse would be:
A. "We will have to discuss some alternatives with the doctor."
B. "Your symptoms might be related to a contagious influenza."
C. "Your symptoms are normal and should decrease with time."
D. "We will have to run some tests to find out what is going on."

ALTERNATE FORMAT

77. The nurse must calculate intake and output for the patient with continuous bladder irrigation. At the beginning of the shift, the patient had 150 mL of irrigation fluid in the bag. By the end of the shift, 1250 mL (of a 2000 mL bag) remains. The total catheter output throughout the shift was 1000 mL. How much urine output did the patient have throughout the shift?

_____

78. The nurse is providing care for a patient with benign prostatic hypertrophy. Clinical manifestations, as described by the patient, include:
A. urinary frequency with strong stream.
B. difficulty initiating a stream and nocturia.
C. daytime urinary frequency with incontinence.
D. fever, chills, nausea, and vomiting.

79. The nurse is teaching a patient about testicular self-examination. Which of the following statements by the patient indicates understanding of assessment technique?
- A. "I should roll my testicle between my thumb and forefinger during a warm shower."
- B. "While lying down on the bed, I should gently touch all surfaces of each testicle."
- C. "While standing in front of a mirror, I should check for symmetrical position."
- D. "I should have my partner perform the testicular examination for me."

80. The nurse is providing education about treatment for candidiasis. In response, the patient recognizes which of the following as a means by which the normal vaginal flora can be restored?
    A. Eat 8 ounces of yogurt daily.
    B. Take daily doses of antibiotics.
    C. Use vinegar douches daily.
    D. Use miconazole (Monistat) as ordered.

81. The nurse is caring for a patient whose last menstrual period began on August 29, 2009. Using Nägele's rule, the estimated date of birth is which of the following?
    A. May 4, 2010
    B. May 5, 2010
    C. June 4, 2010
    D. June 5, 2010

82. The nurse is providing education to a pregnant woman about presumptive, probable, and positive signs of pregnancy. The patient demonstrates understanding of the information when she states that which of the following is a presumptive sign of pregnancy?
    A. elevated hCG levels
    B. amenorrhea
    C. Braxton-Hicks contractions
    D. abdominal enlargement

83. The nurse is providing education to a pregnant woman who has been experiencing nausea and vomiting. The patient demonstrates understanding of ways to reduce the nausea and vomiting when she states which of the following?
    A. "I will ask my husband to bring me eggs and bacon in bed every day."
    B. "I will limit my eating to a small breakfast with a large lunch and dinner daily."
    C. "I will have less nausea if I sip Diet 7UP or Diet Pepsi throughout the day."
    D. "If something makes me sick, I will try eating it again another day."

84. The nurse is providing education to a pregnant woman about presumptive, probable, and positive signs of pregnancy. The patient demonstrates understanding of the information when she states that which of the following is a positive sign of pregnancy?
    A. elevated hCG levels
    B. visualization of the fetus by ultrasound
    C. Braxton-Hicks contractions
    D. quickening

85. The nurse working in a prenatal clinic becomes concerned that a patient may be a battered woman based on which of the following statements made by the patient?
    A. "We are really having trouble with money right now because my husband is laid off."
    B. "My guy says I could never make it without him because I'm slow and not too smart."
    C. "I only get to do things with my friends about once a month now that we're married."
    D. "I don't get out much for fun, and I am exhausted because all I ever do is work."

86. A woman gave birth to a healthy baby 2 weeks ago. What type of lochia would the nurse expect to find when assessing this patient?
    A. lochia rubra
    B. lochia sangra
    C. lochia alba
    D. lochia serosa

87. The nurse is caring for a newborn immediately following delivery. At 1 minute, the infant has a heart rate of 128, a good respiratory effort with a strong vigorous cry, active motion of all extremities, and is completely pink. Based on this assessment, the nurse must document the 1-minute Apgar as which of the following?
    A. 7
    B. 8
    C. 9
    D. 10

88. The nurse is providing care for a patient who will undergo a total hip replacement surgery today. The nurse knows that preoperative teaching about DVT prophylaxis has been effective when the patient makes which of the following statements?
    A. "I will have to take warfarin (Coumadin) for about 4 weeks after discharge."
    B. "I will need to wear compression devices at night for at least 2 weeks after surgery."
    C. "If I ambulate within 24 hours after surgery, my risk of DVT is significantly lower."
    D. "I will need to give myself injections of enoxaparin (Lovenox) for about 6 weeks."

89. Which of the following medications may be given during cardiac surgery to reduce the risk of atrial fibrillation?
    A. atropine
    B. metoprolol
    C. enalapril
    D. verapamil

90. The nurse is caring for a patient who is experiencing extreme fatigue related to radiotherapy. When planning this patient's care, the nurse should do which of the following to aid in conservation of energy for the patient?
    A. Avoid entering the room unless absolutely necessary.
    B. Cluster patient care activities to allow for long rest periods.
    C. Ask the patient to ring the bell if he or she needs anything.
    D. Turn and reposition the patient every 2 hours for comfort.

91. The nurse is caring for a female patient who is concerned that she may be at higher than normal risk of breast cancer. Which of the following factors identified by the patient place her at higher than normal risk for development of breast cancer?
    A. 60 years of age
    B. used birth control pills for 25 years
    C. breastfed two children
    D. menopause at 48 years of age

92. **The nurse is caring for a patient who will undergo bone marrow harvesting. The nurse informs the patient that the harvest will occur:**
    A. under local anesthetic at the bedside.
    B. under conscious sedation at the bedside.
    C. under local anesthetic in same-day surgery.
    D. in the operating room under general anesthesia.

93. **The nurse is admitting a patient diagnosed with leukopenia. Which of the following is the most important nursing intervention for this patient?**
    A. Wash hands before and after each patient contact.
    B. Encourage use of mouth swabs instead of a toothbrush.
    C. Monitor blood pressure and pulse every 4 hours.
    D. Allow ample visitation to keep the patient's spirits up.

94. **The nurse is caring for a cachectic cancer patient near the end of life. As a patient advocate, it is most important for the nurse to:**
    A. discuss plans for enteral nutrition with the physician.
    B. encourage the patient and family to consider a PEG tube.
    C. ask about the patient's personal goals for end-of-life care.
    D. provide adequate amounts of artificial nutrition and fluids.

95. **The nurse who is caring for a patient undergoing chemotherapy must be particularly attentive to monitoring for which of the following signs and symptoms of toxicity?**
    A. delayed capillary refill
    B. increased urine output
    C. altered level of consciousness
    D. bradycardia

96. **The nurse has been confronted by management concerning elements of dress and personal adornment seen as inconsistent with agency guidelines. Based on a federal court ruling, management may not legally require the nurse to remove or cover which of the following?**
    A. a religious head-covering
    B. excessive jewelry
    C. tattoos
    D. artificial nails

97. **A nurse considering several offers of employment understands that working on a unit that utilizes primary care delivery will involve:**
    A. passing medications as needed throughout the unit.
    B. working with RNs to provide total care to assigned patients.
    C. delegating various responsibilities to UAP.
    D. working on a team that includes RNs, LPNs, and UAP.

98. **A nurse is considering whether a specific nursing policy should be modified. The best guidance for nursing policy modification would be achieved through which of the following?**
    A. the advice of a more experienced nurse
    B. the advice of a physician who specializes in the content area
    C. relevant research articles from recent peer-reviewed journals
    D. information found in the renal section of a nursing textbook

99. A group of staff nurses is preparing to report on what they learned at a conference about evidence-based practice (EBP). Within their presentation, they should refer to which of the following organizations that has significant impact upon evidence-based practice?
    A. Sigma Theta Tau
    B. The Cochrane Collaboration
    C. American Nurses Association
    D. American Association of Colleges of Nursing

100. A nurse employed in an outpatient clinic knows that which of the following actions would constitute a violation of the Health Insurance Portability and Accountability Act (HIPAA)?
    A. reading a note made by another healthcare provider in a patient's chart
    B. telling a patient that a biopsy came back positive for cancer
    C. leaving test results on a patient's office phone without written consent
    D. failing to change the paper on an exam room table between patients

ANSWERS

1. **(B)**; The nurse must translate micrograms into milligrams: $\dfrac{0.250\ \mu g}{1000\ \frac{\mu g}{mg}} = 250\ mg$

   Then, mathematically, $\dfrac{0.250\ \frac{mg}{dose}}{0.125\ \frac{mg}{tablet}} = 2\ \dfrac{tablets}{dose}$.

2. **(C)**; Variant (Prinzmetal's) angina is characteristically associated with EKG changes related to coronary artery spasm, which results in decreased oxygen supply to the myocardium.

3. **(A, B, C)**; Digoxin (Lanoxin) may be given undiluted or diluted in 4 mL NSS. There is more risk of precipitation with undiluted administration. Digoxin must be administered over a minimum of 5 minutes. The volume of drug to be drawn up is calculated as follows: $\dfrac{500\ mcg}{2\ mL} = 200\ \dfrac{mcg}{mL}$; 250 mcg = 0.250 mg. Therefore, 1 mL must be drawn up in the syringe. Low serum potassium levels may potentiate digoxin toxicity.

4. **(B)**; Thrombolytic drugs break down existing clots and predispose the patient to bleeding. Typically, patients receiving thrombolytic drugs also receive heparin infusion to impair the clotting ability of the blood. The thrombolytic breaks down existing clots while heparin helps to prevent formation of new clots. Therefore, once thrombolytic therapy has been initiated, it is not prudent to perform either venipuncture or arterial puncture.

5. **(D)**; Myocardial cell death occurs as a consequence of myocardial infarction. With unstable angina, cell death does not occur. The pain of angina is typically less severe than AMI, but not always. AMI results from coronary artery occlusion with pain not relieved by nitroglycerin for at least 20 minutes.

6. **(C)**; The serum potassium level is 5.9 mEq/L, and normal serum potassium levels should be 3.5–5.3 mEq/L.

7.

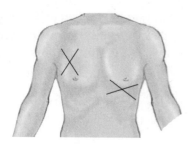

8. **(A)**; Niacin therapy can cause extreme flushing of the face, neck, and ears. Taking 325 mg of aspirin 30 minutes prior to the niacin helps to reduce the unpleasant flushing.

9. **(C)**; First, convert the patient's weight to kg by dividing 175 by 2.2, which equals 79.54 kg. Next, figure out how many mLs = 1 mcg by dividing the total volume (250 mL) by the number of micrograms of dopamine (400,000) to equal 0.000625 mL/mcg. Then apply the information to the following equation:

$$\frac{5\ \mu g \times 79.54\ kg}{minute} \times \frac{60\ minutes}{1\ hour} \times 0.000625\ \frac{mL}{\mu g} = 14.9\ \frac{mL}{hr} \ .$$

10. **(C)**; First, convert the patient's weight to kg by dividing 250 by 2.2, which equals 113.6 kg. Next, figure out how many mLs = 1 mcg by dividing the total volume (250 mL) by the number of micrograms of dobutamine (250,000) to equal 0.001 mL/mcg. Then apply the information to the following equation:

$$\frac{5\ \mu g \times 113.6\ kg}{minute} \times \frac{60\ minutes}{1\ hour} \times 0.001\ \frac{mL}{\mu g} = 34\ \frac{mL}{hr} \ .$$

11. **(D)**; First, calculate the bolus using the following ratio method:

$$\frac{1000\ mL}{20\ grams} = \frac{x\ mL}{4\ grams}, \text{ where } 4000 = 20x. \text{ Therefore, } x = 200\ mL \text{ to infuse over } 30$$

minutes (0.5 hr): 200 mL × 0.5 hour = $400\ \frac{mL}{hr}$ (BOLUS).

Next, calculate the maintenance infusion using the same ratio technique:

$$\frac{1000\ mL}{20\ grams} = \frac{x\ mL}{2\ grams}; \text{ where } 2000 = 20x. \text{ Therefore, } x = 100\ mL \text{ to infuse each hour } or$$

100 mL/hr (maintenance).

12. **(C)**; Primary treatment for Buerger's focuses on smoking cessation and avoidance of second-hand smoke. Smoking cessation counseling is essential because continued smoking will enhance progression of the disease.

13. **(C)**; Clinical manifestations of thoracic aortic aneurysm include substernal chest pain, back and neck pain, dyspnea, cough, and stridor. Respiratory symptoms are due to pressure on the trachea.

14. **(A, B, C, D)**; The patient is at risk for development of venous thromboembolism because of age >40, having had major abdominal surgery, having been admitted to the ICU, and because of prolonged immobility of more than three days.

15. **(D, B, A, C, E)**; The nurse must first verify that the drugs are correct as ordered and then identify the patient by at least two means (name and birth date). Next, the Atro-

vent (bronchodilator) should be administered followed in a few minutes by the Flovent (glucocorticoid). Finally, the patient should gargle to decrease the chances of developing oral candidiasis. It is important that the bronchodilator is administered first to open the airways so that the glucocorticoid will then be distributed through the airways.

16. **(5 mL)**; Use the ratio method to solve $\dfrac{40 \text{ mg}}{2 \text{ mL}} = \dfrac{100 \text{ mg}}{x}$; then $40x = 200$. $\dfrac{200}{40} = x$, so $x = 5$ mL.

17. **(B)**; When the low-pressure alarm on a ventilator sounds, the nurse should immediately look for and reconnect any disconnected tubing between the patient and ventilator.

ALTERNATE FORMAT

18. **(A, B)**; SIMV is a mode of ventilation that is used with patients who are able to breathe on their own to some degree. It is often used as a mode for weaning patients from mechanical ventilation. In this mode, the ventilator is programmed to deliver a set number of breaths per minute at a given tidal volume. Patients can initiate breaths any time. The tidal volume of patient breaths is dependent upon the respiratory effort generated by the patient.

19. **(B, C, D)**; Controlled mandatory ventilation (CMV) is a ventilatory mode that is not widely used because 100% of the ventilatory effort is carried by the ventilator. However, in the case of organ donors who are being prepared for harvest surgery, it is an appropriate mode. Ventilator-initiated breaths are full tidal volume. All breaths are ventilator initiated because the patient is clinically dead. If the ventilator fails, the nurse must immediately bag the patient because there will be no spontaneous respiratory effort.

20. **(A, D)**; The mechanically ventilated patient who will undergo pressure support trials has demonstrated some indication of readiness to wean. When the patient is on a pressure support trial, it is critically important for the nurse to monitor the patient very closely because there is no set rate or tidal volume and, therefore, no alarms to indicate if the patient is compromised. As a stand-alone mode in stable ventilated patients, pressure support simply decreases the work of breathing by maintaining a continuous positive airway pressure, but the patient must still initiate all breaths with a tidal volume that provides effective respiration.

21. **(B, C, D)**; The patient can initiate a breath any time. All ventilated breaths will be full tidal volume. Patient initiated breaths will have variable tidal volumes. The addition of positive end expiratory pressure (PEEP) results in increased intrathoracic pressure because PEEP causes the alveoli to remain expanded at the end of expiration. The increased intrathoracic pressure results in decreased ventricular filling and decreased cardiac output. Therefore, blood pressure assessments should be completed on patients who are having PEEP added during mechanical ventilation. If the patient becomes hypotensive, the nurse would contact the physician for further orders, which may include vasopressor drugs.

22. **(B)**; When the patient coughs forcefully against the ventilator, the high pressure alarm will sound. Frequently, patients require suctioning when the high pressure alarm sounds.

23. **(C)**; The gold standard test for diagnosis of pulmonary embolus is pulmonary angiogram, but it is an expensive, invasive test with significant risks for the patient. Therefore, a spiral CT is performed more frequently and is highly accurate for diagnosing large emboli.

24. **(B, D, G)**; This ABG result reveals uncompensated respiratory alkalosis.

ABG component	Value	What it reveals related to acid-base balance
pH	7.48	*Alkalotic; uncompensated*
pCO$_2$	32	Decreased; contributes to alkalotic pH; *primary problem*
HCO$_3^-$	22	Decreased; acting to buffer alkalosis
pO$_2$	90	Within normal limits

25. **(B)**; The nurse can document that the patient exhibits some degree of arousal if, when the nurse applied nail bed pressure, the hand is withdrawn. This indicates responsiveness to sensory stimulation.

26. **(D)**; Orientation to person is generally the last orientation parameter lost. Lack of orientation to person occurs with severe dysfunction, such as delirium.

27. **(B)**; The nurse can assess attention and concentration by asking the patient to count backward from 100 by 7s. The nurse could ask a less educated patient to name the months of the year in reverse order or the days of the week backwards.

28. **(C)**; Cerebral angiography depends upon the use of contrast media to define the vasculature of the brain. Following the procedure, it is desirable for the patient to increase fluid intake to facilitate excretion of the contrast.

29. **(B)**; The nurse understands that dexamethasone (Decadron) is a glucocorticoid medication and that an expected outcome of treatment with this drug is reduction of intracranial pressure.

30. **(D)**; Tissue plasminogen activator (t-PA), approved by the FDA for treatment of ischemic stroke within 3 hours of onset of symptoms, lyses the clot and restores blood flow to the brain tissue. Clopidogrel (Plavix) is an antiplatelet agent that, when administered along with aspirin, has significantly improved clinical outcomes for patients who have experienced ischemic events. Abciximab (ReoPro) is often used in conjunction with aspirin and heparin to decrease the risk of ischemic complications of endovascular interventions.

31. **(D)**; Status epilepticus is a life-threatening emergency that involves continuous cycles of seizure activity. Medications used to treat status epilepticus include diazepam (Valium), lorazepam (Ativan), and phenobarbital.

32. **(B)**; The nurse should encourage the patient to use an alternate form of birth control because Dilantin decreases the effectiveness of oral contraceptives.

33. **(C)**; Manifestations of transient ischemic attack include focal neurological deficits, like inability to sense one side of the body, *unilateral loss of vision*, loss of speech, or facial droop. Global deficits, like restlessness, confusion, or lethargy, are not characteristic with transient ischemic attacks.

34. **(A)**; Hemorrhagic strokes occur rapidly and without significant warning signs, although some patients experience severe headache at the onset of symptoms. The nurse should anticipate that the patient with suspected hemorrhagic stroke, as identified by ambulance personnel, has symptoms that are significant enough to warrant the potential diagnosis from the field. Therefore, the nurse should anticipate that the patient will have loss of consciousness and severe neurologic impairment upon arrival to the emergency department.

35. **(B)**; The 75-year-old (*>65*) widower (*male*) with pancreatic cancer (*terminal illness*) who talks about using insulin and pain pills (*plan*) is the patient at highest risk for suicide of those presented. The 22-year-old female who lives with her parents and broke up with a boyfriend has one stress but no significant risks for suicide. The 45-year-old married female with a stressful job also has no significant risk for suicide. Although the 35-year-old married man has a potentially terminal illness, he has social support and significant others, which results in reduced risk for suicide.

36. **(A)**; Negative symptoms of psychosis involve loss of normal functioning. They include affective flattening, *alogia* (restricted thought and speech), avolition/apathy (lack of behavior initiation), and anhedonia/asociality (inability to experience pleasure or maintain social contacts).

37. **(B)**; Persons with histrionic personality disorder exhibit excessive emotions and behave in a manner that is attention seeking. Persons with this type of personality disorder view relationships as closer than they actually are; will do something to be the center of attention; are often sexually provocative in dress and behavior; seek out compliments; dress in expensive clothing; and crave novelty, stimulation, and excitement.

38. **(C)**; This patient displays features of obsessive-compulsive personality. Patients with this disorder crave control, value perfection, have excessive devotion to work, experience difficulty relaxing, demonstrate rule-conscious behavior, and have an inability to discard anything.

39. **(A)**; Acute dystonia is an extrapyramidal side effect. Amenorrhea, breast secretion, and sexual dysfunction are endocrine-related side effects of the drug.

40. **(Neuroleptic malignant syndrome)**; Neuroleptic malignant syndrome occurs in about 0.2 to 1% of patients who take antipsychotic medications. The syndrome is fatal in about 10% of cases. Neuroleptic malignant syndrome is characterized by decreased level of consciousness, muscle rigidity, hyperpyrexia, labile hypertension, tachycardia, tachypnea, diaphoresis, and drooling. Treatment involves early detection and discontinuation of the drug as well as stabilizing the patient medically.

41. **(B)**; Acute glomerulonephritis most commonly occurs within 1 to 3 weeks after an untreated streptococcal respiratory infection, so the nurse should be sure to ask whether the patient has recently had a very sore throat.

42. **(B)**; The postoperative nephrectomy patient is most at risk for atelectasis, not only related to general anesthesia but also as a result of having a flank incision that limits postoperative deep breathing.

43. **(B)**; Of the choices listed, prostatic hypertrophy is the likely cause of postrenal failure. By definition, conditions that cause postrenal failure cause obstruction to urine flow after the kidney.

44. **(A)**; The nurse understands that heart failure, hemorrhage (*GI bleed*), and shock are examples of possible etiologic factors in the development of prerenal azotemia.

45. **(D)**; Amphotericin B is a heavy-duty antifungal that is nephrotoxic in more than 80% of patients. This group of drugs is known to be highly nephrotoxic.

46. **(B)**; Antibiotics commonly used for treatment of pyelonephritis include sulfa drugs (Bactrim), cephalosporins (Maxipime, Ceclor), amoxicillin, *levofloxacin*, and ciprofloxacin.

47. **(B)**; The patient with acute glomerulonephritis will have symptoms that may include *oliguria (<400 mL/24 hr)*, *proteinuria*, hematuria, *azotemia (elevated BUN)*, and mild edema.

48. **(C)**; Classic signs of nephrotic syndrome include hyperlipidemia, massive proteinuria, edema, and hypoalbuminemia.

49. **(A)**; Cyanocobalamin (vitamin B_{12}) is referred to as a maturation factor for red blood cells. When individuals lack this vitamin, their erythrocytes become larger and irregularly shaped. The cells also have a shorter life span. AquaMEPHYTON is vitamin K, thiamine is vitamin B_1, and pyridoxine is vitamin B_6.

50. **(A)**; In the body, fibrinolysis is a process by which a clot is broken down over time. This process is effective at breaking down clots that are not immediately life-threatening. Heparin has no effect on existing clots.

51. **(C)**; The nurse who is caring for a patient with DIC should anticipate the need to administer *cryoprecipitate* to replace fibrinogen, platelets for thrombocytopenia, and fresh frozen plasma to replace all clotting factors except platelets.

52. **(B)**; The nurse who is caring for a patient with DIC would expect to find that partial thromboplastin time is prolonged, *prothrombin time is prolonged*, platelet count is decreased, and D-dimer is elevated.

53. **(D)**; Upon physical assessment of the patient with leukemia, the nurse would anticipate finding that the patient suffers from night sweats, gingival bleeding, *ecchymoses*, weakness, fatigue, anorexia, *shortness of breath*, decreased activity tolerance, epistaxis, *pallor*, and splenomegaly or hepatomegaly.

54. **(C)**; Among strategies to prevent sickle cell crisis, the patient should be encouraged to drink 4 to 6 liters of fluid per day, *to avoid overexertion*, to use stress-reduction techniques, and to avoid exposure to the cold. Having a job at a sawmill in the wintertime may not be desirable because of constant exposure to a cold environment.

55. **(D)**; The nurse anticipates assisting with management of pain associated with the hemiarthrosis. These measures would include *joint immobilization*, application of ice, and administration of analgesics (no aspirin because of its effects on coagulation).

56. **(B)**; The nurse must notify the physician immediately if the patient experiences uncontrolled or excessive pain because these are signs of compartment syndrome, a serious complication.

57. **(A)**; A fat embolism may occur following fracture of the long bones. Signs and symptoms include chest pain, dyspnea, tachycardia, *apprehension, petechiae over the trunk and axilla,* altered level of consciousness, and decreased O$_2$ saturation.

58. **(A)**; Allopurinol (Zyloprim) slows or stops production of uric acid by inhibiting an enzyme required for synthesis of uric acid.

59. **(D)**; Fasciotomy involves a deep incision into the fascia to relieve pressure within the compartment. Timing of this treatment is crucial. Done too early, the patient will lose a lot of blood. Done too late, tissue death will occur.

60. **(B)**; ESR is a test that indicates the rate at which red blood cells settle out of unclotted blood. A normal value for females aged 50–85 years is 30 mm/hr, and for males of the same age, the normal value is 20 mm/hr. Elevated levels indicate that an inflammatory process is present.

61. **(B)**; The patient should be instructed to increase foods that are high in fiber when the acute inflammation has subsided. These high-fiber foods include such things as wheat bran, oat bran, shredded wheat, oatmeal, whole wheat bread, *multigrain bread,* cooked *asparagus,* broccoli, squash, *spinach,* lettuce, carrots, peaches, apples, and oranges.

62. **(C)**; The patient with acute diverticulitis should be instructed to avoid foods with small seeds; nuts and foods with skins, like raisins, grapes, and corn; strawberries; raspberries; *blueberries;* figs; rye bread with caraway seeds; *popcorn;* sesame seeds; poppy seeds; *sunflower seeds;* nuts; cucumbers; and okra. Avoidance of these foods will help to decrease exacerbations of diverticulitis.

63. **(B)**; Patients with achalasia develop symptoms related to the failure of the lower esophageal sphincter (LES) to relax properly following swallowing. The patient develops chronic and progressive dysphagia, regurgitation, and chest pain.

64. **(B)**; Patients with ulcerative colitis tend to have severe diarrhea. Activity restriction may help to reduce intestinal peristalsis and limit diarrhea.

65. **(B)**; The nurse must be sure to evaluate for the presence of an adequate gag reflex when the patient returns from an esophagogastroduodenoscopy (EGD). The patient's throat is anesthetized prior to this examination, which involves insertion of a flexible scope through the esophagus (esophago), into the stomach (gastro), and then into the small bowel (duodenoscopy). Therefore, it is important for nurses to assess for presence of the gag reflex when the patient returns to the nursing unit before administering any fluids by mouth.

66. **(C)**; The nurse should identify a new site and insert another peripheral line. It is not a good idea to administer the medication through the TPN line because protecting the patient from line sepsis is of the utmost importance. Insertion of a multi-lumen catheter over a guide wire is not a nursing intervention. Insertion of a peripherally-inserted central catheter requires a physician order.

67. **(C)**; Kidneys of infants are immature and do not have the ability to dilute or concentrate urine or to regulate electrolyte loss. This makes infants prone to developing dehydration.

68. **(D)**; Dumping syndrome is a common problem following gastric resections. It occurs because the food bolus enters the duodenum or jejunum very quickly. Water is pulled

into the lumen of the gut to dilute the food bolus. This fluid shift causes a rapid decrease in blood volume and a reflex response by the sympathetic nervous system that results in *tachycardia*, orthostatic hypotension, dizziness, flushing, and *diaphoresis*. Patients may also have nausea; epigastric pain; cramping; and loud, hyperactive bowel sounds within 5 to 30 minutes after a meal. Diarrhea occurs soon afterward.

69. **(D)**; The infant should be positioned in a prone position with the head and chest elevated 30 degrees to reduce the likelihood of reflux.

70. **(B)**; If the patient reports an odd sensation around the mouth, the nurse must assess for hypocalcemia (by Chvostek's or Trousseau's signs), which could result from inadvertent removal of parathyroid tissue during the surgery.

71. **(C)**; The patient with diabetic ketoacidosis is likely to have pH <7.30; HCO_3 <15 mEq/L; and elevated serum glucose.

72. **(B, C)**; This patient's anterior pituitary gland is working normally (normal TSH), but the thyroid gland is producing excessive amounts of hormone ($\uparrow T_3$ and T_4).

73. **(B)**; This patient has hyperthyroidism secondary to overproduction of TSH.

74. **(D, C, A, B, E, F)**; First, the nurse must verify the insulin order on the MAR. Next, the top of each vial should be disinfected with alcohol. Then, the nurse should draw up the 10 units of regular insulin, followed by the 20 units of NPH insulin. Prior to administration, the nurse must verify the correct patient by at least two forms of identification; finally, the nurse can administer the insulin subcutaneously.

75. **(B)**; This patient may not always be aware of episodes of hypoglycemia because the atenolol (Tenormin) tends to mask the signs.

76. **(C)**; Many patients experience GI symptoms at the onset of metformin therapy; however, the symptoms typically subside with time.

77. **(100 mL)**; 2000 − 1250 = 750 mL of irrigation from the present bag *plus* 150 mL of the previous bag *(= 900 mL total) infused during the shift*. The total catheter output was 1000 mL, so 1000 mL total output − 900 mL irrigation = *100 mL urine* output for the shift.

78. **(B)**; The patient with benign prostatic hypertrophy describes clinical manifestations of the disorder, which include urinary frequency, *nocturia*, weak stream, *difficulty starting and stopping the stream*, and dribbling.

79. **(A)**; The patient should be encouraged to perform testicular self-examination at least once per month by gently rolling each testicle between the thumb and forefinger of each hand. The examination should be done with soapy hands in a warm bath or shower.

80. **(A)**; The patient can help to restore the normal vaginal flora by consuming 8 ounces of yogurt with live active cultures daily.

81. **(D)**; Using Nägele's rule, the calculation would occur as follows: Begin with the first day of the last menstrual period and subtract 3 months (August 29 − 3 months = May 29). Add 7 days (May 29 + 7 days = *June 5, 2010*).

82. **(B)**; Presumptive signs include *amenorrhea*, nausea and vomiting in pregnancy (morning sickness), excessive fatigue, urinary frequency, changes in the breast, and quickening. Braxton Hicks, elevated hCG levels, and abdominal enlargement are probable signs of pregnancy.

83. **(C)**; The patient can limit nausea and vomiting by eating small, frequent meals throughout the day and by avoiding odors or causative factors as well as greasy or highly seasoned foods. *The patient should also consider drinking carbonated beverages.* Patients also should be encouraged to eat some dry crackers or toast before arising in the morning as opposed to a full meal of bacon and eggs. Large meals should be discouraged.

84. **(B)**; Positive signs of pregnancy are those that are completely objective and cannot be confused with any other pathologic state. They include audible fetal heartbeat, palpation of fetal movement by a trained examiner, and *visualization of the fetus by ultrasound.*

85. **(B)**; This statement affirms that the woman does not have much self-esteem. Battered women often are submissive, passive, and dependent. With a need to seek approval from men in their lives, many battered women do not work outside the home, are isolated from family and friends, and are totally dependent on their partner.

86. **(C)**; Lochia rubra is dark red discharge that occurs for the first 2 to 3 days following birth. Lochia serosa is a pinkish discharge that follows from about day 3 to day 10. *Lochia alba*, a creamy or yellowish discharge, persists for another week or two after lochia serosa subsides.

87. **(D)**; The infant's 1-minute Apgar should be rated as a 10 based on the following scoring system: HR >100 = 2; good respiratory effort with a strong cry = 2; active motion of all extremities = 2; vigorous cry = 2; and completely pink skin color = 2 for a total of 10.

88. **(A)**; Patients who have total hip or knee replacement surgery, repair of hip fracture, and major gynecologic surgeries are at higher risk for development of venous thromboembolism and should remain on antithrombotic drug therapy (warfarin or enoxaparin) for 2 to 4 weeks following surgery.

89. **(B)**; Beta blockers may be administered during cardiac surgery to reduce the likelihood of atrial fibrillation. Atropine increases heart rate. Enalapril is an ACE inhibitor. Verapamil is a calcium channel blocker.

90. **(B)**; The nurse should cluster patient care activities to allow for long rest periods. This is the most effective means to help conserve the patient's energy. The nurse must be attentive to the patient's needs but should not constantly enter the patient's room because it would be exhausting for the patient.

91. **(B)**; Hormonal risks for development of breast cancer include *use of birth control pills* or hormone replacement therapy; early menarche (before 12 years of age); late menopause (after 55 years of age); and first pregnancy after 30 years of age. Nonhormonal risk factors include family history; lack of regular exercise; postmenopausal obesity; increased use of alcohol; working the night shift; older than 65 years of age; no full-term pregnancies; never breastfed; higher socioeconomic status; Jewish heritage; and two or more first-degree relatives with breast cancer at an early age.

92. **(D)**; Bone marrow harvesting occurs in the operating room under general anesthesia. It generally involves multiple punctures into the anterior or posterior iliac crest to obtain 500 to 700 mL of marrow.

93. **(A)**; The patient with leukopenia is at risk for infection. Therefore, it is critically important for the nurse to wash hands before and after each patient contact.

94. **(C)**; As a patient advocate, the nurse's most important job in caring for one who is near end of life is to ascertain the patient's goals. This is important because the patient may or may not wish to have artificial nutrition and/or hydration. It is the patient's right to choose.

95. **(A)**; The nurse who is caring for a patient undergoing chemotherapy must monitor the patient for *signs and symptoms of heart failure* and signs of decreased cardiac output. These might include crackles in the lungs, cough, decreased urine output, restlessness, *delayed capillary refill*, etc. Patients who have undergone chemotherapy experience decreased pulmonary function as a lifelong effect associated with long-term treatment.

96. **(A)**; Body piercings, tattoos, and artificial nails are not protected under the right to freedom of expression. Religious head coverings are protected, and management may not legally require them to be removed.

97. **(B)**; Primary care involves all-RN staffing. Having one RN pass medications on the unit is consistent with the functional model of care delivery. Delegating responsibilities to a UAP is consistent with team nursing. Organizing RNs, LPNs, and UAP into teams is consistent with team nursing.

98. **(C)**; Current research articles in peer-reviewed journals constitute the evidence upon which clinical practice guidelines and, ultimately, decisions about nursing practice should be based. The advice of a more experienced nurse may or may not be based on evidence. Physicians may be considered experts on medical practice but not nursing practice. Although the information found in nursing texts is increasingly based on evidence, texts may contain some information based on convention rather than evidence.

99. **(B)**; The Cochrane Collaboration is a global collective that conducts systematic reviews of research studies and generates evidence summaries from which the clinical practice guidelines used by healthcare professionals are derived. The American Association of Colleges of Nursing (AACN) is a consortium of baccalaureate nursing programs, Sigma Theta Tau is the honor society for nursing, and American Nurses Association is a national nursing organization—none of which are explicitly facilitators of EBP.

100. **(C)**; Leaving a message containing sensitive medical information where others might hear it (without written consent) constitutes a violation of patient confidentiality. In the course of providing patient care, it is often necessary for nurses to read notes written by other healthcare providers. RNs do not convey diagnoses because that is a medical responsibility. HIPAA does not address patient safety.

Keep Track

- Percent correct. (Divide the number of questions you answered correctly by the total number of questions you answered.) _____

- Number of questions you missed due to a reading error: _____

- Number of questions you missed due to errors in analysis: _____

- Number of assessment questions you missed: _____

- Number of lab value questions you missed: _____

- Number of drug/treatment questions you missed: _____

Nugget List

Chapter number _____ Topic _____

Sources

CHAPTER 7

Question 3: Image from *Arrhythmia Recognition: The Art of Interpretation*, courtesy of Tomas B. Garcia, MD.

CHAPTER 9

General, question 9: Image from *Arrhythmia Recognition: The Art of Interpretation*, courtesy of Tomas B. Garcia, MD; **drugs and treatments, question 8:** image from *Arrhythmia Recognition: The Art of Interpretation*, courtesy of Tomas B. Garcia, MD.

CHAPTER 13

General, question 2: Adapted from Hoyson, P. M. & Serroka, K. A. (2008). *NCLEX-RN review: 1,000 questions to help you pass* (chap. 23, question 6). Jones and Bartlett: Sudbury, MA; **general, question 3:** Hoyson, P. M. & Serroka, K. A. (2008). *NCLEX-RN review: 1,000 questions to help you pass* (chap. 23, question 8). Sudbury, MA: Jones and Bartlett; **general, question 13:** adapted from Chernecky, C., Stark, N., & Schumacher, L. (2008). *NCLEX-RN Review Guide: Top Ten Questions for Quick Review* (sec. V, question 29). Sudbury, MA: Jones and Bartlett; **general, question 14:** adapted from Chernecky, C., Stark, N., & Schumacher, L. (2008). *NCLEX-RN Review Guide: Top Ten Questions for Quick Review* (sec. V, question 33). Sudbury, MA: Jones and Bartlett; **general, question 15:** adapted from Chernecky, C., Stark, N., & Schumacher, L. (2008). *NCLEX-RN Review Guide: Top Ten Questions for Quick Review* (sec. V, question 38). Sudbury, MA: Jones and Bartlett; **general, question 16:** adapted from Chernecky, C., Stark, N., & Schumacher, L. (2008). *NCLEX-RN Review Guide: Top Ten Questions for Quick Review* (sec. V, question 40). Sudbury, MA: Jones and Bartlett; **general, question 17:** adapted from Chernecky, C., Stark, N., & Schumacher, L. (2008). *NCLEX-RN Review Guide: Top Ten Questions for Quick Review* (sec. V, question 44). Sudbury, MA: Jones and Bartlett; **general, question 19:** adapted from Chernecky, C., Stark, N., & Schumacher, L. (2008). *NCLEX-RN Review Guide: Top Ten Questions for Quick Review* (sec. V, question 56). Sudbury, MA: Jones and Bartlett; **general, question 20:** adapted from Chernecky, C., Stark, N., & Schumacher, L. (2008). *NCLEX-RN Review Guide: Top Ten Questions for Quick Review* (sec. V, question 69). Sudbury, MA: Jones and Bartlett; **general, question 21:** Chernecky, C., Stark, N., & Schumacher, L. (2008). *NCLEX-RN Review Guide: Top Ten Questions for Quick Review* (sec. V, question 70). Sudbury, MA: Jones and Bartlett; **general, question 22:** adapted from Chernecky, C., Stark, N., & Schumacher, L. (2008). *NCLEX-RN Review Guide: Top Ten Questions for Quick Review* (sec. V, question 111). Sudbury, MA: Jones and Bartlett; **general, question**

23: adapted from Chernecky, C., Stark, N., & Schumacher, L. (2008). *NCLEX-RN Review Guide: Top Ten Questions for Quick Review* (sec. V, question 177). Sudbury, MA: Jones and Bartlett; **general, question 27:** Hoyson, P. M. & Serroka, K. A. (2008). *NCLEX-RN review: 1,000 questions to help you pass* (chap. 23, question 28). Jones and Bartlett: Sudbury, MA; **physical assessment, question 1:** Hoyson, P. M. & Serroka, K. A. (2008). *NCLEX-RN review: 1,000 questions to help you pass* (chap. 23, question 2). Jones and Bartlett: Sudbury, MA; **drugs and treatments, question 6:** Hoyson, P. M. & Serroka, K. A. (2008). *NCLEX-RN review: 1,000 questions to help you pass* (chap. 23, question 7). Jones and Bartlett: Sudbury, MA; **drugs and treatments, question 7:** adapted from Chernecky, C., Stark, N., & Schumacher, L. (2008). *NCLEX-RN Review Guide: Top Ten Questions for Quick Review* (sec. V, question 87). Sudbury, MA: Jones and Bartlett; **drugs and treatments, question 8:** adapted from Chernecky, C., Stark, N., & Schumacher, L. (2008). *NCLEX-RN Review Guide: Top Ten Questions for Quick Review* (sec. V, question 90). Sudbury, MA: Jones and Bartlett; **drugs and treatments, question 9:** adapted from Chernecky, C., Stark, N., & Schumacher, L. (2008). *NCLEX-RN Review Guide: Top Ten Questions for Quick Review* (sec. V, question 108). Sudbury, MA: Jones and Bartlett; **drugs and treatments, question 10:** adapted from Chernecky, C., Stark, N., & Schumacher, L. (2008). *NCLEX-RN Review Guide: Top Ten Questions for Quick Review* (sec. V, question 127). Sudbury, MA: Jones and Bartlett; **drugs and treatments, question 11:** adapted from Chernecky, C., Stark, N., & Schumacher, L. (2008). *NCLEX-RN Review Guide: Top Ten Questions for Quick Review* (sec. V, question 132). Sudbury, MA: Jones and Bartlett; **drugs and treatments, question 15:** adapted from Chernecky, C., Stark, N., & Schumacher, L. (2008). *NCLEX-RN Review Guide: Top Ten Questions for Quick Review* (sec. V, question 163). Sudbury, MA: Jones and Bartlett; **drugs and treatments, question 16:** Chernecky, C., Stark, N., & Schumacher, L. (2008). *NCLEX-RN Review Guide: Top Ten Questions for Quick Review* (sec. V, question 217). Sudbury, MA: Jones and Bartlett; **drugs and treatments, question 17:** adapted from Chernecky, C., Stark, N., & Schumacher, L. (2008). *NCLEX-RN Review Guide: Top Ten Questions for Quick Review* (sec. V, question 218). Sudbury, MA: Jones and Bartlett.

CHAPTER 20

General, question 1: Adapted from Hoyson, P. M. & Serroka, K. A. (2008). *NCLEX-RN review: 1,000 questions to help you pass* (chap. 20, question 2). Jones and Bartlett: Sudbury, MA; **general, question 9:** adapted from Hoyson, P. M. & Serroka, K. A. (2008). *NCLEX-RN review: 1,000 questions to help you pass* (chap. 20, question 10). Jones and Bartlett: Sudbury, MA; **general, question 28:** adapted from Hoyson, P. M. & Serroka, K. A. (2008). *NCLEX-RN review: 1,000 questions to help you pass* (chap. 20, question 23). Jones and Bartlett: Sudbury, MA; **general, question 29:** Chernecky, C., Stark, N., & Schumacher, L. (2008). *NCLEX-RN Review Guide: Top Ten Questions for Quick Review* (sec. II, question 91). Sudbury, MA: Jones and Bartlett; **physical assessment, question 1:** adapted from Hoyson, P. M. & Serroka, K. A. (2008). *NCLEX-RN review: 1,000 questions to help you pass* (chap. 20, question 1). Jones and Bartlett: Sudbury, MA; **physical assessment, question 11:** adapted from Hoyson, P. M. & Serroka, K. A. (2008). *NCLEX-RN review: 1,000 questions to help you pass* (chap. 20, question 26). Jones and Bartlett: Sudbury, MA; **interpretation of lab values, question 6:** Hoyson, P. M. & Serroka, K. A. (2008). *NCLEX-RN review: 1,000 questions to help you pass* (chap. 20, question 28). Jones and Bartlett: Sudbury, MA.